Topics in Anaesthesia and Critical Care

H.K.F. VAN SAENE, L. SILVESTRI, M.A. DE LA CAL (EDS)
Infection Control in the Intensitive Care unit
1998, 380 pp, ISBN 3-540-75043-6

J. MILIC-EMILI (ED)
Applied Physiology in Respiratory Mechanics
1998, 246 pp, ISBN 3-540-75041-X

G. GUARNIERI, F. ISCRA
Metabolism and Artificial Nutrition in the Critically Ill
1999, 130 pp, ISBN 88-470-0042-4

J. MILIC -EMILI, U. LUCANGELO, A. PESENTI, W.A. ZIN
Basics of Respiratory Mechanics and Artificial Ventilation
1999, 268 pp, ISBN 88-470-0046-7

M. TIENGO, V.A. PALADINI, N. RAWAL
Regional Anaesthesia, Analgesia and Pain Management
1999, 362 pp, ISBN 88-470-0044-0

I. SALVO, D. VIDYASAGAR
Anaesthesia and Intensive Care in Neonates and Children
1999, 324 pp, ISBN 88-470-0043-2

G. BERLOT, H. DELOOZ, A. GULLO
Trauma Operative Procedures
1999, 210 pp, ISBN 88-470-0045-9

Anestesia e Medicina Critica

G. SLAVICH
Elettrocardiografia Clinica
1997, 328 pp, ISBN 3-540-75050-9

G.L. ALATI, B. ALLARIA, G. BERLOT, A. GULLO, A. LUZZANI,
G. MARTINELLI, L. TORELLI
Anestesia e Malattie Concomitanti - Fisiopatologia e clinica del
periodo perioperatorio
1997, 382 pp, ISBN 3-540-75048-7

B. ALLARIA, M.V. BALDASSARE, A. GULLO, A. LUZZANI,
G. MANANI, G. MARTINELLI, A. PASETTO, L. TORELLI
Farmacologia Generale e Speciale in Anestesiologia Clinica
1997, 312 pp, ISBN 88-470-0001-7

A. GULLO
Anestesia Clinica
1998, 506 pp, ISBN 88-470-0038-6

Regional Anaesthesia
Analgesia and Pain Management

Springer

Milano
Berlin
Heidelberg
New York
Barcelona
Hong Kong
London
Paris
Singapore
Tokyo

M. Tiengo
V.A. Paladini
N. Rawal (Eds)

Regional Anaesthesia Analgesia and Pain Management

Basics, Guidelines and Clinical Orientation

Series edited by
Antonino Gullo

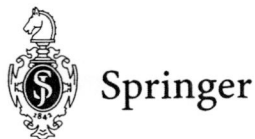 Springer

M. TIENGO, MD
Professor Emeritus
University of Milan, Milan - Italy

V.A. PALADINI, MD
Department of Anaesthesia, Intensive Care and Pain Therapy
University of Trieste, Cattinara Hospital, Trieste - Italy

N. RAWAL, MD
Department of Anaesthesiology and Intensive Care
Orebro University Hospital, Orebro - Sweden

Series of *Topics in Anaesthesia and Critical Care* edited by
A. GULLO, MD
Department of Anaesthesia, Intensive Care
and Pain Therapy
University of Trieste, Cattinara Hospital, Trieste - Italy

© Springer Verlag Italia, Milano 1999

ISBN 978-88-470-0044-5   ISBN 978-88-470-2240-9 (eBook)
DOI 10.1007/978-88-470-2240-9

Library of Congress Cataloging-in-Publication Data: Applied for

Cover design: Simona Colombo, Milan
Typesetting and layout· Compostudio, Milan

SPIN: 10697697

Foreword

Local-regional anaesthesia and pain therapy represent two areas of common interest for all physicians. A thorough preparation in functional anatomy and general pharmacology, including familiarity with local anaesthetics and analgesics is considered fundamental background for further study or clinical application of such techniques. Knowledge of the mechanisms of action, efficacies and side effects of the relevant drugs is essential, as is appreciation of possible drug interactions to evaluate toxic effects.

Local-regional anaesthesia and pain management are being increasingly used in diverse medical specialties, including those requiring manual dexterity. Many medical specialities such as obstetrics, orthopedics and traumatology, particularly with geriatric patients, and many scientific societies have developed guidelines to assist in choosing the most efficient and appropriate clinical approach, especially when the use of invasive techniques is required. Such guidelines direct the treatment of acute post-operative pain, the management of pain associated with cancer, and the medical support of terminally ill patients who present a series of overlapping symptoms such as pain, anxiety, and fear, and who often require personalized therapeutic care. Given the difficulty of these issues, it is important to consider the manner in which a physician obtains the patient's authorization for new therapies. Patient consent is most critical when the clinician, for scientific or ethical reasons, chooses a therapy that is experimental or in which the medical staff's experience is insufficient. In this context in particular, and in all cases in which local-regional anaesthesia and analgesia are utilized, legal issues assume prominent levels as a result of the expectations that the patient has regarding both the illness and the physician's competence.

Therefore, in contemporary medicine, and in particular in the fields of local-regional anaesthesia and pain treatment, correct evaluation of the medical outcome becomes essential, especially in relation to the cost-benefit balance: obviously not only in terms of resources consumed (i.e. budget), but also and more importantly for the quality of life of the patient.

November, 1998   *Antonino Gullo, MD*

Contents

REGIONAL TECHNIQUES

ORGANIZATION OF PAIN SERVICE

Contributors

Adriansen H.
Department of Anaesthesiology, University Hospital of Antwerp, Edegem, Belgium.

Amanzio M.
Department of Neuroscience and CIND Center for the Neurophysiology of Pain, University of Turin Medical School, Turin, Italy.

Babinet-Berthier A.
Department of Anaesthesiology, Hôpital Tenon, Paris, France.

Ballerio R.
Center for Cardiopulmonary Pharmacology, Institute of Pharmacological Sciences, University of Milan, Milan, Italy.

Barbolan B.
Department of Anaesthesia, Intensive Care and Pain Therapy, University of Trieste, Cattinara Hospital, Trieste, Italy.

Benedetti C.
Anesthesia Pain Services, The Ohio State University, James Cancer Hospital, Columbus, USA.

Benedetti F.
Department of Neuroscience and CIND Center for the Neurophysiology of Pain, University of Turin Medical School, Turin, Italy.

Berti M.
Department and Chair of Anaesthesiology, University of Milan, IRCCS San Raffaele Hospital, Milan, Italy.

Bianchi M.
Department of Pharmacology, University of Milan, Milan, Italy.

Bonnet F.
Department of Anaesthesiology, Hôpital Tenon, Paris, France.

Branca L.
Department of Anaesthesia and Intensive Care, General Hospital, Locri, Italy.

Broggi G.
Department of Neurosurgery, C. Besta Neurological Institute, Milan, Italy.

Calzà L.
Pathophysiology Center for the Nervous System, Hesperia Hospital, Modena, Italy.

Casati A.
Department and Chair of Anesthesiology, University of Milan, IRCCS San Raffaele Hospital, Milan, Italy.

Castelletti I.
Department of Obstetrics and Gynecology, Anaesthesia and Intensive Care Unit, University of Turin, Italy.

Cestelli A.
A. Monroy Department of Cell Biology, Palermo, Italy.

Chang D.H.-T.
University of Sidney, Royal North Shore Hospital, St. Leonards, Australia.

Di Bello L.
Department of Anaesthesia, Intensive Care and Pain Therapy, University of Trieste, Cattinara Hospital, Italy.

Di Liegro I.
"A. Monroy" Department of Cell Biology, Palermo, Italy.

Dones I.
Department of Neurosurgery, C. Besta Neurological Hospital, Milan, Italy.

Fanelli G.
Department and Chair of Anesthesiology, University of Milan, IRCCS San Raffaele Hospital, Milan, Italy.

Favalli L.
Department of Pharmacology, University of Pavia, Italy.

Ferrari Baliviera E.
Department of Anaesthesia and Intensive Care, S. Filippo Neri Hospital, Rome, Italy.

Ferrario P.
Department of Pharmacology, University of Milan, Milan, Italy.

Ferrero M.E.
Department of General Pathology, University of Milan, Italy.

Ferroli P.
Department of Neurosurgery, C. Besta Neurological Hospital, Milan, Italy.

Finco G.
Department of Anaesthesiology and Intensive Care, Pain Therapy Centre, University of Verona, Policlinico Hospital, Verona, Italy

Franzini A.
Department of Neurosurgery, C. Besta Neurological Hospital, Milan, Italy.

Fulgenzi A.
Department of General Pathology, University of Milan, Italy.

Gammaldi R.
Department of Anaesthesia and Intensive Care, Buon Consiglio Hospital, Fatebenefratelli, Naples, Italy.

Glynn C.J.
Oxford Pain Relief Unit, Nuffield Department of Anaesthetics, University of Oxford, Churchill Hospital, Oxford, UK.

Gottin L.
Department Anaesthesiology and Intensive Care, Pain Therapy Centre, University of Verona, Policlinico Hospital, Verona, Italy.

Govoni S.
Department of Pharmacology, University of Pavia, Italy.

Ischia S.
Department of Anaesthesiology and Intensive Care, Pain Therapy Centre, University of Verona, Policlinico Hospital, Verona, Italy.

Kouyanou K.
Psychiatric Hospital of Attica, Athens, Greece and Department of Psychological Medicine, Institute of Psychiatry, London, UK.

Lugani D.
Department and Chair of Anesthesiology, University of Milan, IRCCS San Raffaele Hospital, Milan, Italy.

Margaria E.
Department of Obstetrics and Gynecology, Anaesthesia and Intensive Care Unit, University of Torino, Italy.

Mather L.E.
University of Sidney, Royal North Shore Hospital, St. Leonards, Australia.

Masoero E.
Institute of Pharmacology, University of Pavia, Italy.

Mennini F.S.
Faculty of Business and Economics, CEIS, University Tor Vergata, Roma, Italy.

Mercieri M.
Anesthesia Pain Services, The Ohio State University, James Cancer Hospital, Columbus, USA.

Nicosia F.
Department of Anaesthesia and Intensive Care, National Cancer Institute, Genoa, Italy.

Nolli M.
Department of Anaesthesia and Intensive Care, General Hospital, Cremona, Italy.

Osman M.
Department of Anaesthesiology, Hôpital Tenon, Paris, France.

Paladini V.A.
Department of Anaesthesia Intensive Care and Pain Therapy, University of Trieste, Cattinara Hospital, Trieste, Italy.

Palazzo F.
Institute of Biomedical Technologies, CNR, Rome, Italy.

Panerai A.E.
Department of Pharmacology, University of Milan, Milan, Italy.

Petruzzelli P.
Department of Obstetrics and Gynecology, Anaesthesia and Intensive Care Unit, University of Turin, Italy.

Piacevoli Q.
Department of Anaesthesiology and Intensive Care, B. Filippo Hospital, Rome, Italy.

Polati E.
Department of Anaesthesiology and Intensive Care, Pain Therapy Centre, University of Verona, Policlinico Hospital, Verona, Italy.

Pozza M.
Pathophysiology Center for the Nervous System, Hesperia Hospital, Modena, Italy.

Rawal N.
Department of Anaesthesiology and Intensive Care, Òrebro University Hospital, Orebro, Sweden.

Sacerdote P.
Department of Pharmacology, University of Milan, Milan, Italy.

Sala A.
Center for Cardiopulmonary Pharmacology, Institute of Pharmacological Sciences, University of Milan, Milan, Italy.

Savettieri G.
Institute of Neuropsychiatry, Palermo, Italy.

Savoia G.
Department of Anaesthesia and Intensive Care, Buon Consiglio Hospital, Fatebenefratelli, Naples, Italy.

Scibelli G.
Department of Anaesthesia and Intensive Care, Buon Consiglio Hospital, Fatebenefratelli, Naples, Italy.

Servello D.
Department of Neurosurgery, C. Besta Neurological Hospital, Milan, Italy.

Tiengo M.
Professor Emeritus, University of Milan, Milan, Italy.

Viappiani S.
Center for Cardiopulmonary Pharmacology, Institute of Pharmacological Sciences, University of Milan, Milan, Italy.

Zamperoni A.
Department of Anaesthesia, Intensive Care and Pain Therapy, University of Trieste, Cattinara Hospital, Italy.

Zanni M.
ORL Department, General Hospital, Carpi, Italy.

Zarini S.
Center for Cardiopulmonary Pharmacology, Institute of Pharmacological Sciences, University of Milan, Milan, Italy.

PATHOPHYSIOLOGY OF PAIN
AND GENETIC ADVANCE

Chapter 1

Integrated axon-synapse unit in the central nervous system

A. Cestelli, G. Savettieri, I. Di Liegro

One of the most daunting questions in developmental neurobiology concerns the mechanisms which allow cohorts of neurons to develop the intricate, yet stereotypic pattern of connections in the adult nervous system: it has been estimated that 10^{11} neurons of human brain establish a network of 10^{14} synaptic contacts. We must consider, however, that most neurons are generally grouped into classes with a characteristic pattern of connectivity and this mere fact allows the wiring of complex neural networks to be controlled by the reiteration and diversification of a relatively small number of prototypic connection patterns. On the other hand, it is a matter of fact that axon projection to the corresponding targets, which is a key element in the assembly of the nervous system, links the early inductive interactions that establish neuronal identity to the later steps of synapse formation. It is worth remembering that in the last decade it has been demonstrated that the exocytic trafficking system, which is the heart of the synaptic machinery, represents one of the most fascinating examples of conservation of a complex biological system throughout evolution, from yeast to vertebrates [1]. Neurons extend axons and dendrites through an outstanding variety of environments using a specialized structure which each of them has at its end, the growth cone [2, 3]. Growth cones detect and respond to information from their immediate environment by extending filopodia and lamellae that are endowed with a panoplia of receptors.

The present review focuses on the four main elements which contribute to the formation of an integrated axon-synapse unit in the nervous system:
– the establishment of neuronal polarity which determines the orientation and the rate of extension of growth cones;
– the molecules (growth factors, cell and extracellular matrix adhesion proteins) in the local environment of an extending axon which control growth cone behavior;
– the intracellular machinery which integrates multiple extracellular signals to produce the coordinated and directed response of growth cone navigation;
– the mechanisms which select and eventually refine the initial connections into highly tuned and functioning neural circuits.

Neuronal polarity

The developmental events leading to the establishment of neuronal polarity have been well characterized in hippocampal neurons in culture [4]. Shortly after plating, the neuronal perikaryon is surrounded by a wide lamellipodium (stage 1). Within the the next 4-12 h, the lamellipodium thickens in certain areas and several short neurites (typically 15-25 μm in length) extend: these neurites have been referred to as minor proocesses, because at this stage their features are not yet obviously axonal or dendritic (stage 2). Some 12-24 h later, only one of the processes elongates: this neurite is the cell axon and its selective elongation is the first morphological evidence of neuronal polarity (stage 3). Within the next 3-4 days in culture, the elongation of the remaining minor processes which acquire the morphological features mark them as dendrites (stage 4). The last stage (stage 5), which starts on the seventh day in culture, does not involve a change in polarity, but implies continued maturation of both axonal and dendritic processes, including dendritic branching, the onset of synaptogenesis, and the formation of dendritic spines.

With regard to the establishment of neuronal polarity, the morphological appearance, dynamics and function of growth cones are equivalent to those of membrane extensions that decorate the leading edges of migrating cells. This means that increased growth cone size reflects membrane addition and this can generate the advancement force of a trailing neurite, and, in fact, in most stage 2 neurons the emergence of the axon can be predicted when the following criteria are satisfied: a) a large and dynamic growth cone; b) an abundant organelle trafficking in the corresponding neurite. In a recent paper it has been demonstrated that peroxisomes, mitochondria, post-Golgi vesicles, ribosomes and some proteins, which normally localize in axonal and dendritic processes, all appear polarized to one of neurites of stage 2 cells [5]. Moreover, since similar asymmetric distribution is also observed in already polarized (stage 3) cells, bulk cytoplasmic flow may also play a role in the stabilization of the early axon.

In addition, neuronal polarization also requires more sophisticated mechanisms, such as molecular sorting. Molecular sorting ensures that proteins, lipids, and organelles segregate into the different plasma membrane and cytoplasmic domains of polarized cells (i.e. axonal and dendritic in neurons and apical and basolateral in epithelia) [6, 7]. In fully polarized neurons, membrane proteins are recognized as axonal or dendritic by specific signals present in their primary structure: in the cytoplasmic terminal for dendritic proteins [8] and in the transmembrane ectodomain for axonal proteins [9]. In neurons which are undergoing polarization, early dendrites can become the cell axon if the first axon is damaged [5]: this supports the hypothesis that, during development, neuronal polarization is an adventitious phenomenon and that at this early stage all growth cones of a single neuron receive and retrieve similar amounts of membrane, enough to maintain neurite attachment and a balance between elongation and retraction. In addition, a recent paper provides strong evidence that targeting of basolateral (in epithelial cells) and dendritic (in neurons) proteins depends on a common mechanism, while the sorting of proteins to the axon requires signals that are not present in apical proteins of polarized epithelial cells [10].

As we shall see in the following sections, at a certain point of development, only a single growth cone, after a fortuitous longer or tighter attachment to the substratum or contact with a higher concentration of growth factor, can become more stabilized than others and this creates a local change which, in turn, signals the cell body for augmented polarized flow of membrane, cytoskeletal and cytosolic proteins, lipids, and organelles. Stabilization of this early polarization will then result in axonal formation.

Roles of growth factors, cell and extracellular matrix adhesion proteins in axonal pathfinding

Axonal pathfinding during development is highly stereospecific and depends upon the interaction among receptor molecules present in the growth cone and extrinsic cues, such as soluble factors, secreted by intermediate and final targets, glycosyl phosphatidylinositol (GPI)-anchored or transmembrane glycoproteins on the surface of cells, and components of extracellular matrix (Fig. 1). Correct navigation is likely to require the presence of a large number of cues that can both stimulate or inhibit axonal growth. In most cases, the guidance of axons to their final destination can be considered as a series of short-range projections to intermediate targets under the influence of local guidance cues. As we shall see in a later section, axons respond to these cues by means of a motile sensory apparatus at the growth cone.

One class of molecules that has been recently implicated in the development of axonal projections is the neurotrophin family of growth factors. Neurotrophins are small, secreted proteins which promote the survival of various classes of neurons in critical periods of nervous system development [11]; mem-

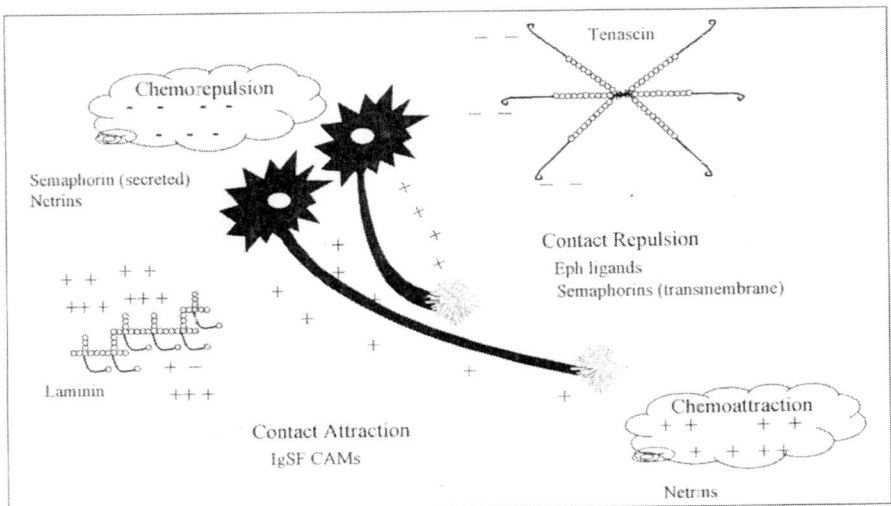

Fig. 1. Axon pathfinding guidance molecules. *IgSF CAMs*, immunoglobulin superfamily cell adhesion molecules

bers of this family include nerve growth factor (NGF), brain-derived neurotrophic factor (BDNF), neurotrophin-3 (NT-3), and neurotrophin 4/5 (NT-4/5). A few recent studies have provided evidence that neurotrophins can also exert a significant effect on axonal projections in the CNS.

A long-standing hypothesis concerning the pattern of axonal projections holds that developing axons require target-derived factors for their stabilization and that ingrowing axons compete for limiting amounts of such target-derived trophic factors, one of the most important classes of which being the neurotrophin. It has also been proposed that, during thalamocortical development, more active thalamic afferents have a competitive advantage. A prediction of this hypothesis is that an excess of target-derived neurotrophins should eliminate competition among thalamic afferents, and, indeed, it has been shown [12] that infusion of BDNF or NT-4/5 into the visual cortex of kittens during the critical period prevents the segregation of geniculocortical axons into ocular dominance columns.

The ability to obtain a response to neurotrophin does not, however, necessarily mean that these factors have the same function in vivo. In a recent study neurotrophin "receptor bodies" were infused into developing visual cortex [13]. Receptor bodies are fusion proteins consisting of the ligand-binding domain of a receptor (in this case, one of the neurotrophin receptors, Trk-A, Trk-B, or Trk-C) fused to the Fc portion of human Immunoglobulin G (IgG). It was found that infusion of Trk-B-IgG, but not Trk-A-IgG or Trk-C-IgG, into the visual cortex of kittens blocked the segregation of lateral geniculate nucleus axons into ocular dominance columns. This means that a Trk-B ligand, most likely BDNF or NT-4/5, participates in the eye-specific segregation of geniculate axons.

One class of molecules implicated in the generation of neural networks in neurohistogenesis is that of the neural members of the immunoglobulin superfamily (IgSF). These molecules belong to different subfamilies on the basis of their overall domain arrangement and mode of plasma membrane anchoring [14, 15]. In line with their structural diversity, axonal IgSF members are involved in different aspects of neurohistogenesis; for instance, they play a role in radial and tangential migration of neural precursors, in neurite fasciculation and in contact-dependent axonal guidance and stimulation of neurite extension, as well as in contact-dependent inhibition of neurite growth. The overlapping expression of IgSF proteins on several axonal systems during development suggests that some of these molecules may cooperate functionally. Their direct molecular interactions have been investigated by measuring the aggregation of protein-coated fluorescent microspheres and their binding to transfected eukaryotic cells, as well as by ELISA, by co-capping analyses and by chemical cross-linking experiments. Such studies have been extended by neurite outgrowth assays in combination with antibody interference experiments that examined neurite outgrowth on transfected eukaryotic cells or on neural substrates, and, finally, by examination of the consequences of both loss- and gain-of-function mutants [14]. Through these methodologies, molecules of the IgSF have been demonstrated to be involved in multiple *trans* and *cis* interactions, either homophilically or heterophilically. For example, the F11 glycoprotein not only interacts with the extracellular matrix (ECM) proteins tenascin (TN)-R and TN-C, but also with axonal adhesion receptors, such as L1/NgCAM (neuron-glia cell adhesion molecule), NrCAM (NgCAM-related cell adhesion molecule), and receptor protein tyrosine phosphatase (RPTP) β/ζ [14]. The most complex interaction pattern was found for the axonal glycoprotein NgCAM, which binds to at least six different proteins: TAG-1 (transiently expressed axonal glycoprotein-1)/ axonin-1, DM-GRASP (immunoglobulin-like restricted axonal surface protein that is expressed in the dorsal funiculus and ventral midline of the chick spinal cord), laminin, phosphacan, neurocan and, homophilically, to itself.

This multivalency is in accord with the modular-domain organization of IgSF molecules and confers to the construction of the nervous system architecture a resemblance to immune system function, which also depends on complex molecular interactions among molecules of the IgSF. This complexity is further increased by context effects: for example, F11 and its ECM ligand TN-R are responsible for repulsion in cerebellar neurons [16], whereas they modulate axonal outgrowth response in tectal neurons [17].

In addition, recent findings have shown that mutations in the IgSF adhesion molecule L1 gene are associated with severe neurological deficits [18, 19].

Since its identification as a member of the IgSF, NCAM (neural cell adhesion molecule) remains the prototypic CAM: alternative splicing generates the main size classes of 180, 140, and 120-kDa. The transmembrane 180 and 140 isoforms are expressed by neurons, while glial cells express mainly 140-kDa NCAM, and myotubes express a variant of the 120-kDa GPI-anchored NCAM [20]. Antibody perturbation studies provided the first evidence that NCAM could stimulate axonal growth responses and a direct demonstration was obtained by culturing neurons over monolayers of transfected fibroblasts expressing physiologically relevant levels of individual NCAM isoforms [21]. Interestingly, these studies provided the first direct evidence that post-translational processing could modulate the ability of this molecule to stimulate axonal growth responses: this regulation revolves around the ability of a large linear homopolymer of sialic acid (called polysialic acid or PSA) to attenuate cell interactions and thereby create plasticity in the positioning and movement of cells and/or their processes. PSA is expressed on growing axons and is generally lost during development, except in some regions. Its pattern of expression in the adult brain is consistent with its role in synaptic plasticity [22]. As enzymatic removal of PSA increases the adhesive function of NCAM, its role was initially thought to be inhibiton of NCAM function. On the other hand, enzymatic removal of PSA dramatically reduces the ability of NCAM to stimulate axonal growth, suggesting that it is a positive rather than a negative modulator of NCAM function. To settle these discrepancies, several possible modes of PSA action can be considered, the most obvious being *trans* mechanisms, in which the hydrated volume of PSA would interfere in the approach of two different membranes, and *cis* mechanisms, in which PSA would prevent interactions among molecules within the plane of the same membrane, thus inhibiting formation of stable NCAM clusters that would otherwise be induced by *trans* homo- and heterophilic binding. This then keeps NCAMs in a more dynamic pool, allowing them to participate in the interactions that promote cell migration, axonal growth, and synaptic plasticity. For example, PSA removal from motoneurons entering the plexus is associated with errors in pathfinding by their axons. The same treatment in retinal ganglion cells growing into the tectum leads to a significant alteration in fascicle size. Moreover, the activity-dependent expression of PSA at the synapse suggests a role for this molecule in activity-induced synaptic plasticity. Indeed, it has recently been demonstrated that its enzymatic removal completely prevents the induction of long-term potentiation (LTP) and long-term-depression (LTD) in the CA1 region of hippocampal slice cultures, while it does not affect other cellular and synaptic parameters such as resting and action potentials [22].

The 10-amino acid variable alternatively spliced exon (VASE) changes the structure of the fourth Ig domain of NCAM and this also modulates the axonal growth properties of the whole molecule: use of the VASE exon in either the cellular substrate or responding neuron inhibits the axonal growth response stimulated by NCAM and can account for the loss of neuronal responsiveness to NCAM that has been documented for several populations of neurons [23]. The use of the VASE exon increases during development, and around 50% of NCAM transcripts have VASE in the adult rat. However, as for downregulation of PSA expression, appearance of the VASE sequence is spatially restricted, and in general it does not appear in brain areas that continue to exhibit synaptic plasticity.

The involvement of IgSF CAMs in processes ranging from cell migration to axonal growth and synaptic plasticity makes it difficult to believe that they function simply by modulating cell adhesion. As we shall see in the next section, these molecules activate second messenger cascades. The outgrowth of neuronal processes has also been measured in the presence of various combinations of antagonists and agonists of different, known intracellular signaling pathways: by this approach it was possible to establish a general outline of the temporal order of activation of these molecules, with the tyrosine kinase being the earliest component of the system and the latest being the opening of N-type and L-type calcium channels [24].

The first evidence that fibroblast growth factor (FGF) receptor might be the tyrosine kinase immediately activated by CAMs came with the observation that this recepor shares homology with a small number of CAMs, including NCAM, N-cadherin, and L1, and on this basis it was postulated that these CAMs activate the FGF receptor signaling cascade [24]. There are now three sets of comprehensive experiments supporting the hypothesis that these three CAMs stimulate axonal growth via a FGF receptor-dependent mechanism. Firstly, antibodies that inhibit FGF receptor function inhibit axonal growth responses stimulated by transfected NCAM, N-cadherin, and L1 [25]. Secondly, expression of dominant-negative FGF receptors in neuronal cells specifically inhibits the axonal growth responses stimulated by CAMs [26]. And thirdly, both soluble NCAM and L1-Fc chimeras can stimulate a rapid phosphorylation of the FGF receptor in neural cells, and this is a hallmark of receptor activation [26].

In addition to FGF receptor, a variety of other receptor protein tyrosine kinases (RPTKs) modulate axon growth and regulate target invasion: the largest group of RPTKs is the Eph family, which has 14 members that have been classified into two subgroups (A and B) on the basis of the homology of their extracellular domains [27, 28]. Ligands for these receptors, termed ephrins (for Eph receptor interacting proteins) are membrane-attached proteins themselves and fall into two classes (again, A and B) relating to sequence conservation and the way they are attached to membranes: class A via a GPI anchor, whereas class B has both transmembrane and cytoplasmic regions. These groupings also roughly correspond to the binding specificities of ligands for receptors. Expression of Eph family members in the developing embryo is dynamic and is particularly marked in neural structures: corresponding receptor and ligand classes are often detected in reciprocal and apparently mutually exclusive distributions, suggesting that they may divide the embryo into discrete functional domains [29]: receptor – ligand interactions are expected to occur via cell – cell contact, potentially at boundaries at which domains of receptor- and ligand-expressing cells meet.

The first functional evidence for a role of Eph receptors in axon guidance came from the purification and cloning of ephrin A-5 and the following demonstration that it is the tectal protein responsible for the collapse of retinal axon growth cones [28]. In vitro assays have demonstrated that ligand activation of Eph receptors in neuronal cells initiate antiadhesive responses, characterized by repulsion of axons and collapse of growth cones.

Although much has been learned about the action of RPTKs in the response of cells to extracellular signals, less is known about the regulation and function of receptor-type protein tyrosine phospatases (RPTPs) in these processes. Their function appears to be similar to that of cell adhesion molecules in sensing environmental cues during the process of axon guidance. All RPTPs are composed of an extracellular domain, which shares structural similarities with cell adhesion molecules (suggesting that they play a role in cell – cell communication by directly coupling cell recognition events to signal-transducing pathways inside the cell), a single transmembrane domain, and a cytoplasmic portion, which usually contains two tandemly arranged protein phosphatase domains. RPTPβ is expressed on the surface of glial cells and may regulate the growth of axons via reverse signaling through a protein complex on an adjacent cell, analogous to the Eph receptor – ephrin system [29]. In search for a ligand of RPTPβ it was found that it binds with high affinity and specificity to the GPI-anchored protein contactin/F11 and that this binding leads to cell adhesion and neurite outgrowth. According to this model, RPTPβ expressed on the surface of glial cells binds to a neuronal recognition complex, suggesting a bidirectional link between cell adhesion molecules and RPTPs.

Semaphorins constitute the second large family of proteins which act as repulsive axon guidance cues for specific populations of neurons [30]: as an example, the human genome encodes more than 20 distinct semaphorins, which include both secreted and transmembrane glycoproteins, and this suggests that some of them influence growth cone guidance at a distance, while others act locally (Fig. 1). The evidence that semaphorins function as repulsive signals is extensive. Chicken collapsin-1, a secreted semaphorin and the ortholog of the mammalian semaphorin III/D (Sema III) can function in vitro as a collapsing factor for sensory growth cones. Recently, neuropilin has been shown to be a receptor for Sema III, since it is required for Sema III chemorepulsive and growth cone collapsing functions: antibodies directed against neuropilin inhibit Sema III functions on sensory neurons in vitro, and, more importantly, growth cones of sensory neurons cultured from mice lacking an intact neuropilin gene do not collapse in the presence of Sema III [31].

In the last decade, the role of ECM in brain development has been the subject of intensive research [32] and this although, in the adult CNS, outside blood vassels, and the meningeal surfaces, it is hard to recognize the traits of an ECM. With the exception of synaptic sites, at the electron microscope it is impossible to visualize traces of well-organized, electron-dense material that reveals the presence of ECM. Despite this general lack of convincing proof, several investigators have been intrigued by the ability of many molecules to influence neuronal and glial cell behavior in vitro. Besides glycosaminoglycans (GAGs) and proteoglycans (PGs), other ECM components, such as laminin and fibronectin which modulate cell adhesion and neurite outgrowth in vitro, are transiently expressed in the developing CNS: all together, these data support the hypothesis that ECM does exist in the developing CNS and is a dynamic structure (Fig. 1).

A great variety of developmentally expressed PGs have been implicated in the regulation of neurite outgrowth. PGs are capable of providing signals that either stimulate or inhibit neurite outgrowth. Among the PGs, heparan sulfate (HS) PGs of both neuronal and astrocytic origin are the most closely associated with neuritogenesis. These compounds, which are among the most highly charged molecules in nature, can exert their effects by activating other proteins, such as laminin, NCAM, FGF-2, all of which may stimulate axon outgrowth when complexed with HSPGs [33].

A great body of literature has shown that laminin-1 promotes neurite outgrowth in many neuronal cell types from both PNS and CNS [34]. Moreover, laminin immunoreactivity is transiently expressed in vitro along the pathway of growing axons [35], reflecting the role of this molecule in axon growth and guidance. However, information regarding the differentiation-promoting effects (as distinct from axonal promoting effects) of laminins is still scarce [36].

TN-C, which is a member of a small family of ECM glycoproteins, has been shown in culture to inhibit axon growth by several types of CNS neurons: in vivo [37] its distribution in regions such as barrel fields in the somatosensory cortex is consistent with the possibility that it delineates barriers that restrict axonal growth.

Netrins, laminin-related molecules, represent a family of ECM molecules with a phylogenetically conserved role in axon pathfinding in vertebrates. *Caenorabditis elegans*, and *Drosophila melanogaster* [38]. In rodents, commissural neurons, which are born dorsally in the spinal cord, extend axons circumferentially toward the floor plate, through the receptor DCC (deleted in colorectal cancer) in response to netrin-1 secreted by floor plate cells. In addition to their apparently attactive role, netrins have been implicated as repellents of axons that migrate away from the midline in both *C. elegans* and vertebrates. Furthermore, genetic and biochemical evidence suggests that the attractive and repulsive actions of netrin proteins might involve different functional domains of the netrin molecule and may be mediated by distinct receptor mechanisms.

The diversity of responses show how the interactions of multiple neuronal surface components with several cell surface and ECM molecules can lead to a multiplicity of effects on axonal growth.

Intracellular transduction of extracellular signals

As discussed, the accurate and polarized targeting of a variety of membrane proteins plays a central role in the precise localization of the sites of releasing and receiving the signals that regulate the outgrowth of neurites and the formation as well as the functioning of synaptic connections. During development, these signals must be processed and integrated to ensure continuous adjustment of routes and targets and the selective stabilization of synapses. Moreover, in the adult organism, integration of signals at the synapse seems to be the basis for learning and memory.

We have discussed elsewhere the biochemical mechanisms responsible for neurotrasmission in the postsynaptic elements and for the modulation of neurotransmission itself [39]. Here we will focus on the mechanisms that might modulate nerve terminal growth and synapse establishment and maintenance by retrograde signaling from the growth cone and from the mature axon-synapse unit up to the cell nucleus.

The intracellular spreading (or transduction) of extracellular signals relies on molecular circuits involving a cascade of phosphorylation/dephosphorylation events leading to pleiotropic modulation of the activity of different molecules. Soluble factors as well as adhesion molecules activate these circuits after binding to membrane receptors.

The neurotrophins NGF, BDNF, NF-3 and NF 4/5 that, as discussed above, are required for stabilization and survival of specific classes of neurons bind a group of cognate receptor tyrosine kinases (trk A, B and C: 11). In addition, the four neurotrophins bind a low-affinity receptor, known as $p75^{NTR}$ (low affinity neurotrophin receptor) that is a member of the tumor necrosis factor (TNF) receptor family and transduces ligand-dependent apoptotic signals [40-45]. The main role previously assigned to $p75^{NTR}$ was to enhance binding of neurotrophins to the Trk receptors and, hence, signaling through them [46]. During development, when neurons must compete for limiting amounts of target-derived trophic factors, enhancement of affinity for neurotrophins can be a significant advantage indeed. However, biochemical evidence that $p75^{NTR}$ "presents" NGF to TrkA is only indirect and a cross-linked $p75^{NTR}$-Trk-NGF complex has never been described [40]. More recently, Frade et al. showed that, in chick, NGF causes the death of retinal neurons that express p75^{NTR} but not TrkA [47]; a similar observation has been reported in oligodendrocytes [48]. Neurotrophins can thus elicit cell responses by binding only p75^{NTR}, in the absence of TrkA-C, thus implying the existence of a p75^{NTR}-specific intracellular transduction pathway. The first proof that this is in fact the case came from the finding that binding of any of the neurotrophins to p75^{NTR} in T9 glioma cells or in NIH3T3 embryonal fibroblasts activates sphingomyelinase and increases the release of ceramide [49]. It was also demonstrated that NGF binding to p75^{NTR} induces nuclear translocation of the transcription factor NF-kB and its binding to DNA [44, 50]. On the basis of these findings, Bredesen and Rabizadeh [43] proposed that p75^{NTR} displays an intrinsic receptor effect (IRE) and a distinct ligand-dependent effect (LiRE). The former may be a pro-apoptotic effect that depends on the interaction of unbound, monomeric p75^{NTR} with another molecule which might be cytosolic, membrane-bound, or extracellular. On the other hand, binding of any of the neurotrophins and multimerization of p75^{NTR} would inhibit pro-apoptotic effects and trigger other signaling pathways [43]. The existence of a multiplicity of factors which interact with the intracellular domain of other members of the TNF receptor family suggests that p75^{NTR} has its own intracellular effectors, too. By using the yeast two-hybrid system a potential signal-transducing protein (NGF-receptor interacting factor, NRIF), associated with the cytoplasmic domain of p75^{NTR}, has been indeed identified [44]. Interestingly, association of this zinc finger protein with p75^{NTR} is ligand-dependent and specific for NGF [44]. Taken together, the recent finding that NGF receptors can trigger intracellular signaling pathways, leading to apoptosis, allows renewed consideration of the well-known early observation that removal of trophic factors induces cell death in the developing nervous system. One can now envisage that, when neurons sense trophic factor deprivation, a sequence of events is triggered, which includes among the final steps activation of apoptosis-specific proteases, now termed caspases. Activation of caspases might represent in turn the commitment point after which neurons cannot be rescued anymore from death by addition of neurotrophins [45]. As cell death implies de novo protein synthesis, at least in some classes of neurons, there must be some transcription factor which induces expression of death genes. One of these proteins seems to be the product of the cellular proto-oncogene *c-jun* which is phosphorylated after activation of the kinase JNK (Jun N-terminal kinase); the JNK activity is induced by a variety of environmental stresses and, interestingly, in many cases it seems to be a necessary but not sufficient prerequisite to death; this means that the decision to undergo programmed cell death must rely on other signals acting in concert with *c-jun* activation [45]. From this point of view, it is worth noting that Trk receptors, at least in PC12 cells, use the same tyrosine residue for coupling to the Ras signaling pathway and to the phosphatidylinositol (3'-OH) kinase (PI-3K). Both couplings appear to occur through src-homology cognate (SHC) and Grb-2 (growth factor receptor-bound protein) adaptor proteins; however, in the first case, Grb-2 further couples to "Son of Sevenless" (SOS: the GDP-GTP exchange factor for Ras), thus activating the Ras pathway, whereas in the second case, Grb-2 docks on a novel protein which couples it to PI-3K [40]. Activation of PI-3K pathway is critical for PC-12 survival, whereas PI-3K inhibitors are not able to induce apoptosis in superior cervical sympathetic neurons maintained in NGF [51]. On the other hand, death of sympathetic neurons, after NGF removal, can be blocked by overexpressing PI-3K or its downstream effector serine/threonine kinase AKT, despite activation of the JNK pathway [45, 51]. Thus, activation of the PI-3K pathway is sufficient to promote survival and can act independently of *c-Jun*. Moreover, PI-3K is not absolutely required for neuronal survival and it seems likely that NGF can activate multiple, and possibly redundant, pathways for survival. We can envisage that the relative roles of, for instance, Ras and PI-3K pathways will depend on the relative concentrations and state of activity of adaptor proteins and/or downstream effectors and, in general, on the precise physiological state of a given neuron. In this sense, the observation that, in Schwann cells, NGF can switch on genes via activation of p75[NTR] and NF-kB, without inducing cell death [44] is of utmost importance. NF-kB is a master factor which regulates the expression of a variety of genes, some of which could be involved in cell survival. In addition to neurotrophins, brain-specific activators of NF-kB also include neurotransmitters such as glutamate (via both AMPA/KA and NMDA receptors), suggesting its involvement in synaptic plasticity [52]. Some studies on neuronal excitation indicate that NF-kB activity might be regulated as a consequence of neurotransmission. Inducible NF-kB activity has been found in synaptosomes from cortex and hippocampus [52-54]. This unexpected localization suggests a synapse-to-nucleus signaling system in which transcriptional factors, activated as a consequence of local synaptic transmission, transduce a signal to the nucleus via retrograde transport (discussed below). This observation might be representative of a more general phenomenon, as a similar peripheral localization has also been reported for some nuclear steroid hormone receptors [55]. Moreover, activation of transcription factors by synaptic activity might represent the obvious link among neurotrophin- and activity-dependent plasticity in the developing as well as in the adult nervous system. Neocortical and hippocampal GABA-containing interneurons, for instance, are susceptible to activity-dependent regulation of soma size, numbers of synaptic contacts, and levels of GABA or neuropeptide expression [42]. In vitro, these effects of neuronal activity on morphology and gene expression may be mimicked, at least in part, by neurotrophins such as BDNF. In the neocortex and hippocampus, synthesis and secretion of BDNF by pyramidal neurons are activity-dependent events. As pyramidal neurons are target cells for the GABA-containing neurons, it has been suggested that BDNF is an activity-dependent, target-derived trophic factor for the GABA-producing interneurons [42].

Interestingly, NF-kB is also known to upregulate genes encoding adhesion molecules such as L1 [44]. Once expressed at the growth cone surface, adhesion molecules, upon interaction with their specific ligands present on other cells or in ECM, will transduce signals via pathways largely similar to the ones described above.

Adhesion is largely mediated by the cytoskeleton; it is therefore not surprising that the intracellular transduction of extracellular signals, arising from cell-cell and cell-ECM contacts, involves structural elements of the cytoskeleton and cytoskeleton-associated proteins as both signal-tranducing factors and targets to be modified as a consequence of the signal (Fig. 2).

During growth cone guidance, significant rearrangements occur which involve the two major cytoskeleton components of the growing axon: filamentous actin (F-actin) and microtubules [56]. Ultrastructural studies reveal that F-actin is localized preferentially in the peripheral cytoplasm, whereas microtubules cross the central cytoplasmic domain of axons. Moreover, at least two F-actin populations are distinguishable in the periphery of the growth cones: a) highly crosslinked networks, in the lamellipodia; b) highly polarized (distal plus-ends) bundles of actin filaments arrays that extend into the filopodia [56] (Fig. 2). The growth cone is at the same time a highly motile structure and a complex sensor able to recognize extracellular signals and to translate them into polarized growth. The peripheral cytoplasmic domain of the growth cone is the region that undergoes the main modifications responsible for movement: a) assembly of filaments at the leading edge; b) retrograde flux of actin toward the central core of microtubules [56, 57]. Both processes depend in part on the existence of actin-associated motor proteins known as unconventional myosins [58, 59]; at least 12 distinct classes of unconventional myosins are now known [58, 59]; nerve growth cones, in which myosin V has been inactivated instantaneously by treatment with specific antibodies, exhibit defects in filopodial extension, suggesting that myosin V plays a role in F-actin deposition, either by mediating

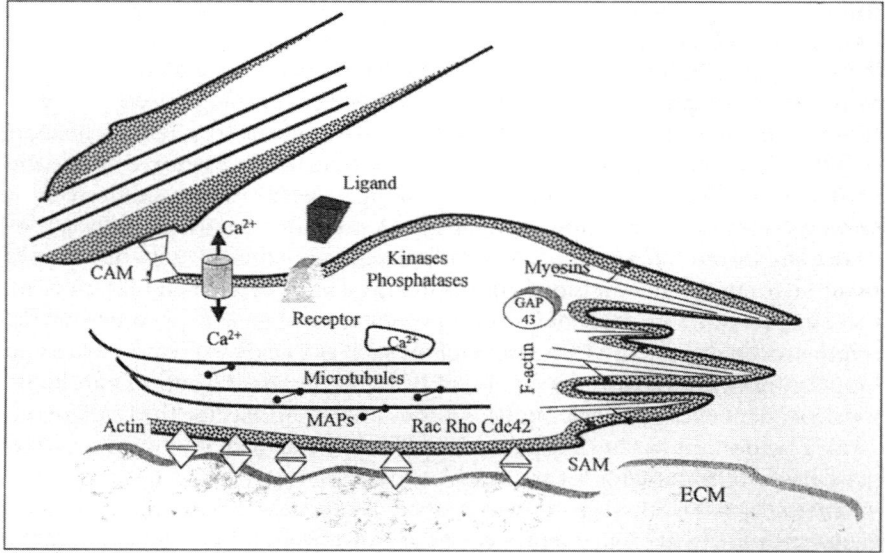

Fig. 2. Transduction pathways in a navigating growth cone: *CAM*, cell adhesion molecule; *MAPs*, microtubule associated proteins; *SAM*, substrate adhesion molecule; *ECM*, extracellular matrix

vesicle transport (and hence transport of new cytoskeleton subunits) up to the base of the filopodium or by pushing F-actin filaments and the plasma membrane one against the other [58]. Myosins are probably also involved in the retrograde F-actin flow: myosin inhibition results, indeed, in a slowing of retrograde F-actin flux, accompanied by an increase in the growth of filopodia which can, in turn, be blocked by inhibitors of actin polymerization [56]. Chick brain myosin 5a (M5a) is associated with punctuate structures and with small organelles that colocalize with both microtubules and actin filaments in growth cones, suggesting its association with synaptic vesicles [59].

The growth of the axon leading edge thus derives either from an increase of actin polymerization or from a decrease in actin retrograde flow [56]. The processes that regulate F-actin assembly at the leading edge also involve proteins able to bind monomeric actin (G-actin), such as profilin and thymosin β4 [60], plus-end capping proteins [60, 61] and actin-related proteins such as protein 2/3 (Arp 2/3) [62].

Microtubules are the second major cytoskeletal component of the growth cone and provide both structural support and the substrate for axonal transport of organelles. The mechanism through which arrays of microtubules in the axons are obtained is still the subject of controversy [63-65]. Two opposing theories have been proposed to explain how cytoskeletal filaments are deposited in axons; according to one model [64], filaments are transported as preformed polymers; according to the other one [65], the monomeric components of the three classes of cytoskeletal proteins (tubulin, actin and neurofilament proteins) are transported in some unassembled or oligomeric form along the axon and then added, where necessary, at the ends of the polymers. Both models acknowledge that individual filaments do not extend all the way from the cell body to the synaptic endings [63]. At the growth cone, microtubules establish dynamic contacts with the actin network, a process that is mainly due to dynamic instability of the microtubule itself and probably modulated by a variety of microtubule-associated poteins (MAPs) [56, 66-68], as demonstrated for MAP2c [68]. In addition, the transient contacts with F-actin are regulated by the activity of microtubule-associated motors, such as kinesin and dynein superfamily proteins [69, 70]. It is worth noting that axons contain a third class of cytoskeletal components: intermediate filaments (IFs) that form a flexible scaffold, essential for structuring the cytoplasm [71]. In most adult neurons of both the central and peripheral nervous system, the predominant type of IF are neurofilaments (NFs); several lines of evidence led to the concept that NFs control the increase of the diameter of the axon; however, the mechanisms that underlie this effect have not been yet fully resolved [71]. More recently, it was realized that the scaffold of IFs is achieved through a family of newly identified IF-associated proteins (IFAPs) that form cross-bridges between IFs and other cytoskeletal elements, such as microfilaments and microtubules [71]. The discovery that the neuronal protein BPAG 1 (bullous pemphigoid antigen 1) n/dystonin can coalign NFs with actin filaments in cultured cells strengthens its possible role as cytoskeletal cross-linking protein and provides an explanation for the defects found in mutant mice [72].

All these findings suggest that the axonal cytoskeleton is a dynamic structure, even if somehow stationary, and that a variety of associated proteins may cross-link the various cytoskeletal polymers and anchor this complex network to the membrane skeleton [73].

Most importantly, organelle and vesicle transport, on the one hand, and the organization of peripheral cytoskeleton, on the other, can be modified by the addition of extracellular ligands to the cells. In 3T3 fibroblasts, it has been demonstrated that the rearrangement of the actin network involves activation of members of the (Ras-homology) Rho family of small GTPases [74] and that Rho activation induces the assembly of stress fibers and focal adhesions [74-76]. Rho seems to act as a molecular switch that controls a specific signal transduction pathway going from membrane receptors to cytoskeletal organization, via recruitment of scaffolding proteins of the ezrin/radixin/moesin (ERM) family, Other members of the Rho family are specifically invoved in the formation of lamellipodia (Ras and Cdc42 homology: Rac) or filopodia (cell division cycle 42: Cdc42); as in the case of Rho, Rac and Cdc42 activation is upstream to the formation of integrin-based adhesion complexes [74-76]. Moreover, there is continuous crosstalk among different members of the various families of small GTPases: a) Ras can activate Rac, inducing formation of lamellipodia; b) Rac can be activated also by Cdc42, thus connecting filopodia and lamellipodia formation; c) Rac can activate Rho. Interestingly, the results of mutational analyses suggest that the activation of Rac and/or Cdc42 leads to actin polymerization and to the activation of JNK via a bifurcating pathway that relies on two different docking proteins [74]. Among the downstream targets of Rho proteins, the Ser/thr-kinase p65^{PAK} (p21-activated kinase), a kinase that might be responsible for regulation of the MAP kinase pathway and, thus, of JNK activation has received much attention [74]. Concerning the elements that are upstream to the small GTPases, more than 15 guanine nucleotide exchange factors (GEFs) have been described, but the mechanisms by which these GEFs are activated by membrane receptors is still unclear [75]. The precise roles of the 10 or so GTPase-activating proteins (GAPs) and of the 3 guanine nucleotide dissociation inhibitors (GDIs) identified to date, all of which are potential inhibitors of Rho small GTPases [74], also still need to be clarified. Although most of information concerning the Rho family comes from fibroblasts, many interesting observations have been made in nerve cells. In neuroblastoma N1E-115 cells, activation of Rac and Cdc42 promotes formation of lamellipodia and filopodia, respectively. Unexpectedly, Rho activation in neurons induces neurite retraction and cell rounding; in this case as well, however, the biochemical cause seems to involve formation of contractile actin-myosin filaments [74]. Very recently, a yeast two-hybrid screen approach led to the identification of two novel proteins that regulate RhoA-mediated control of contractility and neuronal morphology: a) a putative Rho-specific GEF; b) a protein called p116Rip (Rho inhibitor protein), acting as a negative regulator of RhoA [77].

In summary, we can envisage that a growth cone traveling toward an attractive substrate establishes functional linkages between the ECM and cell surface-adhesion receptors via modifications of the actomyosin cytoskeleton that underlies the plasma membrane. The anchoring process stabilizes the cortical cytoskeleton and reduces actin retrograde flux, At the same time, tension is generated between the central and peripheral domains of the axon tip, promoting microtubule extension and further protrusion of the leading edge [56]. In other words, the growth cone can use CAMs and cytoskeleton-associated proteins to mediate substrate cytoskeleton coupling, thus regulating rate and direction of axon growth. But how are these events induced? As we discussed above, NCAM, L1 and N-cadherin signaling involves activation of FGF receptor, a tyrosine kinase coupled to a cascade involving phospholipase $C\gamma$ ($PLC\gamma$) and leading to Ca^{2+} influx [23, 24, 56]. In addition to this pathway, selective nonreceptor tyrosine and Ser/Thr-kinase signaling has been suggested to be involved in both NCAM- and L1-mediated neurite outgrowth [56]. Finally, a link between CAM signaling and cytoskeleton remodeling could be provided by the phosphoinositide metabolism. Hydrolysis (by the $PLC\gamma$ activated by CAM/FGF receptor interaction) of phosphatidylinositol-4,5-bisphosphate (PIP2) promotes activation of the actin-binding proteins profilin and gelsolin (which are inactive when in PIP2-bound form) as well as the production of the second messengers inositol-1,4,5-trisphosphate (IP3) and diacylglycerol (DAG). IP3 induces the release of Ca^{2+} from intracellular stores, thus increasing the cytosolic concentration of a further second messenger [78, 79]. Gelsolin is a Ca^{2+}-activated F-actin-severing protein and profilin is a protein able to promote actin assembly at the plus end of microfilaments. The combined action of all of these factors may lead to remodeling of the cytoskeleton, modulation of membrane traffic, and transduction of the signals up to the cell nucleus. A leading example in this sense is the Ca^{2+}/cAMP-response element binding protein (CREB) which is activated by phosphorylation induced by a variety of neuronal protein kinases, such as protein kinase A (PKA), Ca^{2+}-calmodulin-dependent protein kinase II (CaMKII) and MAP kinase-activated protein (MAPKAP) kinase II [78]. Increased phosphorylation of CREB stimulates the formation of a complex with CREB-binding protein (CBP) and the recruitment of RNA polymerase to specific promoters [78]. CBP on its own is also a potent signal integrator able to stimulate c-fos transcription, when phosphorylated by PKA and MAPK. Moreover, CBP has been suggested to have a role as a histone acetyltransferase, involved in transcription initiation [78]. Interest in the CREB/CBP system is still growing, as it has been suggested to be involved in memory storage [78].

Similar considerations probably also hold for the effects of stimulation of many classes of receptors. For example, stimulation of rat cortical neurons with soluble ephrin-A5 (EphA5) induces redistribution of F-actin from the peripheral to the central domain of the growth cone and the collapse of the growth cone itself [28]. Interestingly, ephrin-B2 (EphB2) induces the collapse in the absence of F-actin redistribution [28]. Holland et al. [80] found that EphB2 associates with the RasGAP and the SH2/SH3 domain adaptor protein Nck.

An axon-specific protein which seems to modulate many of the events discussed above is growth associated protein (GAP)-43 (also known as FI, B-50 or neuromodulin), a protein tightly attached to the cytoplasmic face of the nerve-terminal membrane via a hydrophobic sequence in its N-terminus [81]. In transgenic mice, overexpression of GAP-43 promotes spontaneous formation of new synapses, whereas null mutations of the gene disrupts axonal pathfinding [81]. GAP-43 has been proposed to modulate the set point of trimeric G proteins, influencing their responsiveness to other intra- and extracellular signals. The trimeric G proteins Go and Gi are abundant in growth cone membranes and their activation generally inhibits growth cone motility [81]. Other studies suggest that GAP-43 might affect the state of peripheral cytoskeleton: in the growth cone, indeed, GAP-43 is associated with F-actin, α-actinin, talin, and fo-drin (the brain isoform of spectrin). Moreover, GAP-43 undergoes transient PKC-mediated phosphorylation in response to extracellular signals that depo-larize the membrane [81]. In some cases, phosporylation is persistent and cor-relates with LTP of synaptic efficacy [81].

Stabilization of synapses

As discussed in the previous sections and shown in Fig. 2, a growth cone navigat-ing toward its targets continuously makes, modifies and breaks contacts, while re-ceiving a panoply of different signals derived from: a) cell-cell and cell-ECM ad-hesion; b) soluble factors such as neurotrophins and other growth factors; and, sometimes, c) transient electrical activity [82, 83]. What do growing axons use as a point of reference, when, during navigation, they must decide to still grow or to arrest? How do growth cones sense and react to the gradient of either repellent or attractant molecules? Despite 100 years of discussion on the synapse [84], the biochemical mechanisms that govern the appropriate formation of synaptic con-tacts and regulate the choice of which of them will be stabilized, weakened or eliminated during development, and even in the adult nervous system, are still far from being completely elucidated. Moreover, the concept itself of "choice" is a matter of debate. According to the theory of selective stabilization (discussed in [85] by Changeux), during development, the combination of different epigenet-ic factors "selects" the best synaptic contacts, while inducing elimination of many others. This might mean that neuronal activity does not create novel connec-tions but contributes significantly to elimination of many of them and that the processes of learning and memory rely, at least in part, on elimination rather than on addition. On the other hand, in the last few years, other authors have supported the suggestion that "a central function of experience during develop-ment is to gradually build circuitry by the activity-dependent elaboration of neu-ritic branches and synapses" [86]. In any case, the most important indication that emerges from the tremendous mass of experimental results obtained to date is that neurons, if either physiologically or experimentally challenged, are able to regulate their synaptic efficacy in many ways and that "synapses form, retract, strengthen, and weaken both as neural circuitry is refined in early development and as a basis for learning and memory, throughout life" [87].

References

1. Ferro-Novick S, Jahn R (1994) The molecular machinery of secretion is conserved from yeast to neurons. Proc Natl Acad Sci 90:2559-2563
2. Tessier-Lavigne M, Goodman CS (1996) The molecular mechanisms of axon guidance. Science 274:1123-1133
3. Stoeckli ET, Lendmesser LT (1998) Axon guidance at choice points. Curr Opin Neurobiol 8:73-79
4. Dotti CG, Sullivan CA, Banker GA (1988) The establishment of polarity by hippocampal neurons in culture. J Neurosci 8:1454-1468
5. Bradke F, Dotti CG (1997) Neuronal polarity: vectorial cytoplasmic flow precedes axon formation. Neuron 19:1175-1186
6. Higgins D, Burack M, Lein P, Banker G (1997) Mechanisms of neuronal polarity. Curr Opin Neurobiol 7:599-604
7. Eaton S, Simons K (1995) Apical, basal, and lateral cues for epithelial polarization. Cell 82:5-8
8. Ehlers MD, Mammen AL, Lau LF, Huganir RL (1996) Synaptic targeting of glutamate receptors. Curr Biol 8:484-489
9. Tienari PJ, De Strooper B, Ikonen E, Simons M, Weidemann A, Czech C, Hartman T, Ida N, Multhaup G, Masters GL, Masters CL, van Leuven F, Beyreuther K, Dotti CG (1996) The β-amyloid domain is essential for axonal sorting of amyloid precursor protein. EMBO J 15:5218-5229
10. Jareb M, Banker G (1998) The polarized sorting of membrane proteins expressed in culture hippocampal neurons using viral vectors. Neuron 20:855-867
11. Lewin GR, Barde YA (1996) The physiology of neurotrophins. Annu Rev Neurosci 19:289-317
12. Cabelli RJ, Hohn A, Shatz CJ (1995) Inhibition of ocular dominance column formation by infusion of NT-4/5 or BDNF. Science 267:1662-1666
13. Cabelli RJ, Shelton DL, Segal R, Shatz CJ (1997) Blockade of endogenous ligands of TrkB inhibits formation of ocular dominance columns. Neuron 19:63-75
14. Brummendorf T, Rathjen FG (1995) Cell adhesion molecules 1: immunoglobulin superfamily. Protein Profile 2:963-1108
15 Walsh FS, Doherty P (1997) Neural cell adhesion molecules of the immunoglobulin superfamily. Annu Rev Cell Biol 13:425-456
16. Pesheva P, Gennarini G, Goridis C, Schachner M (1993) The F3/11 cell adhesion molecule mediates the repulsion of neurons by the extracellular matrix glycoprotein J1-160/180. Neuron 10:69-82
17. Norenberg U, Hubert M, Brummendorf T, Tarnok A, Rathjen FG (1995) Characterization of functional domains of the tenascin-R (restrictin) polypeptide-cell attachment site, binding with F11, and enhancement of F11-mediated neurite outgrowth by tenascin-R. J Cell Biol 130:473-484
18. Wong EV, Kenwrick S, Willelms P, Lemmon V (1995) Mutations in the cell adhesion molecule L1 cause mental retardation. Trends Neurosci 18:168-172
19 Cohen NR, Taylor JSH, Scott LB, Guillery RW, Soriano P, Furley AJW (1998) Errors in corticospinal axon guidance in mice lacking the neural cell adhesion molecule L1 Curr Biol 8 26-33
20 Walsh FS, Doherty P (1991) Structure and function of the gene for neural cell adhesion molecule Semin Neurosci 3:271-284
21. Walsh FS, Doherty P (1997) Neural cell adhesion molecules of the immunoglobulin superfamily. Annu Rev Cell Dev Biol 13.425-456

22. Kiss JZ, Rougon G (1997) Cell biology of polysialic acid Curr. Opin Neurobiol 7:640-646
23. Doherty P, Walsh FS (1994) Signal transduction events underlying neurite outgrowth stimulated by cell adhesion molecules. Curr Opin Neurobiol 4:49-55
24 Doherty P, Walsh FS (1996) CAM-FGF receptor interactions: a model for axonal growth. Mol Cell Neurosci 8:99-111
25 Brittis PA, Silver J, Walsh FS, Doherty P (1996) FGF receptor function is required for the orderly projection of ganglion cell axons in the developing mammalian retina. Mol Cell Neurosci 8:120-128
26. Saffell JL, Williams EJ, Mason IJ, Walsh FS, Doherty P (1997) Expression of a dominant negative FGF receptor inhibits axonal growth and FGF receptor phosphorylation stimulated by CAMs. Neuron 18:232-242
27. Eph Nomenclature Committee (1997) Unified nomenclature for Eph family receptors and their ligands. Cell 90:403-404
28. Holland SJ, Peles E, Pawson T, Schlessinger J (1998) Cell-contact-dependent signalling in axon growth and guidance: Eph receptor tyrosine kinases and receptor protein tyrosine phosphatase β. Curr Opin Neurobiol 8:117-127
29. Gale NW, Holland SJ, Valenzuela DM, Flenniken A, Pan L, Henkemeyer M, Strebhardt K, Hirai H, Wilkinson DG, Pawson T, Davis S, Yancopoulos GD (1996) Eph receptors and ligands comprise two major specificity subclasses and are reciprocally compartimentalized during embryogenesis Neuron 17:9-19
30. Kolodkin AL, Ginty DD (1997) Steering clear of semaphorins: neuropilins sound the retreat. Neuron 19:1159-1162
31. Kitsukawa T, Shimizu M, Sanbo M, Hirata T, Taniguchi M, Bekku Y, Yagi T, Fujisawa H (1997) Neurophilin-semaphorin III/D-mediated chemorepulsive signals play a crucial role in peripheral nerve projection in mice. Neuron 19·995-1005
32. Carlson SS, Hockfield S (1996) Central nervous system. In: Comper WD (ed) Tissue Function. Extracellular matrix. Vol I. Harwood Academic, Amsterdam, pp 1-23
33. Small DH, San Mok S, Williamson TG, Nurcombe V (1996) Role of proteoglycans in neural development, regeneration, and the aging brain. J Neurochem 67:889-899
34. Cestelli A, Savettieri G, Salemi G, Di Liegro I (1992) Neuronal cell cultures: a tool for investigations in developmental neurobiology. Neurochem Res 17:1163-1180
35. Cohen J, Burne JF, McKinlay C, Winter J (1987) The role of laminin and the laminin/fibronectin receptor complex in the outgrowth of retinal ganglion cell axons. Dev Biol 122:407-418
36. Savettieri G, Mazzola GA, Rodriguez Sanchez MB, Caruso G, Di Liegro I, Cestelli A (1998) Modulation of synapsin I gene expression in rat cortical neurons by extracellular matrix. Cell Mol Neurobiol 18:369-378
37. Faissner A, Kruse J (1990) J1/tenascin is a repulsive substrate for central nervous system neurons. Neuron 5:627-637
38. Cook G, Tannahill D, Keynes R (1998) Axon guidance to and from choice points. Curr Op Neurobiol 8:64-72
39. Savettieri G, Cestelli A, Di Liegro I (1996) Biochemistry of neurotransmission: an update. In: Gullo A (ed) Anaesthesia, pain, intensive care and emergency medicine. Springer-Verlag, Berlin Heidelberg New York, pp 43-73
40. Tolkosky A (1997) Neurotrophic factors in action. Trends Neurosci 20:1-3
41. Schimmang T, Represa J (1997) Neurotrophins gain a hearing. Trends Neurosci 20:100-102
42. Marty S, da Penha Berzaghi M, Berninger B (1997) Neurotrophins and activity-dependent plasticity of cortical interneurons. Trends Neurosci 20:198-202
43. Bredesen DE, Rabizadeh S (1997) p75NTR and apoptosis: Trk-dependent and Trk-independent effects. Trends Neurosci 20:287-290

44. Carter BD, Lewin GR (1997) Neurotrophins lie or let die: does p75^{NTR} decide? Neuron 18:187-190

45. Bergeron L, Yuan J (1998) Sealing one's fate: control of cell death in neurons. Curr Opin Neurobiol 8:55-63

46. Chao MV (1994) The p75 neurotrophin receptor. J Neurobiol 25:1373-1385

47. Frade JM, Rodriguez-Tebar A, Barde YA (1996) Induction of cell death by endogenous nerve growth factor. Nature 383:166-168

48. Casaccia-Bonnefil P, Carter BD, Dobrovsky RT, Chao MV (1996) Death of oligodendrocytes mediated by the interaction of nerve growth factor with its receptor p75. Nature 383:716-719

49. Dobrowsky RT, Werner MH, Castellino AM, Chao MV, Hannun YA (1994) Activation of the sphingomyelin cycle through the low affinity neurotrophin receptor. Science 265:1596-1599

50. Carter BD, Kaltschmidt C, Kaltschmidt B, Offenhauser N, Bohm-Matthaei R, Baeuerle PA, Barde YA (1996) Selective activation of NF-kB by nerve growth factor through the neurotrophin receptor p75. Science 272:542-545

51. Phipott KL, McCarthy MJ, Kippel A, Rubin LL (1997) Activated phosphatidyl inositol 3-kinase promote survival of superior cervical neurons. J Cell Biol 139:309-815

52 O'Neill LAJ, Kaltschmidt C (1997) NK-kB: a crucial transcription factor for glial and neuronal cell function. Trends Neurosci 20:252-258

53 Kaltschmidt C, Kaltschmidt B, Baeuerle PA (1993) Brain synapses contain inducible forms of the transcription factor NF-kB. Mech Dev 43:135-147

54. Meberg PJ, Kiney WR, Valcourt EG, Ruttenberg A (1996) Gene expression of the transcription factor NF-KB in hyppocampus: regulation by synaptic activity. Mol Brain Res 38:179-190

55. Blaustein JD, Lehman MN, Turcotte JC, Greene G (1992) Estrogen receptors in dendrites and axon terminals in the guinea pig hypothalamus. Endocrinology 131:281-290

56. Suter DM, Forscher P (1998) An emerging link between cytoskeletal dynamics and cell adhesion molecules in growth cone guidance. Curr Opin Neurobiol 8:106-116

57. Welch MD, Mallavarapu A, Rosenblatt J, Mitchison TJ (1997) Actin dynamics in vivo. Curr Opin Cell Biol 9:54-61

58 Titus MA (1997) Unconventional myosins: new frontiers in actin-based motors. Trends Cell Biol 7:119-123

59. Mermall V, Post PL, Mooseker MS (1998) Unconventional myosins in cell movement, membrane traffic, and signal transduction. Science 279:527-533

60. Carlier MF (1998) Control of actin dynamics. Curr Opin Cell Biol 10:45-51

61. Ayscough KR (1998) In vivo functions of actin-binding proteins. Curr Opin Cell Biol 10:102-111

62. Welch MD, Iwamatsu A, Mitchison TJ (1997) Actin polymerization is induced by Arp 2/3 protein complex at the surface of Listeria monocytogenes. Nature 385:265-269

63. Bray D (1997) The riddle of slow transport-an introduction. Trends Cell Biol 7:379

64. Baas PW, Brown A (1997) Slow axonal transport: the polymer transport model. Trends Cell Biol 7:380-384

65 Hirokawa N, Terada S, Funakoshi T, Takeda S (1997) Slow axonal transport: the subunit transport model. Trends Cell Biol 7:384-388

66. Heidemann SR (1996) Cytoplasmic mechanisms of axonal and dendritic growth in neurons Int Rev Cytol 165:235-296

67. Delacourte A, Buée L (1997) Normal and pathological Tau proteins as factors for microtubule assembly Int Rev Cytol 171 167-224

68. Cunningham CC, Leclerc N, Flanagan LA, Janmey PA, Kosik KS (1997) Microtubule-as-

sociated protein 2c reorganizes both microtubules and microfilaments into distinct cytological structures in an actin-binding protein-280-deficient melanoma cell line. J Cell Biol 136:845-857

69   Hirokawa N, Noda Y, Okada Y (1998) Kinesin and dynein superfamily proteins in organelle transport and cell division. Curr Opin Cell Biol 10:60-73

70.   Hirokawa N (1998) Kinesin and dynein superfamily proteins and the mechanism of organelle transport. Science 279:519-526

71.   Houseweart MK, Cleveland DW (1998) Intermediate filaments and their associated proteins: multiple dynamic personalities. Curr Opin Cell Biol 10:93-101

72.   Yang Y, Dowling J, Yu QC, Kouklis P, Cleveland DW (1996) An essential cytoskeletal protein connecting actin microfilaments to intermediate filaments. Cell 86:655-665

73.   Nixon RA (1998) The slow axonal transport of cytoskeletal proteins. Curr Opin Cell Biol 10:87-92

74.   Hall A (1998) Rho GTPases and the actin cytoskeleton. Science 279:509-514

75.   Schlaepfer DD, Hunter T (1998) Integrin signalling and tyrosine phosphorylation: just the FAKs? Trends Cell Biol 8:151-157

76.   Howe A, Aplin AE, Alahari SK, Juliano RL (1998) Integrin signaling and cell growth control. Curr Opin Cell Biol 10:220-231

77.   Gebbink MF, Kranenburg O, Poland, M, van Horck FP, Houssa B, Moolenaar WH (1997) Identification of a novel, putative Rho-specific GDP/GTP exchange factor and a RhoA-binding protein· control of neuronal morphology. J Cell Biol 137:1603-1613

78.   Bito H, Deisseroth K, Tsien RW (1997) Ca⁺⁺-dependent regulation in neuronal gene expression Curr Opin Neurobiol 7:419-429

79.   Mikoshiba K (1997) The InsP3 receptor and intracellular Ca^{2+} signaling. Curr Opin Neurobiol 7:339-345

80.   Holland SJ, Gale NW, Gish GD, Roth RA, Songyang Z, Cantley LC, Henkemeyer M, Yancopoulos GD, Pawson T (1997) Juxtamembrane tyrosine residues couple the Eph family receptor EphB2/Nuk to specific SH2 domain proteins in neuronal cells EMBO J 16:3877-3888

81.   Benowitz LI, Routtenberg A (1997) GAP-43: an intrinsic determinant of neuronal development and plasticity. Trends Neurosci 20:84-91

82.   Gallo G, Letourneau PC (1998) Axon guidance: GTPases help axons reach their targets Curr Biol 8:R80-R82

83   Brosamle C (1998) The making, changing, and breaking of contacts. Trends Neurosci 21:91-94

84.   Sheperd GM, Erulkar SD (1997) Centenary of the synapse: from Sherrington to the molecular biology of the synapse and beyond Trends Neurosci 20:385-392

85.   Changeux JP (1997) Letter to the editor. Trends Neurosci 7:291-293

86.   Purves D, White L, Riddle D (1997) Letter to the editor. Trends Neurosci 7:293

87.   Davis GW, Goodman CS (1998) Genetic analysis of synaptic development and plasticity: homeostatic regulation of synaptic efficacy. Curr Opin Neurobiol 8.149-156

Chapter 2

Neurochemical memory in pain circuits

L. Calzà, M. Pozza, M. Zanni

The pathophysiology of pain syndromes refers to two groups of experimental models aimed to mimic inflammatory and neuropathic pain [1]. In the first case, an overstimulation of peripheral nociceptors leads to pain sensation and to abnormal sensory modalities characterized by changes in quality sensation, like allodynia or increased response to painful stimuli such as hyperalgesia. In the second case, a lesion of peripheral or central pain pathways causes persistent pain that also comprises aberrant somatosensory processes, such as the phantom limb. In inflammatory pain, pain fibres are intact and no anatomical rearrangements in spinal and supraspinal tracts are present. In contrast, in neuropathic pain all tracts involved in pain transmission undergo severe anatomical rearrangements that take part in pain syndrome generation and evolution.

However, clinical conditions can hardly be seen in such a schematic view, due to the complex nature of pathological events leading to pain and to the progression of the diseases that cause pain. In cancer pain, for example, inflammatory pain can predominate at the early stages of the disease, but since local invasions take place a neuropathic component can also be present due to lesion of peripheral nerves or terminal branches. Moreover, in nonmalignant conditions such as rheumatoid arthritis in which a severe rearrangement of joint soft tissues and bone involving arthicular nerve ending takes place, inflammatory and neuropathic pain can co-exist.

Thus, development of experimental models of pain reflecting more directly clinical conditions should be a major goal in basic research, and the interpretation of experimental data should focus on the proposed model. In the recent past, we extensively used the arthritis model provoked by complete Freund's adjuvant (CFA) injection as chronic pain model. CFA-induced arthritis is a chronic inflammation, including joints, that is produced by a single intradermal injection of ground, heat-killed *Mycobacterium butyricum*. This model has been extensively used for studying inflammatory pain, but we believe that it can represent a more complex condition, in which inflammatory pain can evolve also including a neuropathic component.

Fos expression during acute and chronic pain

During the past 10 years, Fos histochemistry has been extensively used in the study of pain pathophysiology. It is known that cell surface stimuli, including transmitter receptor activation, trigger multiple signalling pathways linked to nuclear control elements [2, 3]. In 1987, Hunt et al. [4] described the induction of c-fos-like proteins in spinal cord neurones following sensory stimulation. These experiments suggested that in pain circuits synaptic transmission may induce rapid changes in gene expression in certain post synaptic neurones, leading to fos transcription. The fos proto-oncogene encodes a DNA-binding protein (Fos) that functions as a component of the transcription factor activator protein-1 (AP-1) [5]. In mammals, several gene promoters contain the AP-1 binding domain. According to Kandel's view on memory storage, early-activated genes including fos are part of the cellular programme that guarantees synaptic plasticity and the ability of neurones to alter the strength of their synaptic connectivity with activity and experience [6, 7]. Thus, the appearance of Fos and Fos-related antigens (Fras) in spinal cord neurones following a noxious stimulus could anticipate a long-lasting modification of protein synthesis providing a molecular trace of pain experience and phenotype changes.

The activation of immediate early genes by external stimuli in neurones is rapid and transient. However, repeated stimulation or also a single stimulus can lead to chronic induction of these genes, so that detectable and even high levels of Fos and Fras remain in specific neural populations for a long period. This has been proved using pharmacological tools. Dopaminergic drugs and psychoactive molecules, such as chronic morphine, induces chronic Fras [8, 9]. However, chronic functional stimuli, such as dehydration, repeated stress, or mechanical and chemical injuries and denervation are also able to induce a long-term Fras expression [10].

Pain stimuli can induce prolonged expression of Fos and Fras in pain pathways as well and this is probably involved in long-lasting phenotype changes in pain circuits. For example, increased opiate synthesis in the spinal cord during inflammation is Fos-mediated. In acute and chronic inflammation, enkephalin and dynorphin synthesis dramatically increases in the spinal cord [11-13]. Both preprodynorphin [14] and preproenkephalin [15] genes contain the AP-1-like binding site in the 5' upstream region, suggesting a direct role of early genes in pain-mediated activation of spinal opiate synthesis. The use of antisense technology provided further evidence for the role of fos. Pretreatment with c-fos mRNA antisense prevents Fos protein and preprodynorphin mRNA increase due to the intraplantar injection of formalin [16]. Chronic arthritis induced by CFA injection causes Fos increase in spinal cord, which remains elevated for up to 3-5 weeks [17, 18]. At this time, inflammation has already decreased and no signs of spontaneous pain are observed. In contrast, endogenous opioids and opiate receptors are still up-regulated, and the naloxone test revealed that the opiatergic tone affects pain threshold [19]. Thus, even without evident behavioural indices of spontaneous pain, prolonged Fos activation is coupled to increased opioid and opioid receptor synthesis in the spinal cord.

Although less investigated, other brain areas could retain a molecular memory of pain experience. In particular, during CFA-induced arthritis, stress circuits

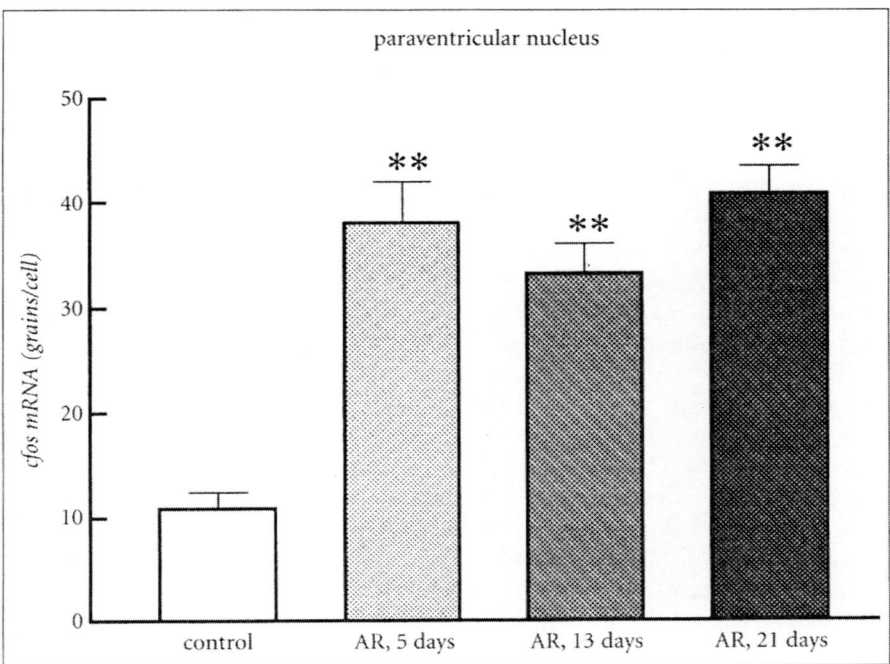

Fig. 1. c-fos mRNA expression in the paraventricular nucleus of the hypothalamus as evaluated 5, 13 and 21 days after induction of arthritis (*AR*). The experiment was performed by in situ hybridization. One-way analysis of the variance and Dunnett's post-hoc test: $**p<0.01$

that include brainstem catecholaminergic areas are activated. An increase in *fos* mRNA occurs in the paraventricular nucleus of the hypothalamus (Fig. 1) already 5 days after CFA injection and the mRNA level remains elevated up to 21 days after CFA injection. Both magnocellular neurones, containing the neurohormones oxytocin and vasopressin, and parvocellular neurones, including those expressing corticotrophin-releasing hormone, express Fos mRNA. This is particularly interesting because of the key role played by the paraventricular nucleus in body homeostasis, stress response and immune reaction. During different stress paradigms, including psychosocial and physical stress, the paraventricular nucleus of the hypothalamus provides the prompt adaptation of body homeostasis to altered metabolic and emotional requirements, through endocrine and neural mechanisms. Fos activation during stress and noxious stimuli [20, 21] is coupled to a complex series of phenotype adjustments including hormone, peptide and enzyme synthesis [22, 23]. Stress-induced analgesia depends on the hypothalamic control of the hypophyseal-adrenocortical system exerted by the paraventricular nucleus [24], and the adjustment of sympathetic tone during stress is provided by the bidirectional connections between the paraventricular nucleus of the hypothalamus and the catecholaminergic neurones in the brainstem. Thus, prolonged Fos activation during arthritic pain could sustain a prolonged alteration of brain circuits providing endocrine, emotional and autonomic integration during stressful conditions, including pain.

Transition from acute to chronic pain: a phenotypic switch in pain circuits?

Increasing evidence during recent years has suggested that the neurochemical and functional phenotype of neurones undergo modification during the evolution of painful states and these changes could in turn be responsible for transition among different types of pain.

In a series of studies over the past 10 years, Hokfelt et al. investigated the neurochemical changes occurring in large and small diameter neurones in dorsal root ganglia after peripheral nerve transection, focusing on peptides and their receptors [25, 26]. Part of these results are summarized in the lower panel of Fig. 2, where the arrows indicate the increase or decrease in the number of large and small neurones expressing peptides and peptide receptors in dorsal root ganglia after sciatic nerve transection. This means that a certain number of neurones start, or stop, to synthetize a new set of proteins/peptides after the nerve damage. For example, the level of the peptide galanin dramatically increases in large and small neurones after the axotomy [27] and experiments using the peptide antagonist [28] or antisense probes [29] suggested that galanin is upregulated after axotomy to counteract the development of neuropathic pain. According to Hokfelt [26], two pain defence systems exist: one is confined to the dorsal root ganglia, it involves galanin and it counteracts neuropathic pain; the second one is due to spinal opioids and it is active in inflammatory pain.

We have quantitatively analysed changes in neuropeptides and/or their mRNAs in the dorsal root ganglia and their nerve terminals in the dorsal horn as well as in local interneurons in the dorsal spinal cord during induction and maintenance of chronic inflammation induced by CFA [13]. After induction of experimental arthritis, there is an increased responsiveness to stimuli applied to the joint with a time-course that mirrors the development of spontaneous pain behaviour in awake animals [30]. The continuous stimulus of primary sensory neurones, which is coupled to an increased release of neurokinin A and substance P (SP) in the dorsal horn, is a key mechanism in the development and maintenance of spinal hyperexcitability [31]. Our results are summarized in Figure 2. At a short-time interval (5 days) following the CFA injection, i.e. as soon as signs of inflammation appear, there is a decrease in immunostaining for SP, calcitonin gene-related peptide (CGRP), and galanin in fibres in the superficial layers of the spinal cord, likely reflecting the peptide release from sensory neurones. Peptide content then gradually increases, so that after 21 days a recovery (CGRP, galanin) or even increase (SP) can be observed when compared to control rats. At this time (21 days), CGRP, SP and galanin peptide content as well as CGRP and galanin mRNA expression have increased in the dorsal root ganglia (DRGs). In the spinal cord, not only opioid peptide (DYN and ENK) synthesis

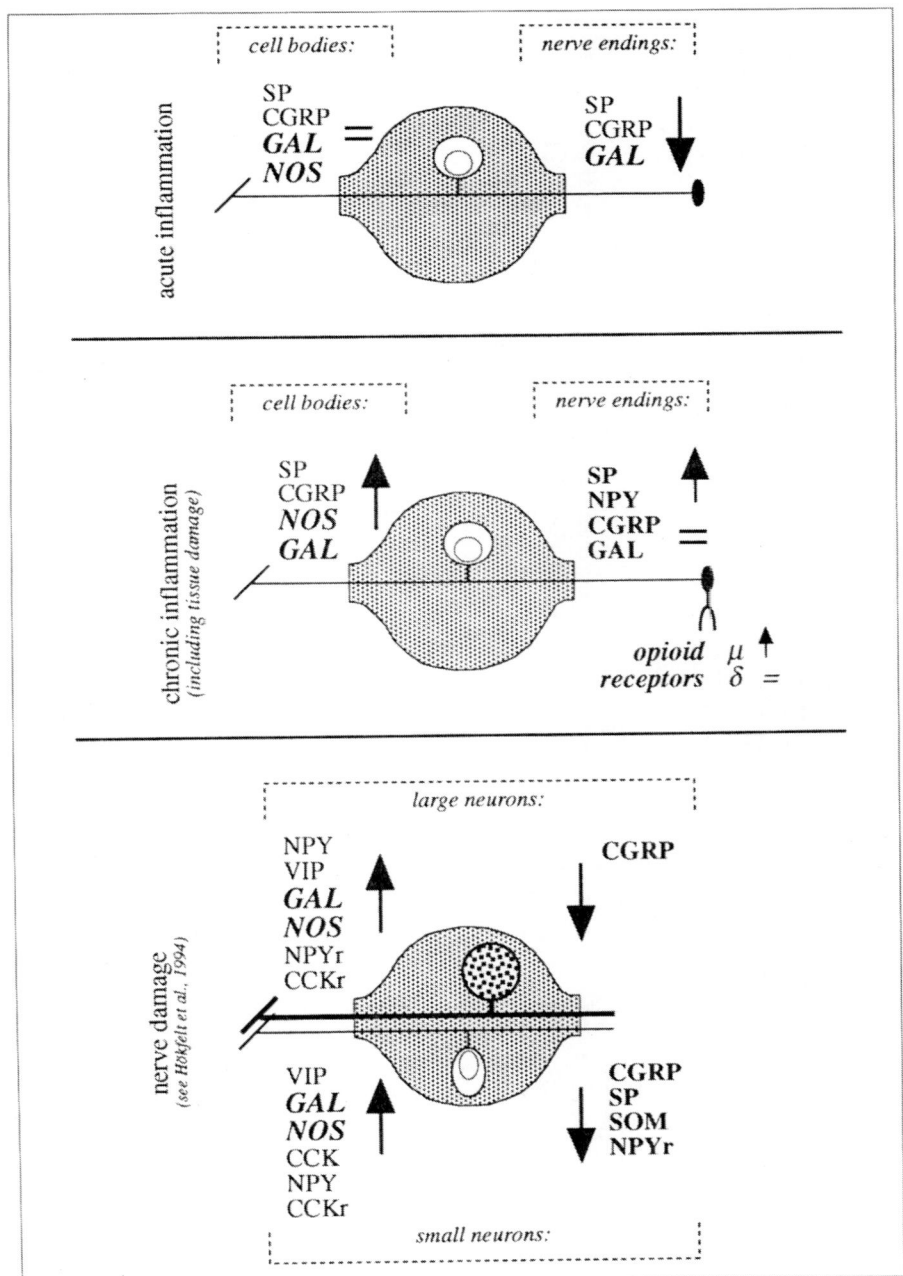

Fig. 2. The main changes in peptide and enzyme content in dorsal root ganglia during inflammation and nerve damage. *CCK*, cholecystokinin, *CCKr*, cholecystokinin receptor, *CGRP*, calcitonin gene-related peptide; *GAL*, galanin; *NOS*, nitric oxide synthase, *NPY*, neuropeptide Y; *NPYr*, neuropeptide Y receptor; *SP*, substance P; *VIP*, vasoactive intestinal peptide

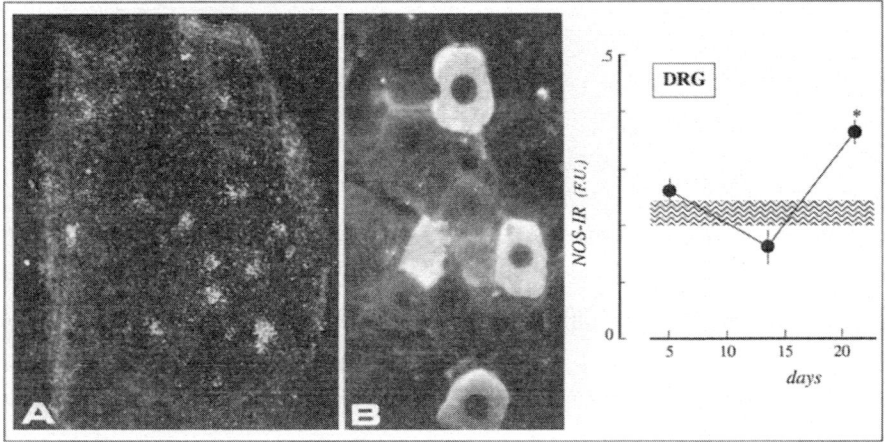

Fig. 3. (a) Nitric oxide synthase (NOS) mRNA expressing neurons and NOS-immunoreactive neurons (b) in lombar dorsal root ganglia (DRG). The graph shows changes in NOR immunoreactivity in DRG during chronic arthritis, compared to control animals (horizontal bar). The results are expressed as microphotometric units. One-way analysis of the variance and post-hoc Dunnett's test: *p<0.05

in local interneurons is strongly up-regulated during chronic inflammation and pain 21 days after CFA-injection, but also SP and galanin synthesis. Moreover, we also described changes in nitric oxide synthase mRNA [32] and enzyme (Fig. 3) during different phases of CFA-induced arthritis. Neuronal NO synthase mRNA expression and neuronal NO synthase immunoreactivity increased in neurones of lumbar dorsal root ganglia in arthritic rats compared to those of normal rats, whereas neuronal NO synthase mRNA expression decreased in lamina X and lamina I-II of the lumbar spinal cord. The modulation of neuronal NO synthase synthesis in the spinal cord and dorsal root ganglia that we have found in polyarthritis when the disease reaches its peak corresponds exactly to the one described for models of neuropathic pain. In fact, a reduction in spinal NO synthase activity and an increase in neuronal NO synthase expression in dorsal root ganglia have been described for various models of neuropathic pain [33-35]. In contrast, either an increase and no changes in acute inflammation and pain without tissue damage have been described in the spinal cord [36, 37].

We then suggested that the initial stages of our arthritic model may be characterized by an inflammatory type of pain, whereas later stages may also include a neuropathic component. According to this, mRNA expression of the peptide galanin in dorsal root ganglion of polyarthritic rats 21 days after CFA injection is also higher [13] as it happens in models of neuropathic pain [25, 26]. This possibility is suggested in view of the severe rearrangement of articular and bone tissues involving joint nerve endings after CFA injection [38]. NOS involvement in neuronal phenotype changes that are found in the transition from acute to chronic pain raises a number of intriguing questions, ranging from the role of nitric oxide in joint inflammation development and maintenance [39], to local blood flow regulation [40] and from a role of NO in spinal nociception [41] to sensory memory coupled to glutamatergic mechanism in dorsal root ganglia and spinal cord [42].

How these phenotypic changes affect the sensory process is not yet fully understood. A great contribution on this has been provided by Woolf et al. [43]. They recently described that during inflammation Aβ fibres also acquire the capability to increase the excitability of spinal cord neurones, due to a phenotypic switch in a subpopulation of neurons in DRG that start to synthetize SP during inflammation [44].

Acknowledgements. This study was supported by EU BIOMED 2 BMH4-CT95-0172 and by the Pathophysiology Center for the Nervous System, Hesperia Hospital, Modena, Italy.

References

1. Merskey H, Bogduk N (eds) (1994) Classification of chronic pain. IASP Press, Seattle
2. Robertson LM, Kerppola TK, Vendrell M, Luk D, Smeyne RJ, Bocchiaro C, Morgan JI, Curran T (1995) Regulation of c-fos expression in transgenic mice requires multiple interdependent transcription control elements. Neuron 14:241-252
3. Hughes P, Dragunow M (1995) Induction of immediate-early genes and the control of neurotransmitter-regulated gene expression within the nervous system. Pharmacol Rev 47:134-178
4. Hunt SP, Pini A, Evan G (1987) Induction of c-fos-like protein in spinal cord neurons following sensory stimulation. Nature 328:632-634
5. Curran T, Morgan JI (1994) Fos: an immediate-early transcription factor in neurons. J Neurobiol 26:403-412
6. Goelet P, Castellucci VF, Schacher S, Kandel ER (1986) The long and the short of long-term memory-a molecular framework. Nature 322:419-422
7. Abel T, Martin KC, Bartsch D, Kandel ER (1998) Memory suppressor genes: inhibitory constraints on the storage of long-term memory. Science 279:338-341
8. Hope BT, Nye HE, Kelz MB, Self DW, Iadarola MJ, Nakabeppu Y, Duman RS, Nestler EJ (1994) Induction of a long-lasting AP-1 complex composed of altered Fos-like proteins in brain by chronic cocaine and other chronic treatments. Neuron 13:1235-1244
9. Nye HE, Nestler EJ (1996) Induction of chronic Fos-related antigens in rat brain by chronic morphine administration. Mol Pharmacol 49:636-645
10. Pennypacker KR, Hong J-S, McMillian MK (1995) Implications of prolonged expression of Fos-related antigens. Trends Pharmacol Sci 16:317-321
11. Iadarola MJ, Brady LS, Draisci G, Dubner R (1988) Enhancement of dynorphin gene expression in spinal cord following experimental inflammation: stimulus specificity, behavioural parameters and opioid receptor binding. Pain 35:313-326
12. Dubner R, Ruda MA (1992) Activity-dependent neuronal plasticity following tissue injury and inflammation. Trends Neurosci 15:96-103
13. Calzà L, Pozza M, Zanni M, Manzini CU, Manzini E, Hokfelt T (1998). Peptide plasticity in primary sensory neurons and spinal cord during adjuvant-induced arthritis in the rat: an immunocytochemical and in situ hybridization study. Neuroscience 82:575-589

14. Civelli O, Douglass J, Goldstein A, Herbert E (1985) Sequence and expression of the rat prodynorphin gene. Proc Natl Acad Sci USA 82:4291-4295

15 Zhu YS, Branch AD, Robertson HD, Inturrisi CE (1994) Cloning and characterization of hamster proenkephalin gene. DNA Cell Biol 13:25-35

16. Hunter JC, Woodburn VL, Durieux C, Pettersson EKE, Poat JA, Hughes J (1995) C-fos antisense oligodeaxynucleotide increases formalin-induced nociception and regulates preprodynorphin expression. Neuroscience 65:485-492

17. Abbadie C, Besson JM (1994) Chronic treatments with aspirin or acetaminophen reduce both the development of polyarthritis and Fos-like immunoreactivity in rat lumbar spinal cord. Pain 57:45-54

18. Calzà L, Pozza M, Manzini CU, Mascia MT, Manzini E (1996) C-fos activation and NOS mRNA regulation in pain pathways during adjuvant-induced arthritis in the rat. In: Bonucci E (ed) Biology and pathology of cell-matrix interactions Cleup, Padova, pp 318-326

19. Zanni M, Pozza M, Arletti R, Magnani F, Calzà L (1998) Long-term regulation of opioids in the spinal cord of arthritic rats. Society for Neuroscience Meeting, Los Angeles

20. Ceccatelli S, Villar MJ, Goldstein M, Hokfelt T (1989) Expression of fos-like immunoreactivity in transmitter charcterized neurons after stress Proc Natl Acad Sci USA 86:9569-9573

21 Smith DW, Day TA (1994) C-fos expression in hypothalamic neurosecretory and brainstem catecholamine cells following noxious somatic stimuli Neuroscience 58:765-775

22. Calzà L, Giardino L, Zanni M, Gallinelli A, Toschi L (1991) Neuropeptide Y as a central relay in the control of the body homeostasis In: Genazzani AR, Nappi G, Petraglia F, Martignoni E (eds) Stress and related disorders from adaptation to dysfunction. Parthenon Publishing, Carnforth, pp 239-246

23 Calzà L, Giardino L, Ceccatelli S (1993) Stress-related increase of NOS mRNA in the paraventricular nucleus of young and old rats. Neuroreport 4.627-630

24. Filaretov AA, Bogdanoc AI, Yarushkina NI (1996) Stress-induced analgesia. The role of hormones produced by the hypophyseal-adrenocortical system. Neurosci Behav Physiol 26:572-578

25. Hokfelt T, Zhang X, Wiesenfeld-Hallin Z (1994) Messenger plasticity in primary sensory neurons following axotomy and its functional implications. Trends Neurosci 17:22-30

26 Hokfelt T, Zhang X, Xu X-Q, Ji R-R, Shi T, Corness J, Kerekes N, Landry M, Rydh-Rinder M, Broberger C, Wiesenfeld-Hallin Z, Bartfai T, Elde R, Ju G (1997) Transition of pain from acute to chronic cellular and synaptic mechanisms. In: Jensen TS, Turner JA, Wiesenfeld-HallinZ (eds) Proceedings on the 8th World Congress on Pain. IASP Press, Seattle, pp 133-154

27. Hokfelt T, Wiesenfeld-Hallin Z, Villar M J, Melander T (1987) Increase of galanin-like immunoreactivity in rat dorsal root ganglion cells after peripheral axotomy. Neurosci Lett 83:217-220

28. Verge VM, Xu XJ, Langel U, Hokfelt T, Wiesenfeld-Hallin Z, Bartfai T (1993) Evidence for endogenous inhibition of autotomy by galanin in the rat after sciatic nerve section. demonstrated by chronic intrathecal infusion of a high affinity galanin receptor antagonist. Neurosci Lett 149.193-197

29. Ji RR, Zhang Q, Bedecs K, Arvidsson J, Zhang X, Xu XJ, Wiesenfeld-Hallin Z, Bartfai T, Hokfelt T (1994) Galanin antisense oligonucleotides reduce galanin levels in dorsal root ganglia and induce autotomy in rats after axotomy. Proc Natl Acad Sci 91:12540-12543

30. Kidd BL, Morris VH, Urban L (1996) Pathophysiology of joint pain. Ann Rheumatic Dis 55:276-283

31. Schaible H-G, Jarrott B, Hope PJ, Duggan AW (1990) Release of immunoreactive sub-

stance P in the spinal cord during development of acute arthritis in the knee joint of the cat: a study with antibody microprobes. Brain Res 529:214-223

32. Pozza M, Bettelli C, Magnani F, Mascia MT, Manzini E, Calzà L (1998) Is neuronal nitric oxide involved in adjuvant-induced joint inflammation. Eur J Pharmacol (in press)

33. Choi Y, Raja SN, Moore LC, Tobin JR (1996) Neuropathic pain in rats is associated with altered nitric oxide synthase activity in neural tissue. J Neurol Sci 138:14-20

34. Verge VMK, Xu Z, Xu X-J, Wiesenfeld-Hallin Z, Hokfelt T (1992) Marked increase in nitric oxide synthase mRNA in rat dorsal root ganglia after peripheral axotomy: in situ hybridization and functional studies. Proc Natl Acad Sci 89:11617-11621

35. Steel JH, Terenghi G, Chung JM, Na HS, Carlton SM, Polak JM (1994) Increased nitric oxyde synthase immunoreactivity in rat dorsal root ganglia in a neuropathic pain model. Neurosci Lett 169:81-84

36. Lam HHD, Hanley DF, Trapp BD, Saito S, Raja S, Dawson TM, Yamagushi H (1996) Induction of spinal cord neurol nitric oxide synthase (NOS) after formalin injection in the rat paw. Neurosci Lett 210:201-204

37. Traub RJ, Solodkin A, Meller ST, Gebhart GF (1994) Spinal cord NADPH-diaphorase histochemical staining but not nitric oxide synthase immunoreactivity increases following carrageenan-produced hindpaw inflammation in the rat. Brain Res 668:204-210

38. Esser RE, Hildebrand AR, Angelo RA, Watts LM, Murphey MD, Baugh LE (1995) Measurement of radiographic changes in adjuvant-induced arthritis in rats by quantitative image analysis. Arthritis Rheum 38:129-138

39 Cochran FR, Selph J, Sherman P (1996) Insights into the role of nitric oxide in inflammatory arthritis. Med Res Rev 16:547-563

40. Gross SS, Wolin MS (1995) Nitric oxide: pathophysiological mechanisms. Ann Rev Physiol 57:737-769

41. Meller ST, Gebhart GF (1993) Nitric oxide (NO) and nociceptive processing in the spinal cord. Pain 52:127-136

42. Coderre TJ (1993) The role of excitatory amino acid receptors and intracellular messengers in persistent nociception after tissue injury in rats. Mol Neurobiol 7:229-246

43 Woolf CJ, Doubell TP (1994) The pathophysiology of chronic pain-increased sensitivity to low threshold Ab-fibre inputs. Curr Opin Neurobiol 4:525-534

44. Neumann S, Doubell TP, Leslie T, Woolf CJ (1996) Inflammatory pain hypersensitivity mediated by phenotypic switch in myelinated primary sensory neurons. Nature 384: 360-364

Chapter 3

Withdrawal reflex: philosophy and physiology

M. TIENGO

*To the memory of Vito Valterra, the illustrious mathematician who, in 1932, published his
"Mathematical Theory of the Struggle for Life", a splendid mathematical analysis of survival strategies where the fundamental model is the withdrawal reflex.
"The chief function of the central nervous system is to send messages to the muscles which
will make the body move effectively as a whole". E.D. Adrian, Nobel Prize 1932.*

The term "withdrawal reflex" is intended to mean any reflex whose end purpose
is to protect the organism or one of its tissues from being damaged (Fig. 1). One
example is the corneal reflex described as "irritation of the cornea causing the
reflex closure of the lids" [1].

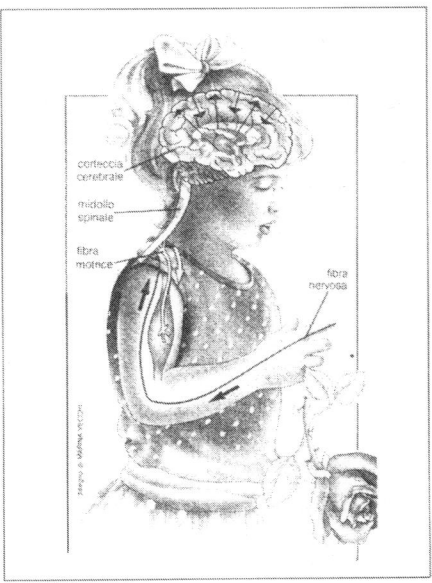

Fig. 1. Withdrawal reflex Child pricked with a rose thorn. The reflex withdrawal is controlled
both by physical (analgesia endogenous system) and by mental (attention, anxious, depression) factors

Reflex action in the leg or arm, provoked by a painful stimulus, is commonly used in pain studies. K.D. Craig writes: "With some exceptions, traumatic injury, such as lacerations or burns, provokes a vigorous withdrawal reflex, as well as protective movements and stereotyped patterns of verbal and nonverbal expressive behavior recognizable as pain onlookers" [2].

Philosophical roots

Aristotle did not consider muscular tissue as the organ of movement. In fact, in his *De Anima,* he expounds his concept whereby the instruments of animal movement are the bones which are moved by the nerves.

Galen (131-200 A.D.) was the first person to attribute movement to the muscles. In fact, in his book entitled *De Motu Musculorum,* he recognizes muscles as being the organs of movement. The nerves embedded in the muscles grow out of the brain and spinal cord. If a nerve is interrupted, no muscular movement is possible. A sectioned or compressed nerve deprives the muscle of feeling and movement. Therefore, in Galen's conception, nerves are conductors that run from the brain "like streams" and provide the muscles with a force that allows them to function and contract.

To Galen's credit, he introduced both the term and concept of muscular tone. In fact, in his *De Motu Musculorum,* he recognizes that muscles have four types of movement: contraction, extension, passive movement and tonic maintenance. Muscle tone is the "pneuma" effect, that is, the force which, according to historical philosophy, represents the cohesion between the macrocosm and the microcosm. This would explain why a muscle becomes flaccid when its nerves have been severed: that is, when its "pneuma" has been cut off. But, according to Galen, the pneuma that the brain provides for the nerves comes from the supreme source: the soul. The physiological notion regarding tone thus has a philosophical origin where it is conceived as being a permanent will of the soul.

Another concept introduced by Galen is "voluntary movement". This is the type of movement a person can originate and control when wishing to do something or to stop doing something. With voluntary movement, the person can, therefore, initiate, accelerate, slow down, and stop a movement, and repeat the whole process. Galen considered that voluntary movement had a central origin and that it depended on the brain. However, since the brain was still under the control of the soul, movement had a transcendent origin. Galen had trouble explaining how the intelligent soul is able to move the body according to a specific end purpose. In other words, what remained an enigma for Galen was whether the soul acted directly on the body or by means of some instrument that acted as an intermediary between the soul and the movement.

Regarding the mechanism of muscular contraction, Galen could not provide an explanation. All we know is that he made a distinction between nerves and tendons. He devided the nerves in two categories: soft nerves (for sensitivity) which connected the brain to the sensitive parts of the body and hard nerves (for movement) which connected the spinal cord to the various movable parts of the body. Therefore, as Galen saw it, body movement was always dominated by the soul. This thesis persisted down through the centuries, and we find Malebranche supporting it with his theory that only God, the Creator of bodies, could provide muscles with motive force.

The first treatise regarding muscular activity *De Musculi Fabrica* was written by Fabrizio d'Acquapendente (1537-1619). The treatise states that the *brain* is the *primum movens*. It also says that the bones are mute – that is, they do not provide movement; the muscles are mute and provide movement at the same time, while the nerves are channels that conduct the animal spirit emanated by the brain to the muscles. We have no proof that Descartes (1595-1650) had ever read *De Musculi Fabrica*, but it seems quite unlikely that he did not know about Acquapendente's celebrated theories.

Descartes initiated a theory regarding the mechanism of movement. In his theory, he was the first person to replace the confused notion of "sympathy" with an almost mathematical notion of mechanism and made a distinction between animal movement and psychic animation. "We can see", writes Descartes, "that when a part of the body is injured it no longer obeys our will". In his *De Homine*, Descartes provides two examples of withdrawal reflex in the form of illustrations. The first, very well known, example shows a boy reacting in pain as a flame burns his foot. The second, lesser known, illustration shows the same situation except that the person burns his arm (Fig. 2). In refusing to attribute body movement control to the soul, and sustaining that the soul cannot direct-

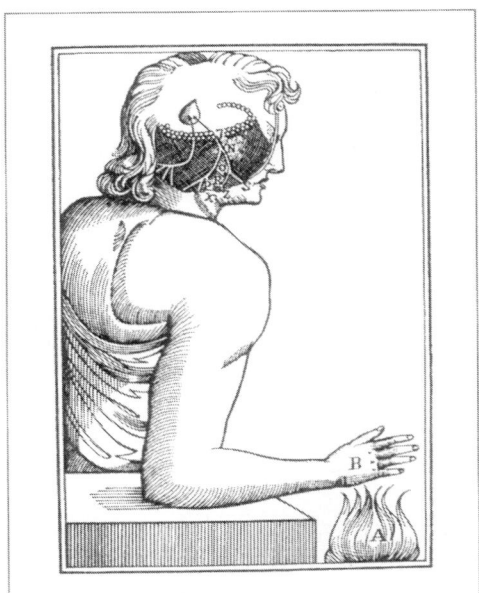

Fig. 2. Withdrawal reflex. A flame burns his hand (Franz Descartes, 1670 De Homine)

ly stimulate any movement whatsoever, Descartes writes: "There is no need for the soul. All it takes to produce movement is thought. However, thought is produced by the soul". There is no general agreement as to whether Descartes had actually defined reflex action as it is understood today. The question is whether Descartes' general theory regarding involuntary or automatic movement places automatism in relation to the phenomenon that we, today, call reflex action. Descartes considers a large number of reflex movements pertinent to automatic muscular phenomena, such as swallowing, the flexing of an arm or leg when subjected to a strong heat stimulus (like a flame), pupil adjustment, coughing and sneezing. However, notwithstanding Descartes' careful study of nerve and muscle physiology, we still wonder if we really can give him credit for having defined the reflex action concept as it is understood today. We have to admit, however, that, given the mechanistic spirit of his physiology, he was fairly close to this understanding. In fact, Fearing claims Descartes' concept of automatism implicitly contained the idea of reflex action [3]. The discussion was renewed at the turn of this century when the study of reflex action dominated physiology. Fulton observed that "the notion of reflex action dates back to Descartes but not the term" [4]. Minkowski, referring to Descartes' description of how the pupil of the eye automatically narrows when exposed to light, sustains that Descartes established the notion of reflex action (Fig. 2). Emile Du Bois Raymond, in his commemoration address at the funeral of Johannes Muller (1851), stated that Descartes already had described withdrawal reflex correctly one century before Prokaska and, by analogy, had borrowed the term from the reflected image to indicate something which is reflected back [5]. On the other hand, after thoroughly analyzing Descartes' writings, Canguilhem holds the completely opposite view, stating that none of Descartes' documents mention either the term or the concept of reflex action.

Thomas Willis (1621-1675), who taught natural philosophy at Oxford and medicine in London, was a very fine anatomist and an exceptional clinician. Like Descartes, Willis was interested in healing and preventing disease [6]. But he had the advantage over Descartes of being both a learned philosopher and a medical doctor with considerable practical experience. Canguilhem sustains that Willis is really the first person to have instituted the concept of reflex action. Willis may not have invented the term "reflex action", but he did establish the basic theories and all the logical requirements of the physiological concept of reflex action. According to Canguilhem, the origin of the reflex function is found in the *De Motu Musculari* work (1670) which describes the three "principles" of movement: the *origin* of the action, that is, the first indication of the movement to be carried out which is in the brain; the *nervous excitation and transmission* to the mobile particles inside the nerves; and the *muscle motive force*, that is, the force of contraction. However, the muscle reflex action must be preceded by something that causes the reflex action, such as a scratch. Willis selects the same examples given in *De Motu Musculari* that Descartes describes in his *De Homine* and his "Traité des Passions": the foot-sole skin reflex, the pupil reflex and the eyelid reflex.

Experimental evidence

In the eighteenth century, physiologists and doctors were primarily interested in muscular contraction. The word "reflection", a term used in physics, seems to have been used analogously by Unzer (1727-1799) to indicate muscular contraction in response to a sensorial stimulus [7]. The transformation from a sensorial impression to a conscious perception requires continuity between the nerves and the brain. The impression is "reflected" from the brain through the nerves to the muscles where it causes movement. Thus, for Unzer, the notion of reflection and reflected impression becomes essential for explaining animal movement. However, there also could be an internal sensorial impression which is not accompanied by any representation, that is, without going through the brain. In this case, reflection takes place but without any conscious representations. When the legs of a decapitated frog are stimulated, they continue to contract. To investigate this phenomenon more thoroughly, Unzer studied the sensorial stimulation behavior of hundreds of decapitated animals. In his mechanistic concept for illustrating how animal forces worked, Unzer used the windmill metaphor proposed by Leibniz rather than Descartes' watch metaphor. Only human beings have a soul, and the sensorial impression travels up the nerves to the brain where it becomes a conscious perception. The nagging question during the eighteenth century was whether or not a person, upon being beheaded, continued to have conscious sensorial perception, as was the case with decapitated frogs. This was the period when beheading by guillotine was in vogue, and it was rather disquieting to see how the facial muscles would contract after the head was separated from the body. Some accounts have it that a few victims actually got up and took two or three steps after having been beheaded.

In this climate, Jiri Prochaska (1749-1820), professor of anatomy and physiology at the University of Prague, conducted splendid research on decapitated animals. As we read in Brazier, Prochaska believed in "sensorium commune" where an automatic turn-around took place [8]. He thought this turn-around might be located in the medulla or in the cord itself, but he did not agree with Unzer that this could be in the ganglia. However, he did agree that the nerves might have an intrinsic "vis insita" force that enabled them to function when isolated from the brain. He was more down to earth than his teacher Unzer and proposed that the purpose of unconscious movement (like reflex action) was the preservation of the individual [9]. It is generally accepted that the term "reflex" was coined by Prochaska. In this era, all of those who studied the nervous system were concerned with the consitution of "vis nervosa", as named by Albrecht von Haller to denote outflow from the brain to the muscles. Prochaska used the same term – but in a rather different sense – the capability of the nerve to receive impressions and trasmit them. He realized that this might take place unconsciously and therefore without participation by the brain. He described this transmission as a "reflection" taking place in what he called the "sensorium commune" (...). The unconscious transmission from sensory to motor Prochaska had in mind were mostly respiratory and cardiac responses, although he noted the withdrawal of a limb by a decapitated animal and concluded that part of the "sensorium commune" must therefore lie in medulla spinalis.

Lacking any anatomical references, progress in neurophysiology during the eighteenth century proceeded very slowly and with great hesitation. In 1811, Bell expounded his spinal reflex theory – "a natural response to pain" – and, in 1822, Magendie provided the experimental evidence [10]. This was an important discovery for both physiology and clinical neurology and went down in history as the "Bell and Magendie Law". This law says that the posterior spinal roots transport sensorial impulses from the periphery to the central nervous system, while the anterior roots which come out of the medulla conduct the motor impulses toward the periphery. However, Magendie himself states that the rear roots sometimes contain motor elements and the anterior roots sometimes show that they contain sensitive elements. As the physiologist Luigi Luciani (1840-1919) later writes, it was this contradictory evidence regarding the functions of the roots that caused the value of this law to be disputed for many years, until experimentation by Loget, Claude Bernard and other neurophysiologists demonstrated the validity of Bell and Magendie's observations [11].

Johannes Muller (1801-1858), whose birth at the beginning of the ninenteenth century almost symbolized the advent of a new era, very definitely contributed to modernizing the conception of physiology. He showed that "each sensorial system responds to different stimuli in just one invariable, characteristic way" and, therefore pain must follow nerve paths that are distinctly separate from tactile paths [12]. Muller had celebrated debates with Weber who sustained that pain was produced by an excessive amount of feeling and that it reached the brain along the same tactile paths. It is said that these polemics ended in a duel between them. In his fundamental treatise "Handbuch der Physiologie des Menschen", published in 1826 when he was only 25 years old, Muller provides a long, thorough scientific description of muscular function, movement and reflex action. He observes that the most surprising fact is that there are muscles that obey voluntary orders and others that do not.

Muller's extraordinary and refined didactic capabilities are shown in Table 1, the index of his "Handbook of Physiology", which refers to the physiology of muscular activity and reflex action.

The first chapter of section II "Voluntary and involuntary movement" contains a paragraph on "reflex movement". As Muller writes, this movement occurs when the sensitive nerves are excited and the centrifugal and centripetal currents passing through them go through the brain and the spinal medulla. There are two main groups: organic-system reflex actions (coughing due to irritation of the breathing system, vomiting due to irritation of the gastric mucosa, sneezing, intestinal spasms, etc.), and organic-system reflex actions that cannot be contolled with the will (heart, internal and glandular secretions, etc.). Finally, Muller considers the reflex actions caused by "passions" and refers to Spinoza's mathematical classification, whereby there are exciting passions and depressing passions from which one withdraws or flees, following one's survival instinct. This

Table 1. Table of contents from: J. Müller (1845), Manuel de Physiologie, Ed. Francaise, J.B. Bailliere, Paris, IV, I:1-119

Section I. Organs and causes of animal movement
- Chapter I. Different types of movement and motor organs. MUSCULAR TISSUE. Chemical properties of muscles. Physical properties of muscles
- Chapter IV. Causes of animal movement. Influence of blood

Section II. The different muscle movements
- Chapter I. Voluntary and involuntary muscle movements. Movement caused by external and internal, heterogeneous irritation. Automatic movement. Automatic movement that depends on the sympathetic nerve. Automatic movement that depends on the central organs. Intermittent type of animal system automatic movement. Continuous type of animal system movement. Reflex movement. Movement caused by passions
- Chapter II. Complex voluntary movement. Simultaneous series of movements. Association of movement with ideas. Association of movements with movements. Association of ideas with movements. Instinctive movement
- Chapter III. Marching and running locomotion. Jumping. Swimming. Flying. Wriggling, Climbing

---

also includes a protective reflex action due to some harmful cause. Facial expressions are also considered integrated muscular reflex actions resulting from depressing passions of the soul, which include pain.

Johannes Muller's successor as professor of physiology at the University of Berlin was Emile Du Bois Raymond (1818-1896). He became a member of the Berlin Academy of Sciences in 1854 and was celebrated for his work regarding neuromuscular electrophysiology [13]. The contribution made by this outstanding physiologist in the field of muscular reflex action was quite notable. Agreeing with what Canguilhem had noted in his text, Raymond credited Descartes with having "ingeniously anticipated both the term and concept of reflex action". As a matter of fact, from the previously mentioned illustrations contained in the *De Homine* work, as well as from the accurate description of eyelid reflex action provided by Descartes' in his "Traité des passions", I would sustain that Descartes had introduced – albeit unknowingly – the actual general concept of the withdrawal reflex into the field of physiology.

Another of Muller's students, Eduard Friedrich Pflugler (1829-1910), who was one of the nineteenth century's most eclectic physiologists, established a series of laws governing all the reflex movements [14]. These laws, called Pfluger's Reflex Laws, are:

1. moderate excitation, transmitted to a reflex center, is reflected in the stimulation of homolateral muscles;
2. a stronger stimulation also goes to the center of the opposite side, symmetrically to the first one, causing homolateral as well as opposite-side contractions (law of symmetry);
3. a still stronger stimulation reaches the medullar centers located above the involved metamere (law of irradiation);
4. the stimulation can increase still further, and reach the bulb, and produce

generalized reflexes throughout the body or, instead of partial contractions, it can cause convulsions (law of reflex generalization).

In the second half the nineteen century, M.A. Foster, professor of physiology at Cambridge University and Sherrington's teacher, wrote a "Treatise on Physiology" which was also published in Italian in 1883 [15]. In this work he considers the reflex actions of the spinal medulla and states that the medulla provides the best and most numerous examples of reflex action. In fact, the reflex action can be considered the spinal medulla's function par excellence, and its gray matter can be considered as being a multitude of reflex centers. "Each reflex action essentially consists of transforming afferent impulses into efferent impulses". Foster then states and describes the four principles of reflex action.

"In order to have a reflex action, the required mechanism includes a) a communicating external or internal sensitive surface, b) a sensing nerve or, using a more proper or general term, an afferent nerve, with c) a central nerve cell or group of united nerve cells, d) which, by means of a nerve, motor nerves or efferent nerves, in relation to e) with a muscle, various muscles or a few other elements of irritatable tissue that can respond by means of a change in their condition, to the arrival of afferent impulses. The afferent impulses starting from c) pass along b) and arrive at e) and produce a recognizable effect. A reflex action essentially consists of the transforming afferent impulses into efferent impulses by means of the irritable protoplasm of a nerve cell". Foster provides examples by describing the reflex action in connection with coughing, underlining the fact that "there is a very large difference between the size of the stimulus (a hair) and the reflex response (coordinated groups of glottis and breathing muscles)". Note thus, in the second half of the nineteenth century, Foster provided the withdrawal concept that was later to be further developed by his student Sherrington: "The most outstanding feature of the reflex actions in the frogs is their utilitarian character. The differentiated sensorial impulses produced by the application of the stimulus to the skin produce larger movements directed at a single purpose. It is much easier to produce a reflex action by applying a slight pressure on the skin than by applying a strong inductive shock directly to the nerve trunk". Foster was able to see that both the nature of the reflex and the nature of the impulses producing the stimulation depended on:

1. the intensity of the stimulus ("the effects of a weak stimulus applied to an afferent nerve are limited to just a few efferent nerves, whereas the effects of a strong stimulus can extend to a large number of nerves");
2. the location where the stimulus was applied ("the stimulation of a particular point produces special movements");
3. the particular conditions of the medulla ("strychnine increases the speed of the reflex action").

If the circumstances are altered, altogether different movement may be produced. Thus, when a drop of acid is placed on the right side of the frog, its right leg almost will react to remove the acid. Whereas, in exceptional cases, when the right leg is severed or the right foot is prevented from removing the acid, the left foot will be used for this purpose. This would seem to indicate a choice made with intelligence. Moreover, Foster also preludes a concept of integration that was then later introduced by Sherrington at the beginning of the twentieth century. "Certain relationships can be observed between the stimulated sensitive point and the resulting movement. The foot withdraws from the stimulus; that is, the movement is measured to repel or push away the stimulus. In other words, the perturbation produced by the central nerve cells – which, with slight stimulation is restricted to just a few cells and just a few nerve fibers – *overflows*, so to speak, when the stimulus is increased or extended to a number of nearby communicating cells, thus sending the impulses to an ever-larger number of efferent nerves".

Making a distinction between automatism, meaning to "initiate perturbations independently from any external stimulus", and neuromuscular reflex, "transforming afferent sensorial impulses into efferent motor impulses", Foster made some important observations. To begin with, he observed that the spinal medulla presents the best and most numerous examples of reflex action. The spinal medulla can thus be defined as "the prime locus of reflex action". As regards the brain's control over spinal reflexes, Foster writes: "When the brain of a frog has been removed, the reflex actions are much stronger than when the frog was intact. Therefore, there must be something in the brain – a mechanism or something else – that prevents the development of spinal reflex actions. And we know from experience that stimulating certain parts of the brain has a considerable effect on reflex action". Even though this observation had also been made by Prochaska, we can consider this the birth of physiological research on descending inhibition systems and, therefore, on systems of endogenous analgesic systems. This digression on Foster's activity was necessary, as you will see in the conclusions, for defending my theses on Descartes and the affirmations regarding his natural philosophy, in particular that the dualism that he sustained had retarded the start of the grand season of discoveries regarding the physiology of the nervous system.

Working on the neuroglia and carrying on with Wirchoff's same research, Bizzozzero's student Camillo Golgi invented the "black reaction" that finally permitted clear microscopic observation of the cells of the nervous system, to which Waldeyer, in 1891, had given the name "neurons" [16]. Another anatomist, Ramon y Cajal, who in 1906, together with Golgi, received the Nobel Prize, used this discovery to explore the histological structure of the nervous system thoroughly [17]. Paraphrasing the title of the famous work by James Burke, we could say that it was the day which changed the universe. Physiologists finally could understand the morphology of these nerve networks whose functions they had been anxious to learn and about which, up to that time, a lot of hypotheses uniting metaphysics and physiology had been made. In his monumental work, Cajal provides exemplary designs showing the anatomical disposition of the nerve networks of the spinal reflex, spinothalamic pain, and sensorial paths. Medical science's leading physiologists could thus finally see the nerve paths about which so many hypotheses had been made.

The twentieth century opened with the great lesson by Charles Sherrington, who provided a considerable number of important discoveries regarding defense reflexes. Sherrington, who was Foster's physiology professor at the legendary Trinity College in Cambridge, became a physiologist a few years later at the University of Oxford where he continued along this same line of research and reached such a high scientific level that he became known as the founder of modern experimental physiology. In 1906, he put all the evidence he had gathered into a book [18]. This ingenious, revolutionary work, which became famous, introduced the concept of integration into the field of neurophysiology and contributed to raising experimental physiology to heights never before achieved up to that time.

During the 1930s, Sherrington's students Eccles, Liddel, Creed, and Denny-Brown continued with the research work on the physiology of escape reflexes, particularly focusing on how the supraspinal nervous centers inhibit these reflexes. With the study of motorial function, exploration began on the neuronal systems going from the trunk to the medulla and exerting an inhibitory effect. Creed gave an excellent description of the withdrawal reflex. "If a piece of blotting paper is moistened with acid and laid upon the skin of a decapitated frog, it excites a set of movements by which the animal gets rid of the irritating agent. The movements are reflex actions. The response involves a chain of reactions which, starting in the skin, travel by means of the nerves from the skin to the spinal cord and then back to the periphery to the muscles which, in the cited example, are conveniently named "effector organs". After the spinal cord is destroyed, no action is evoked. Cutting the nerve between the skin and the spinal cord also will abolish the reflex action. Similarly, severing the nerve leading from the spinal cord to the muscle precludes any reflex movement. In this type of reflex response, the path traveled is a simple "reflex arc" consisting of a) an inward path which is composed of a receptor organ connected to an afferent nerve fiber; afferent nerve fibers enter the spinal cord by dorsal roots; b) the nervous (or reflex) center in the central nervous system; c) an outward path, composed of an efferent nerve fiber and an effector organ muscle or gland. Efferent nerve fibers leave the spinal cord by the ventral roots" [19].

In 1932, Sherrington and Adrian, professor of physiology at Cambridge, received the Nobel Prize for physiology and medicine. Sherrington's Nobel Lecture was entitled "Inhibition as Coordinative Factor". Eccles and Gibson in 1979 wrote an excellent book on Sherrington [65], in which the mechanism of quantitative adjustment of reflex contraction is presented, a Sherrington diagram of great historical value. Eccles and Gibson write: "The essence of the story is the gradation of reflex excitation in a motor center. Two factors are involved in the strength of the reflex action: the fraction of the motoneuron pool that discharges the impulses, and the frequency with which the individual motoneurons are discharged. In Figure 3 it can be seen on the base line that the level of excitation is classified in four categories: zeros, subliminal, subtetanics, maximal tetanica. With the latter, the frequency of firing gives the maximal tetanic tension of which the motor is capable. The picture shows a motoneuron pool with the four classes identified. The degrees of excitation of the pool neurons are shown graph-

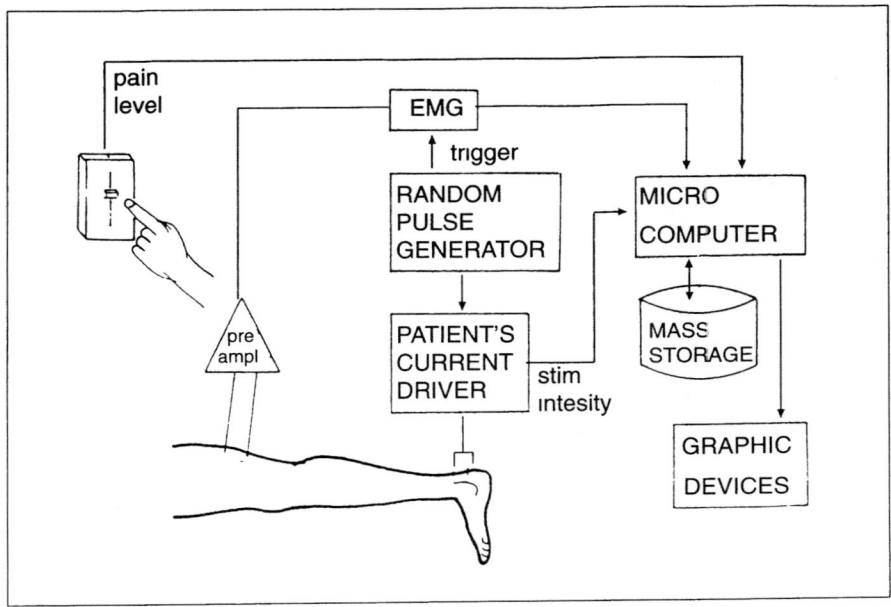

Fig. 3. Schematic representation of the experimental set: a random generator triggers both a current driver, connected with the subject, and an electromyograph for the registration of the reflex response. Pain level is measured by a lever connected with a linear potentiometer and handled by the subject. Stimulation intensity (mA), pain level (in arbitrary units) and EMG signals are acquired on line by a microcomputer providing data storage and analysis, as well as graphic display

ically by dotted lines". The degree of excitation starts from zero, increases through levels devoid of any discharging, goes to the subliminal, the subtetanic levels and then to the maximals. It should be noted that with the maximals, the discharge frequencies continue to increase above the values required for maximum muscle contraction. On the basis of this diagram, Sherrington was able to account for a whole range of reflex responses: for example, responses produced by graded skin pressure, evoking flexor reflexes or by graded stretching evoking postural reflexes. All you have to do is imagine the sloping dotted line in the diagram moved to the right for gradually weakening reflexes and to the left for gradually stronger reflexes. In the former case, there will be fewer or no maximals; the subtetanic fraction will decline and be at lower frequencies, and the larger fraction of the pool will be in subliminals or zero class. In the latter case there will be the reverse adjustment in the pool fraction. As he states "(...) adjustment of amount of contraction (...) proceeds by extensity and intensity (...) The diagram also account for the caracteristic time course of reflex responses produced by a steady excitatory input". Sherrington made many important discoveries regarding the defense reflex [20]. With the study of reflex function, the exploration of neuronal systems which connect the spinal cord and the medulla, causing an inhibitory effect, began.

In March 1985, I organized with J. Eccles, A. Cuello and D. Ottoson the first International Conference on Pain and Motility, at the University of Milan. In collaboration with Dr Roberto Casale (Service of neurophysiological and rehabilitation Medical Center of Montescano), we gave the following presentation (reproduced with the permission of R. Casale and Raven Press) [21].

"Exteroceptive reflexes are commonly defined as an organized and stereotyped motor reaction, often complex, and activated by cutaneous and subcutaneous stimuli. From exteroceptive reflexes come the so-called nociceptive or defensive ones, because they are provoked by stimuli that in animals produce pain [22]. From a neurophysiological point of view, the simplest level of interaction between nociceptive input and motor response, and that which in laboratory tests can be most easily isolated from the network, is the flexion withdrawal reflex of the lower limb. The first to study exteroceptive reflexes, at the beginning of the century, were some of the most important authors of neurological science such as Babinski [23], Sherrington [24], Wernicke [25], and Lloyd [26]. Their interest was to study the physiopathology of movement and the influences that exteroceptive inputs place on the motoneuronal spinal pool. Lloyd observed how the muscular reflex discharge, due to the stimulation of the sensitive nerve in the cat, has two electromyographic components at different onset latencies, showing the involvement of two types of fibers at different rates of conduction. Fundamental works on physiopathological mechanisms of the flexion reflex are those of Hagbarth [27] and of Kugelberg [28] which affirm that there is little doubt that (…) the nervous reflexes elicited from the foot (…) represent the adequate withdrawal movement of the human lower limb to exteroceptive stimuli. Pinelli and Valle [29] were among the first to include the study of polysynaptic flexion reflexes in the evaluation of spasticity in man in both the lower and upper limbs. Pinelli observed a flexion reflex similar to that of Babinski. More recently, Dimitrijevic and Nathan [30, 31] applied it to the study of human spinal spasticity, evaluating phenomena such as habituation and dishabituation".

Flexion withdrawal reflex and nociception studies

In the 1960s we gradually witnessed a change in the researcher's interesta from the motor component of the reflex to its nociceptive aspect. Certainly, one of the scientific events that led to this gradual change of interests was the publication of the spinal gate control theory [32]. As Lloyd had experimented on cats, Hugon [33] and Ertekin and Ackali [34], in the light of this theory, experimented on humans, underlining the nociceptive aspect of the theory and extending to a "significant degree the Melzack-Wall approach to the human subject".

Stimulating the sural nerve in its retromalleolar course with a random pulse consisting of a train of eight to ten shocks at 300 cps we can register from the biceps femoris (caput brevis) muscle two reflex components at different times of onset produced by a stimulus of increasing intensity.

1. Early response of short latency (40-60 ms) and low threshold provoked by tactile nonpainful stimulation, corresponding to a reflex functionally integrated in the postural control of the foot, and called Ra II since it involves group II afferents [35].
2. Delayed response of longer latency (80-150 ms) and higher threshold provoked by a more intense stimulus corresponding to Sherrington's nociceptive reflex. This response was called Ra III since it involves group III afferents. In the early experiment carried out by Hugon [36] the painful nature of stimulation able to provoke the Ra III reflex was confirmed in the verbal report of subjects who underwent the stimulation. The relationship between flexion withdrawal reflex and the pain level was studied by Willer [37], who related the Ra III threshold (expressed in mA) and the pain provoked using a visual analogic scale.

The liminal pain in those experiences was described by the subjects "as a sharp sensation, like a pin-prick localized at the point of stimulation" [33], while the intensity of the stimulus ready to provoke the reflex was approximately 10-13 mA [37]. Further works have provided experimental evidence of the excitatory and/or inhibitory influences acting on spinal neuronal activity.

Stress, attention, anxiety, as well as both painful and nonpainful stimuli such as electrical and vibratory stimulation seem to modify the threshold of the reflex [38-44].

Vibration influences both pain and motility

The study of vibration is particularly interesting, inasmuch as it has followed the concerns of clinical neurophysiology, earlier being dedicated to motility and its disorders, and then, in recent years, to pain.

Vibration was used in clinical neurophysiology because it induces a discharge imitating the static fusimotor activation of the primary ending Ia fiber units that normally occurs under isometric contraction [27]. Vibration activates not only the latter, but also receptive units such as Pacinian corpuscles and rapidly adapting receptors functionally linked with large-diameter fibers [45]. For some years it has been used with the aim of pain control because of this activation and the consequent possibility of modulating nociceptive input at the spinal level [33]. Vibration can inhibit monosynaptic reflexes H and T [46, 47], as well as influencing polysynaptic reflexes [45]; but data on lower limb flexion reflex are not as homogeneous as for H and T reflexes.

Confirming an observation of Delwaide [48], Ertekin and Ackali showed an increase in amplitude and duration of Ra III during vibration. They also observed a facilitatory effect lasting 20 min after vibration ceased. In our laboratory, using a computer-aided system, we are carrying out studies on the effect of vibration on Ra III, and recently we published some data in contrast to Ertekin's observation (Fig. 4) [34]. In this research we examined a group of lumbosciatalgic patients without neurophysiological signs of peripheral nerve impairment

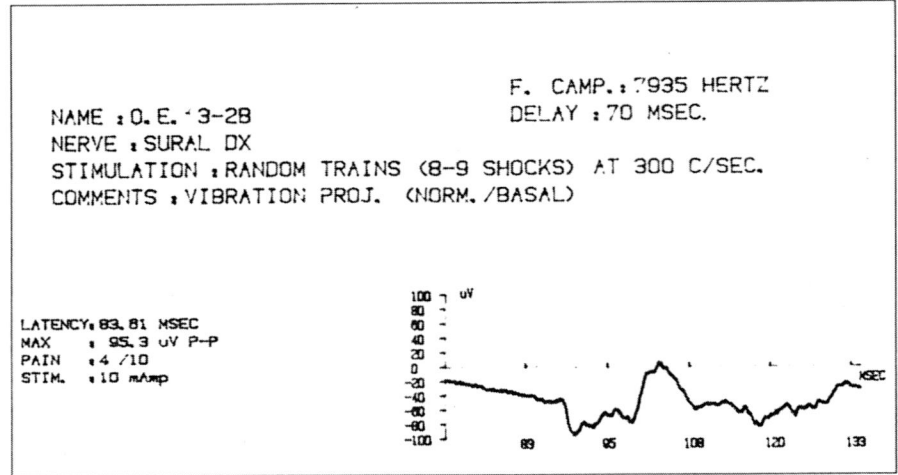

Fig. 4. Sample of graphic display. Top: general data, such as stimulation parameter and technical data, are plotted. Lower left: different wave parameters, such as latency and maximal amplitude; stimulation intensity (mA) and the relative subjective pain intensity (arbitrary units) are shown as well. Lower right: Ra III wave is plotted. Sampling frequency and acquisition delay are plotted in the upper general part

(sural nerve latency, H reflex latency, and amplitude were normal and statistically not different from those of a control group). Harmless, cramping pain was referred at medium intensity in the leg. Vibration stimulus of 100 Hz was applied for approximately 20-25 min to the Achilles tendon after having reached the reflex threshold, and after its amplitude had been stabilized. We measured the pain level with a modified representation of graphic self-pain estimate consisting of a lever attached to a linear potentiometer. Both pain level and stimulation intensity were registered and displayed on the computer screen with the elicited reflex response, and then plotted (Fig. 5).

The application reduced the pain level by 60%-70% with an almost immediate effect and inhibited the Ra III up to its disappearance, increasing the reflex threshold (Fig. 6). Nevertheless, such barrage seemed to be unstable as we registered Ra-III-like randomly high amplitude potentials after this almost total inhibition [49].

The discrepancy between Ertekin's data and ours could be explained, as suggested by Wall and Cronly-Dillon [50], since vibration reduced the effects of low-intensity painful stimulation, whereas it increased that of high intensity.

During Ertekin's experiments, many subjects reported an increase in pain provoked by electrical stimulation during vibration. This leads us to think that the intensity or the electrical stimulus used by this author was higher than our "threshold" stimulus, which was just sufficient to provoke a stable reflex. In the first case, vibration could not interfere with nociceptive input but, on the contrary, could be added to them, clinically increasing the pain and instrumentally increasing the amplitude and length of the reflex. In the second case, vibration could create a barrage, even if incomplete, and would stop provoking an incom-

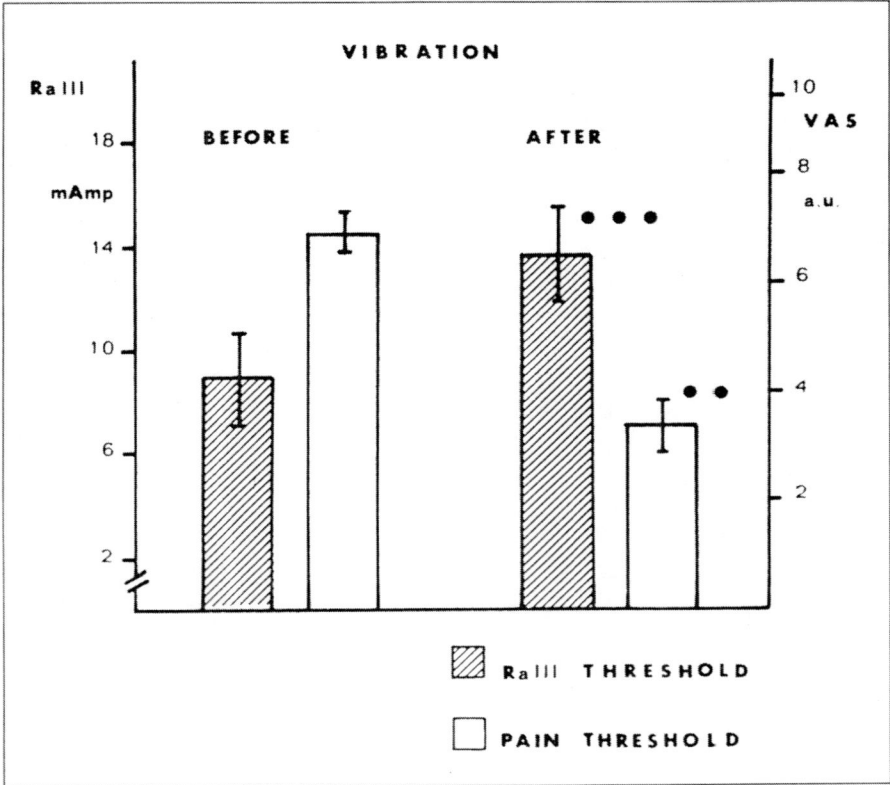

Fig. 5. Histograms represent Ra III wave threshold (striped columns) expressed in mA (left scale), and subjective pain intensity (empty columns) expressed in arbitrary units (right scale) before and after a 20- min 100 Hz vibration treatment in lumbosciatalgic patients. Black dots represent statistical significance [19]

plete barrage only at high frequencies [51], while for those approximate or inferior to 100 Hz such a blockage would be ineffective or at least unstable.

This hypothesis could also be clinically supported by the positive results obtained by other authors [52, 53] in certain pathologies, and by the poor effectiveness we have observed during 1985 in the treatment of certain types of pain in paraplegics and in patients with intense pain [54].

To add to this, Ottoson himself had signaled the increase of pain level in the treatment of cephalic pain when the vibration was placed far from the painful area. In such conditions, factors such as the intensity of the conditioned stimulus and the intensity of spontaneous pain seem to be relevant [55].

Sites, parameters, and time of application of vibration as well as electrical stimulation can be of further relevance.

Finally, we must not forget that the vibratory stimulus at 100 Hz provokes changes in sympathetic tone [39]. Experiments carried out in our laboratory

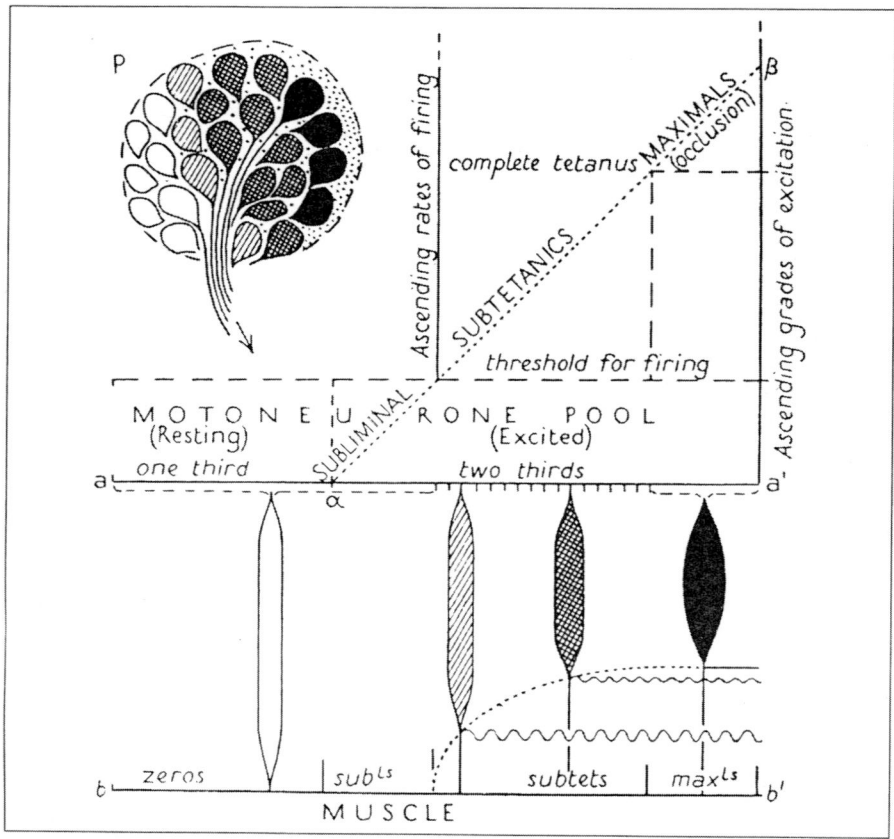

Fig. 6. Scheme or distribution of excitement in a reflex-active motoneuron pool of a muscle. Grade of excitement plotted against numbers of motoneurons (abscissa a a') and motor-units (abscissa b b') α, β denote excitement in active fraction of pool [21]

forced us to maintain whichever exteroceptive stimulus that can produce, at least in the initial phase of application, a sympathomimetic "phasic" response. This sympathomimetic response in some clinically healthy subjects is of huge intensity, altering measurements of nociceptive reflex as well as threshold.

Anthropology of the withdrawal reflex

In collaboration with Prof. Antonio Guerci (Director of Antropological Services, University of Genua, Italy) we currently are developing a research project on the defense response to pain in various anthropological and ethnic situations. The study utilizes the withdrawal reflex model (prevalently, the knee flex reflex) model.

The cultural project of the university department is characterized by the following points:
- strong adherence to biological, physical, environmental, and social facts in the genesis of personality and comportment;
- attentive consideration of the adaptive strategies (biological, anthropological, ethnomedical, ethnological, social), utilized whether in an ontogenetic or a phylogenetic context;
- strong interest in ascertaining the emancipation of the personality from genetic restraints in order to create itself as a psychosocial construction;
- openness to the cultural context as the final intersection of the biological project;
- interest in communication, language, and cognitive processes as the instruments of biosocial adaptation;
- the need to analyze, interpret, and empirically verify the formative models of interaction within diverse cultural contexts;
- the study of the medical strategies, including pain therapy, of peoples different across time and space as a result of their human adaptation to their environment and as a moment of transition from a biological to a cultural approach.

What are current and future possibilities of scientific research on the withdrawal reflex model?

The withdrawal reflex is a highly significant and reliable response model for the study of pain defense, whether in animals or humans.

Bromm writes: "The nociceptive withdrawal reflex is also well established in humans as a measure of pain and pain relief. The strength of the reflex is usually determined by surface electromyogram (EMG) of the referred muscle. Skin conductance reactions (SCR) in response to brief pain stimuli can easily be recorded when they appear with latencies of approximately 2 s all over the body surface. Other vegetative reactions regarded in pain measurement are changes in heart rate, changes in respiratory frequency, and changes in local blood circulation These peripheral reactions are elicited by stimulus-induced neuronal activity within the nociceptive system; as such they may be called nociceptive or nocifensive and can be well investigated in animals. However, from our experiments in the awake human being we know that conscious pain is different. For example, the nociceptor reflex, the most favored animal model in algesimetry, usually appears in humans with stimulus intensities significantly below the subject's response to laboratory pain. Furthermore, the withdrawal reflex is polysynaptic; it underlies fatigue and habituation if repeated stimuli are given. The skin conductance reaction, which is interpreted as a measure of emotion, anxiety or novelty, was found to have the same results" [56].

Given the didactic nature of my presentation, a look at recent research using the withdrawal reflex model is useful. Examples have been drawn from different sectors of medicine, demonstrating the vasteness of application of this model for study.

Recent research

1. M.M. Morgan (Department of Psychology, Washington State University, Vancouver, Washington).
   "Although the sensory coding of nociceptive neurons in the dorsal horn has been studied extensively, surprisingly little is known about how these neurons contribute to nociceptive reflexes. The objective of the present study was to examine the characteristics of dorsal horn neurons capable of initiating hindpaw whithdrawal. To this end, neural and reflex activity were measured simultaneously in response to noxious radiant heat applied to the hindpaw in lightly anaesthetized rats (...). These results suggest that current classification schemes, in particular MR and NS categories, cannot be used as the sole criterion to predict involvement in nociceptive reflexes. However, simultaneous measurement of neural and reflex activity provides an opportunity to determine the characteristics of nociceptive neurons involved in withdrawal reflexes" [57].

2. R. Dirksen, B. Ellenbroek, J. van Egmond, A.R. Cools (Department of Anaesthesiology, University of Nijmegen, The Netherlands).
   "(...) Propofol is a GABA – mimetic general anaesthetic (...). Propofol induced a higher incidence of involuntary muscular contractions and oral movements, but a lower incidence of grooming, in APO-SUS rats rather than in APO-UNSUS rats. Reflex inhibition and narcisis, being defined as the behavior marked by both full absence of purposeful movements and by complete loss of righting reflexes, after propofol did not differ between the two lines (...). Differences in cerebral GABA transmission, especially in the striato – nigro – collicular pathway, did not give rise to difference in the effect of propofol on narcois and hindlimb withdrawal reflex. In contrast, these differences in GABA transmission were accompanied by line – specific differences in the effect of propofol on certain behavioral and cardiovascular parameters" [58].

3. T. Abel, E. Kandel (Howard Hughes Medical Institute Center for Neurobiology and Behavior, Columbia University).
   "(...) In this review we describe the molecular machinery that mediates memory consolidation in each of these systems. One of the surprising findings to emerge, particularly from studies of long-term facilitation in Aplysia, is that memory storage is mediated by not only positive but also negative regulatory mechanisms, in much the same way as cell division is controlled by the proteins encoded by oncogenes and tumor suppressor genes. This suggests the interesting possibility that there are memory suppressor genes whose protein products impede memory storage" [59].

4. Page G.D., France C.R. (Department of Psychology, Ohio University, Athens, Ohio, USA).

"(...) Based on previous evidence that the nociceptive withdrawal reflex may provide an objective index of pain threshold in humans, the present study examined the intensity of sural nerve stimulation required to elicit nociceptive withdrawal in offspring of hypertensives and normatensives. Participants included 60 men and 56 women who were normotensive, 18-23 years of age, and predominately caucasian. To assess the nociceptive withdrawal reflex, ascending and descending intensities of electrical stimulation were applied over the sural nerve while electromyographic activity was recorded from the ipsilateral biceps femoris muscle. Analyses of the intensity of electrical stimulation required to reach the thresholds for nociceptive withdrawal, and subjective pain revealed a pattern of hypoalgesia in individuals at risk for hypertension. First, significantly higher intensities were required to elicit nociceptive withdrawal in offspring of hypertensives versus normotensives. Second, offspring of hypertensives endured significantly more intense stimulation before reporting pain. Third, both parental history of hypertension and resting systolic blood pressure were significant independent predictors of stimulation intensity at nociceptive withdrawal reflex and subjective pain thresholds. These results confirm and extend previous observations of an association between risk for hypertension and hypoalgesia, and suggest that hypoalgesia should be examined as a potential predictor of progressive blood pressure increases in individuals at risk for hypertension" [60].

5. S. Eappen, I. Kissin (Department of Anaesthesia, Brigham and Women's Hospital and Harvard Medical School, Boston, Massachusetts, USA).
"Background: Subarachnoid bupivacaine blockade has been reported to reduce thipental and midazolam hypnotic requirements in patients. The purpose of this study was to examine if local anaesthetically induced lumbar intrathecal blockade would reduce thiopental requirements for blockade of motor responses to noxious and nonnoxious stimuli in rats (...). Methods: After intrathecal and external jugular catheter placement, rats were assigned randomly to two groups in a crossover design study, with each rat to receive either 10 microl of 0.75% bupivacaine or 10 microl of normal saline intrathecally. The doses of intravenously administered thiopental required to ablate the eyelid reflex, to block the withdrawal of a front limb digit, and to block the corneal reflex were compared. In two separate groups of animals, hemodynamic parameters and concentrations of thiopental in the brain were comparate between intrathecally administered bupivacaine and saline. Results: The thiopental dose required to block the described responses was decreased with intrathecally administered bupivacaine versus intrathecally administered saline from (mean±SD) 40±5 to 24±4 mg/kg ($P<0.001$) for the eyelid reflex, from 51±6 to 29±6 mg/kg ($p<0.005$) for front limb withdrawal, and from 67±8 to 46±8 mg/kg ($p<0.01$) for the corneal reflex. The concentration of thiopental in the brain at the time of corneal reflex-blockade for the group given bupivacaine was significantly lower than in the group given saline (24.1 vs 35.8 mg/g, $p=0.02$). Conclusion: This study demonstrates that lumbar intrathecally administered local anaesthetic blockade decreases anaesthetic re-

quirements for thiopental for a spectrum of end points tested. This effect is due neither to altered pharmacokinetics nor to a direct action of the local anaesthetic on the brain; rather, it is most likely due decreased afferent input" [61].

6. H.R. Weng, J. Schouenborg (Department of Physiology and Neuroscience, University of Lund, Sweden).

"Previous studies indicate that the withdrawal reflex system in the rat has a "modular" organization, each reflex pathway performing a specific sensori-motor transformation. Here, we wished to clarify which cutaneous receptors contribute to this system and to determine whether there are differences in this respect between reflex pathways of different muscles. Withdrawal reflexes of the peroneus longus, extensor digitorum longus, and semitendinous muscles were recorded with EMG techniques during high reflex excitability in decere-brate spinal rats (n=26) (...). These findings suggest that some chemonociceptors contribute only weakly, or not at all, to withdrawal reflex pathways. The present data suggest that a selective set of cutaneous receptors contribute to withdrawal reflex pathways and that different withdrawal reflex pathways receive input from essentially the same cutaneous receptor types" [62].

7. T. Hori, T. Oka, M. Hosoi, S. Aou (Dept of Physiology, Kyushu University Faculty of Medicine, Fuuota, Japan).

"Proinflammatory cytokines such as IL-1, IL-6 and TNFα are known to enhance nociception at peripheral inflammatory tissues. These cytokines are also produced in the brain. We found that an intracerebroventricular injection of IL-1β only at non pyrogenic doses in the rats reduced the paw-withdrawal latency on a hot plate and enhanced responses of the wide dynamic range neurons in the trigenminal nuclueus caudalis to noxious stimuli. This hyperalgesia, as assessed by behavioral and neuronal responses, was blocked by pretreatment with IL-1 receptor antagonist (IL-1Ra). The maximal response was obtained 30 min after injection of IL-1β (20-50 pg/kg). On other hand an injection of Il-1β (20-50 pg/kg) into the ventromedial hypotalamus (VMH) prolonged the paw-withrawal latency maximally 10 min after injection. This analgesia, as well as the intra POA IL-1β-induced hyperalgesia, was completely blocked by IL-1Ra or Na salycilate. Our previous study has revealed that i.c.v. injection of PGE2, induces hyperalgesia through EP3 receptors and analgesia through EP1 receptors by its central action. The results, taken together, suggest: 1) that IL-1β at lower doses in the brain induced hyperlagesia through EP3 receptors in the POA; and 2) that the higher doses of brain IL-1β produces analgesia through EP1 receptors, probably, in the VHM" [63].

Conclusions

The withdrawal-effect enigma in the debate regarding body and mind, I feel, is as follows: who orders the activation of the withdrawal effect to rapidly put a living being out of harm's way?

In his book entitled "The Understanding of the Brain", John C. Eccles (1901-1996), who won the Nobel Prize for physiology in 1963, states: "How can we control our muscles to make sure our actions conform to the situations in which we find ourselves? The motorial cortex is an extraordinarily important structure, but it is not what starts off a movement. The pyramidal cells of the motorial cortex, with their large axes that pass through the pyramidal fascia, are important because they provide a direct efferent channel going from the cortex to the motoneurons which, in turn, cause the muscular contractions. This completely direct connection is very important for assuring that the cerebral cortex, by means of the motorial cortex, can very effectively and rapidly evoke the desired movement. However, there are many basic problems yet to be resolved. How can the decision to carry out a muscular movement start off a series of nerve events that lead to the discharging of the pyramidal cells?". Gray Walter (quoted by Eccles) observed that a negative potential appeared at the cortex level, a "waiting wave" preceding the starting stimulus. Korbruner called this negative potential the "preparation potential." On average, the preparation potential begins after 0.8 s and lasts up to 0.1 s before the movement occurs. "What happens in my brain", continues Eccles, "when I decide to perform a movement?". Indeed, after centuries of philosophical inquiry and scientific experimentation the question remains as to what happens during those few hundreds of a second? In multidisciplinary history, studies on pain have opened new avenues which have continued to develop thicker path networks, each requiring further exploration [65-73]. Thus the withdrawal reflex continues to be, in algology, a fascinating scientific and cultural challenge.

References

1. Dorland's Illustrated Medical Dictionary (1985) 27th ed: Saunders, Philadelphia
2. Craig KD (1994) Emotional aspects of pain. In: Wall PD, Melzack R (eds) Textbook of pain, 3rd edn. Churchill Livingstone, Edinburgh, p 264
3. Fearing F (1930) Reflex action, a study in the history of physiological psychology. Williams and Wilkins, Baltimore
4. Fulton JF (1946) Muscular contraction and the reflex control of movement. Williams and Wilkins, Baltimore, pp 3-55
5. Du Bois-Reymond E (1887) Gedachtnisrede auf Johannes Muller. Abhadlungen der Akademie der Wissenschaften, Berlin
6. Willis T (1681) Opera Omnia, Lyon
7. Unzer JA (1771) Erste Grunde einer Physiologie der eigentlichen Thierischen Natur und der Thierischen Korper
8 Brazier MA (1988) A history of neurophysiology in the 17th and 18th centuries. Raven, New York, pp 167-169
9 Unzer JA op. cit.
10. Magendie F (1822) Expérience sur les functions des racines des nerfs qui naissent de la moelle. J Physiol Exp Pathol 3·153-157
11. Luciani L (1901) Fisiologia dell'uomo. Società Editrice Libraria, Milano 2(5):305-384
12. Muller J (1823-1824) Handbuk der Physiologie des Menschen. Coblenz

13. Du Bois-Reymond E (1886-1887) Reden von Emil Du Bois-Reymond Literatur, Philosophie, Zeitsgeschichte Collected by Ernst vun Brucke. Veit, Leipzig

14 Pfuegler E (1859) Unterschungen ueber die Physiologie des Electrotonus, Berlin

15. Foster MA (1883) Trattato di Fisiologia, Ia ed. Francesco Vallardi, Milano

16. Golgi C (1880) Studi istologici sul midollo spinale. Communication made to the third Italian Congress of Psychiatry, Reggio Emilia

17. Ramon Y, Cajal S (1889) Contribución al estudio de la structura de la medula espinal. Rev Trim Histol Norm Pathol 3:4

18. Sherrington CS (1910) Flexion reflex in the limb, crossed extension reflex and reflex stepping and standing. J Physiol 40:28-129

19. Creed RS, Denny-Brown, Eccles JC, Liddel EGT, Sherrington CS (1932) Reflex activity of the spinal cord.Clarendon, Oxford

20. Sherrington CS (1906) The integrative action of the nervous system. Schreibner, New York

21. Casale R, Tiengo M (1987) Flexion withdrawal reflex: a link between pain and mobility In: Tiengo M, Eccles JC, Cuello AC, Ottoson D (eds) Pain and mobility. Advances in pain research and therapy. Raven, New York, pp 77-83

22. Kugelberg E, Eklund K, Griby L (1960) The electromyographic study of the nociceptive reflexes of the lower limb. Mechanisms of the plantar responses. Brain 23:349-410

23. Babinski J (1898) Du phenomène des orteils et sa valeur semiologique. Semaine Med 18:321-322

24. Sherrington JC (1910) op. cit.

25 Wernicke C (1881) Lehrbuch der Gehirnkrankheiten fur Aerzte und Studirende. Vol 1. Kassel

26. Lloyd DPC (1943) Reflex action in relation to pattern and peripheral source of afferent stimulation. J Neurophysiol 6:421

27. Hagbarth KE, Eklund G (1966) Motor effects of vibratory stimuli in man. In: Alquist Wikseel (eds) Muscular afferent and motor control. Granit Nobel Symposium 1, Stockholm, pp 171-196

28. Kugelberg E (1962) Polysynaptic reflexes of clinical importance. Electroencephalogr Clin Neurophysiol 27:S103-S111

29. Pinelli P, Valle M (1960) Studio fisiopatologico dei riflessi muscolari nelle paresi spastiche (sui tests per la misura della spasticità). Arch Sci Med 109:106-120

30. Dimitrijevic MR, Nathan PW (1970) Studies of spasticity in man. Changes in flexion reflex with repetitive cutaneous stimulation in spinal man. Brain 93:743-768

31 Dimitrijevic MR, Nathan PW (1971) Studies of spasticity in man. Dishabituation of the flexion reflex in spinal man. Brain 94:77-90

32. Melzack R, Wall PD (1965) Pain mechanism. a new theory. Science 150:971-979

33. Hugon M (1973) Exteroceptive reflexes to stimulation of the sural nerve in normal man. In: Desmedt JE (ed) New developments in electromyography and clinical neurophysiology. Vol 3. Karger, Basel, pp 713-729

34. Ertekin C, Ackali D (1978) Effect of continuous vibration on nociceptive flexor reflexes. J Neurol Neurosurg Psychiatry 41:532-537

35. Shahani B, Young RP (1971) Human flexor reflexes. J Neurol Neurosurg Psychiatry 34:616-627

36. Hugon M (1967) Réflexes polysynaptiques cutanés et commandes volontaires. Thèse Science Phis, Paris

37. Willer JC (1975) Influence de l'anticipation de la douleur sur les fréquences cardiaques et respiratoires et sur le réflexe nociceptif chez l'homme. Physiol Behav 15:411-415

38. Bathein N (1971) Réflexes spinaux chez l'homme et niveaux d'attention Electroencephalogr.Clin Neurophysiol 30:32-37

39. Boureau F, Willer JC, Dehen H (1977) L'action de l'acupuncture sur la douleur. Bases physiologiques. Nouv Presse Med 6:1871-1874
40. Casale R, Tiengo M (1984) Neurophysiological effects of the administration of a vibratory antalgic stimuli in healthy and lumbosciatalgic patients. Pain [Suppl] 2:57
41. Handewerker HO, Iggo A, Zimmermann M (1975) Segmental and suprasegmental actions on dorsal horn neurons responding to noxious and non-noxious skin stimuli. Pain 1:147-165
42. Willer JC (1977) Comparative study of perceived pain and nociceptive flexion reflex in man. Pain 3:69-80
43. Willer JC, Boureu F, Albe-Fessard D (1979) Supraspinal influences on nociceptive flexion reflex and pain sensation in man. Brain Res 179:61-69
44. Hagbarth KE (1960) Spinal withdrawal reflex in the human lower limbs. J Neurol Neurosurg Psychiatry 23:222-227
45. Knibestol M, Valibo AB (1970) Single unit analysis of mechanoceptor activity from the human glabrous skin. Acta Physiol Scand 80:178-195
46. Lance JW, Nielson PD, Tassinari CA (1968) Suppression of the H-reflex by peripheral vibration. Proc Aust Assoc Neurol 5:45-49
47. Delwaide PJ (1969) Approche de la physiopathologie de la spasticité: réflexe de Hoffmann et vibration appliquées sur le tendon d'Achille. Rev Neurol 121:72-74
48. Delwaide PJ (1973) Human monosynaptic reflexes and presynaptic inhibition. An interpretation of spastic hyperreflexia. In: Desmedt JE (ed) New development in electromyography and clinical neurophysiology. Vol 3. Karger, Basel, pp 509-527
49. Casale R, Giordano A, Tiengo M (1985) Risposte riflesse nocicettive spinali. Variazione della risposta riflessa nocicettiva RaIII e del dolore lombosciatalgico indotte da TENS e vibrazione. Min Anestesiol 51:217-229
50. Wall PD, Cronly-Dillon J (1960) Pain, itch and vibration. AMA Arch Neurol 2:365-375
51. Hagbarth KE (1973) Effects of muscle vibration in normal man and in patients with motor disease. In: Desmedt JE (ed) New development in electromyography and clinical neurophysiology. Vol 3. Karger, Basel, pp 428-443
52. Lundeberg T (1983) Long-term results of vibratory stimulation as a pain relieving measure for chronic pain. Pain 20:13-23
53. Ottoson D, Ekblom A, Hansson P (1981) Vibratory stimulation for the relief of pain of dental origin. Pain 10:37-45
54. Casale R, Buonocore M, Bozzi M, Bodini GC (1986) Variazioni pletismografiche indotte dalla applicazione di uno stimolo vibratorio a 100 Hz nel normale. Boll Soc Ital Biol Sper
55. Bini G, Cruccu G, Hagbarth KE, Shady W, Torebjork E (1984) Analgesic effect of vibration and cooling on pain induced by intraneuronal electrical stimulation. Pain 18:239-248
56. Bromm B (1989) Laboratory animal and human volunteer in the assessment of analgesic efficacy. In: Chapman RC, Loeser JD (eds) Issues in pain measurement. Advances in pain resarch and therapy. Vol 12 Raven, New York, pp 117-143
57. Morgan MM (1998) Direct comparison of heat-evoked activity of nociceptive neurons in the dorsal horn with the hindpaw withdrawal reflex in the rat. J Neurophysiol 79 (1):174-180
58 Dirksen R, Ellenbroek B, van Egmond J, Cools AR (1997) Responses to propofol in relation to GABA functionality of discrete parts of the brain of rats. Pharmacol Biochem Behav 57(4).727-735
59 Abel T, Kandel E (1998) Positive and negative regulatory mechanisms that mediate long-term memory storage. Brain Res Rev 26(2-3) 360-378

60. Page GD, France CR (1997) Objective evidence of decreased pain perception in normotensives at risk for hypertension. Pain 73:173-180
61. Eappen S, Kissin I (1998) Effect of subarachnoid bupivacaine block on anaesthetic requirements for thiopental in rats. Anaesthesiology 88:1036-1042
62. Weng HR, Schouenborg J (1998) On the cutaneous receptors contributing to withdrawal reflex pathways in the decerebrate spinal rat. Exp Brain Res 118:71-77
63 Hori T, Oka T, Hosoi M, Aou S (1998) Pain modulatory actions of cytockines and prostaglandine E2 in the brain. Ann NY Acad Sci 840:269-281
64. Eccles JC, Gibson WC (1979) Sherrington: his life and thought. Springer-Verlag, Berlin Heidelberg New York
65. Popper KR, Eccles JC (1981) L' Io ed il suo cervello, strutture e funzioni cerebrali. Armando, Rome, pp 129-137
66. Searle JC (1983) Intentionality: an essay in philosophy of mind. Cambridge University Press, Cambridge
67. Tiengo M (1992) A quantistic mind interpretation. Seminari sul dolore. Vol. 2. Mattioli, 2:27-29
68. Tiengo M, Moiraghi F (1989) Le radici teoriche di una esperienza scientifica. Seminari sul dolore. Vol 1. Mattioli, pp 35-50
69. Tiengo M (1996) Il dolore nel dibattito cervello-mente. In: Tiengo M, Benedetti C (eds) Fisiopatologia e terapia del dolore. Masson, Milano, pp 523-528
70. Tiengo M (1994) Introduzione. In: Eccles JC (ed) Come l'Io controlla il suo cervello: la mente e i suoi processi. Rizzoli, Milano, pp 7-15
71. Tiengo M (1998) Il dolore il cervello e la mente· l'errore di Cartesio. In: Tiengo M (ed) Atti del I Corso Superiore di Aggiornamento in Fisiopatologia e Terapia del Dolore. Bayer, pp 147-154
72. Tiengo M (1983) Pain and analgesia: from Cartesio to Sherrington. Prologues to first Course of pathophysiology and pain therapy. Milano State University, February
73. Tiengo M (1992) The Alice mirror: a metaphor for pain perception. In: Ventafridda V et al (eds) Highlights on pain and suffering. Mendrisio, Lugano

Chapter 4

Pathophysiology of pain modulation

C.J. GLYNN

The pathophysiology of pain modulation by definition relates to pain in humans, as pain in animals is defined as nociception. This presentation will only provide information and data about pain in humans and will not confuse the issue with nociception (see below for the official definitions). Modulation of pain suggests that the pain is changed for the better, that is to relieve the pain, but it also infers that it is symptomatic management (treatment) of the pain, not treatment of the cause of the pain. The presentation will concentrate on what is often called clinical pain. In humans our understanding of the pathophysiology of pain is based on the modulation of that pain. As a result the pathophysiological mechanisms underlying the pain are inferred from the treatment [1, 2]. This is a circular argument; as a result of successful treatment of a particular pain we infer that the underlying pathophysiological mechanisms of that pain are directly related to this successful treatment. This assumption may not be true for all situations and this observation is fundamental in defining the limits of our understanding of the pathophysiological mechanisms of pain modulation. The evidence for effective treatment (modulation) of pain will be presented and the pathophysiology will be inferred from this modulation.

Pain has been defined by the International Association for the Study of Pain as an unpleasant sensory and emotional experience associated with actual or potential damage or described in terms of such damage [3]. *Nociception* has been defined by the International Association for the Study of Pain as activity induced in the nociceptor, and nociceptive pathways by a noxious stimulus is not pain, which is always a psychological state, even though we may well appreciate that pain most often has a proximate physical cause [3]. Animals *respond* to a noxious stimulus, nociception, humans *perceive* pain. Pain always has two components, a physical and an emotional component; to avoid confusion the pathophysiology and modulation of these two components will be dealt with separately. The relative importance of each of these components is affected by the duration and the environment as well as the sex and the personality of the patient (Fig. 1).

There are two other definitions that should be clarified:
- *neurogenic pain*: pain initiated or caused by a primary lesion, dysfunction or transitory perturbation in the peripheral or central nervous system;
- *neuropathic pain*: pain initiated or caused by a primary lesion or dysfunction in the nervous system [3].

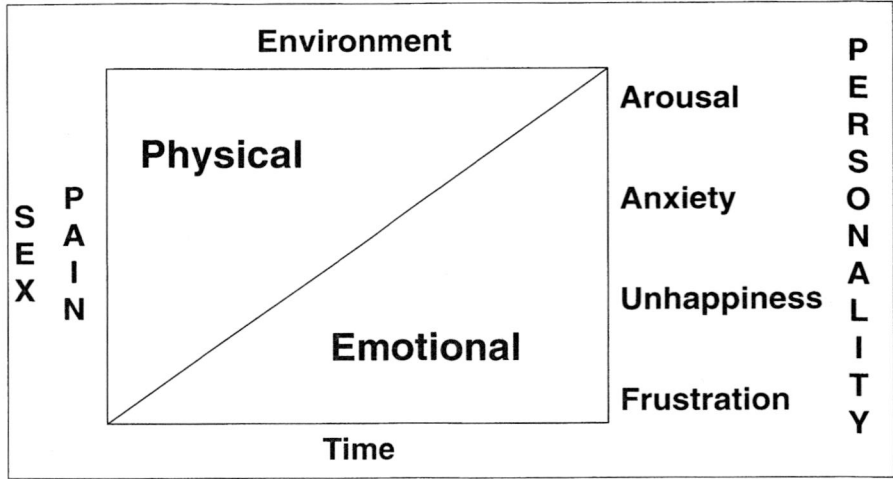

Fig. 1. This figure shows the relationships between the physical and the emotional components of pain, both of these components are always present. The emotional component may be subdivided into three or four unpleasant mood factors which vary according to the type of pain. The perception of pain is further compromised by duration, sex, personality and environment

These two kinds of pain, one of which may be transitory, neurogenic pain and the other which is not considered to be transitory, neuropathic pain, account for a significant proportion of the problems in the treatment of chronic pain. For the purposes of this discussion neuropathic pain will be used to encompass both neurogenic and neuropathic pain. Neuropathic pain differs pathophysiologically from nociceptive pain which is classically associated with trauma and resolves with time as part of the healing process, i.e., post-operative pain. The pathophysiological and modulation differences between nociceptive pain and neuropathic pain will be identified throughout this presentation.

Modulation of the physical component of pain

Conduction analgesia

Conduction analgesia can be defined as that analgesia that is associated with a decrease or blockade of electrical impulses transferred along the axons, the classical example being neural blockade with local anaesthetics. Local anaesthetic blockade is generally successful in the modulation of all peripheral nociceptive and neuropathic pains. Indeed, it is commonly used to confirm or deny a peripheral focus for pain. Occasionally, peripheral nerve blockade may increase neuropathic pain. This is presumably a result of the change in sensory input to the spinal cord and such a pain would be considered to be more central than the site of the blockade. Another reason for the increase in pain following peripheral nerve blockade is the numbness associated with this blockade. Patients with neuropathic pain regularly complain of the altered sensation as pain and the numbness after the local anaesthetic is also interpreted as abnormal, and so as pain.

Transcutaneous electrical nerve stimulation (TENS) is a form of conduction analgesia, in that it puts in another signal that overrides the transmission of pain. It is not very effective in nociceptive pain, particularly if that pain is stimulus related. It is generally considered to be more effective in neuropathic pain. It is not possible with TENS to identify the source of the pain as the modulation may occur at the spinal cord as a result of the altered electrical input.

There is some evidence from bench models that carbamazepine decreases electrical conduction in axons [4] Most of the anticonvulsant drugs used in the treatment of neuropathic pain are membrane stabilisers and as such could all inhibit conduction in peripheral nerves (axons) [5]. These drugs appear to be of little benefit in patients with nociceptive pain; however, there is some recent experimental evidence that suggests these drugs may be of benefit in nociceptive pain.

Pain modulation as a result of conduction analgesia may help to identify the site of the pain and so be of benefit in indicating the possible pathophysiological mechanisms of that pain.

Capsacian cream may be a form of conduction analgesia in that the neurotubules and neurofilaments in the nerves (axons) are believed to be the transport mechanism. The theory behind the use of this cream is that the cream is absorbed, taken up by the nerves and transported in the neurotubules and neurofilaments to the cell body. The Caspian is believed to produce analgesia via the Caspian receptors on the neurone. There is RCT evidence that this cream relieves nociceptive pain (osteoarthritis) and good evidence that it also relieves neuropathic pain (post-herpetic neuralgia). If this proposed mechanism proves to be true then the pathophysiology of the pain modulation suggests more similarity then differences between the pain of osteoarthritis and the pain of post-herpetic neuralgia.

Pharmacological treatment

Nonsteroidal anti-inflammatory drugs

There is abundant evidence that the nonsteroidal anti-inflammatory drugs (NSAIDs) provide analgesia in patients with nociceptive pain. The mechanisms involved in this analgesia are mainly peripheral but it is well known that these drugs do have a central effect as well. The relative importance of this central effect in their analgesic action is unknown. It is said that these drugs are of no benefit in the treatment of neuropathic pain: the evidence for this is based on clinical observation. The author is unaware of any controlled studies that have confirmed this absence of effect in patients with neuropathic pain. Therefore, the pathophysiological mechanisms involved in neuropathic pain are believed not to involve any of

Table 1. Possible peripheral neuromodulators (NSAIDs)

Inhibition of cyclooxygenase-dependent prostanoid formation
Inhibition of intracellular phosphodiesterase
Inhibition of bradykinin levels
Uncoupling of G-protein–membrane protein interactions

the neuromodulators affected by the NSAIDs (Table 1). Conversely, there are many RCTs (randomised controlled trials) confirming the efficacy of NSAIDs in nociceptive pain. The pathophysiological mechanisms involved in the peripheral nociceptive pain are related to neuromodulators inhibited by the NSAIDs. However, the relative importance of each of the individual neuromodulators remains to be defined (Table 1).

COX-2s

This new development of analgesics designed to decrease the side effect profile of the NSAIDs may help elucidate the possible mechanisms of peripheral nociceptive pain. It is believed that these drugs will be of no benefit in the treatment of neuropathic pain, based on the evidence, or lack of evidence with the NSAIDs. One should have an open mind as to the possible benefits of these drugs in neuropathic pain.

Non-opioids

The non-opioid analgesics such as paracetamol have both peripheral and central effects, but their peripheral effects are thought to be the more important. Like the NSAIDs, there is good evidence that these drugs are effective in nociceptive pain and are said to be ineffective in neuropathic pain. The author is unaware of any controlled evidence to support this observation. The analgesic mechanism of action of paracetamol is not known but it is thought to be similar to that of the NSAIDs and so the pathophysiology of the pain relieved by these drugs is unknown.

The information gleamed from the modulation of pain by the NSAIDs and non-opioids underlines the differences in the pathophysiology of nociceptive and neuropathic pain.

Opioids

There is good evidence that the opioids provide effective analgesia in both nociceptive and neuropathic pain. It is said that these drugs are less effective in neuropathic pain than in nociceptive pain [6]. The mechanisms of action of these drugs are mainly central; if there is a peripheral effect of the opioids [7] it is confined to the an intra-articular mechanism [8, 9]. Table 2 shows that some of the possible central pathophysiological mechanisms underlying nociceptive and neuropathic are similar. Subsequent information will indicate that there are differences between the central modulation of neuropathic and nociceptive pain.

The pathophysiological modulation of both neuropathic and nociceptive pain by opioids is most likely via the opioid receptors. In humans the μ receptor is the most important as all the partial agonists and other combinations have failed to provide as good analgesia as the pure μ agonists. There are other receptor agonists in development but their efficacy in man remains to be confirmed.

Table 2. Possible central neuromodulators of opioid analgesia

- Opioid receptors
- Noradrenaline α 2
- Serotonin
- Adenosine
- GABA
- Acetylcholine
- Dopamine
- Neuropeptide Y
- NMDA
- non-NMDA
- Tachykinin
- NO

Antidepressants

A systematic review of antidepressants in neuropathic pain revealed an NNT (number needed to treat) for benefit of 3 with an NNT. for major adverse effect of 22 [10]. The majority of these studies involved the tricyclic antidepressants. Only one involved an SSRI (selective serotonin reuptake inhibitors) (paroxetine) which was not as effective as the tricyclics. There are some clinical observations on the benefit of the SSRIs in the treatment of neuropathic pain but these drugs are considered to be less effective than the tricylics. There are many RCTs confirming greater efficacy of the tricylic antidepressants compared to placebo in the modulation of chronic nociceptive pain.

It would appear from these data that the noradrenergic effect of the antidepressants may be important in the modulation of both neuropathic and nociceptive pain. The serontergic effect would appear to e less important based on the lack of effect of the SSRIs.

Anticonvulsants

A systematic review of the use of anticonvulsants in the management of neuropathic pain revealed that the NNT for benefit was 3 while the NNT for severe adverse side effects was 24 [11]. This study also revealed that sodium valproate was not effective in nociceptive pain (postoperative pain). A recent study in healthy volunteers has shown that lamotrigne and phenytoin may provide analgesia for nociceptive pain [12].

The pathophysiology of modulation of neuropathic pain by the anticonvulsant drugs is believed to a result of their membrane stabilisation via the Na^+ channels. However, some of the newer anticonvulsants have more specific effects on neuromodulators, i.e., gabapentin on GABA, and this may, in the future, help elucidate other possible mechanisms of neuropathic pain. The role of these drugs in the modulation of nociceptive pain remains to be defined.

Unconventional analgesics

Adrenergic blockade

Noradrenaline is considered to be important in the central and peripheral transmission of some neuropathic pain, particularly the complex regional pain syndromes (CRPS). There are more data supporting a peripheral mechanism, guanethidine [13, 14] than central mechanisms (phentolamine [15]). These observations are not supported by controlled data because the conditions are uncommon, the natural history is probably for the pain to resolve, and not all the patients with the same symptoms and signs respond to the same treatment. This lack of controlled data does not mean that a particular treatment does not work for the individual patient. What it means is that we do not know if the particular treatment is a real or a placebo effect. For the individual patient this is an academic question. For the medical profession to understand the neuromodulation, it is important to have controlled data.

It would appear that noradrenaline is an important neuro modulator in some neuropathic pain such as the CRPS but it is not the only neuromodulator involved in all CRPS [13, 15]. It may also be important in the neuromodulation of other neuropathic pain apart from CRPS. These data reinforce some of the differences between neuropathic and nociceptive pain because noradrenergic blockade does not appear to provide any benefit in nociceptive pain. These clinical observations await confirmation from RCT evidence.

α 2-Agonists

Noardrenergic blockade relieves pain associated with in some patients with CRPS, adrenergic α 2-agonists, such as clonidine, also relieve peripheral neuropathic pain [16]. It has also been shown to provide analgesia at the spinal cord level in neuropathic pain [17]. There are occasional case reports of the efficacy of oral clonidine in neuropathic pain but no controlled data. The only evidence that α 2-agonists have any benefit in nociceptive pain is based on the original use of clonidine for migraine. There are no controlled data to support this observation.

The effects of these two adrenergic neuromodulators highlight the difficulty in understanding the pathophysiological mechanisms involved in neuropathic pain. Noradrenergic blockade and noradrenergic agonist both relieve neuropathic pain. This indicates that noradrenaline is important in the pathophysiology of some neuropathic pains but not in all neuropathic pains. There is very poor evidence that noradrenaline has any role in the pathophysiology of nociceptive pain.

NMDA antagonists

The role of NMDA antagonists in the treatment of neuropathic pain has been proposed by a number of authors and there is RCT evidence that ketamine provides better pain relief than magnesium chloride [18]. The difficulties with ketamine are the side effects and the lack of an oral preparation [20]. Another RCT confirmed that intravenous amantadine provided better analgesia than placebo in neuropathic pain [19]. Oral amantadine has also been used successfully in clinical studies. There are numerous clinical observations that NMDA antagonists relieve neuropathic pain but the limitations are the lack of good oral antagonists.

The modulation of neuropathic pain by two different NMDA antagonists indicates that this excitatory amino acid is involved in neuropathic pain. There are no data available to indicate their role in nociceptive pain.

Other suggested neuromodulators

There are many and varied neuromodulators under development. Some of these are listed in Table 3, but most have not been used clinically.

The inhalational general anaesthetics modulate pain via a central mechanism which may be related to the GABA system but may involve any of the central neuromodulators shown in Table 2. Until there are more specific data available it is not possible to infer any pathophysiological mechanisms from these agents.

Table 3. Neuromodulators awaiting clinical trials

- Neurokinin
- Neurotrophins. nerve growth factor
- Tyrosine kinase receptors
- Cannabinoids
- Sodium channel blockade
- Calcium channel blockade· ziconotide
- Cholinergic channel modulation
- Galanin receptor
- 5HT3 receptor antagonist· alosetron
- Prostanoid receptors
- Adenosine receptors

Modulation of the emotional component of pain

Pharmacological treatment

The pharmacological modulation of the emotional component of pain is via the antidepressants, anticonvulsants and the opioids. Morphine has been used to treat every known psychiatric illness successfully because before the 1930s it was the only drug available for such illnesses. Whether the neuromodulation of the emotional component of pain is different to the neuromodulation of the physical component remains to be defined. Therefore it is impossible to differentiate between the pathophysiology of the physical and the emotional components based on the relative responses to these drugs.

Emotional control

It is possible for some patients to control their pain centrally. The pathophysiology of this mechanism is not known. The mechanism of this central control may be related to the mechanisms involved in general anaesthesia which are also unknown.

Conclusions

Pain, be it nociceptive or neuropathic always has two components (Fig. 1). The relative importance of each component needs to be clarified. This makes the interpretation of the pathophysiology of pain modulation from the individual patient's response to treatment more difficult than the interpretation of the pathophysiology of nociception. Pain very rarely has one dimension. The other dimensions shown in Figure 1 are also involved in the pain and the patient's responses to the pain and to the treatment. Thus the individual patient's response to any modulation will be compounded by these two components and by at least these four dimensions.

The pharmacological action of most drugs is not uni-factorial, that is most drugs have more than one effect on the patient. This further complicates the interpretation of the pathophysiology of the modulation of pain. The understanding of the pathophysiology of pain modulation is complicated by the type of pain, the patient and the drug used to successfully treat that pain.

References

1. Meyerson B (1997) Pharmacological tests in pain analysis and in prediction of treatment outcome. Pain 72:1-3
2. Canavero S, Bonicalzi V (1998) The neurochemistry of central pain: evidence from clinical studies, hypothesis and therapeutic implications. Pain 74:109-114
3. Merskey H, Bogduk N (1994) Classification of chronic pain. IASP Press, Seattle, pp 210-213
4. Burchiel KJ (1988) Carbamazepine inhibits spontaneous activity in experimental neuromas. Exp Neurol 102:249-253
5. Chapman V, Suzuki R, Chamarette HLC, Rygh LJ, Dickenson AH (1998) Effects of systemic carbamazepine and gabapentine on spinal neuronal responses in spinal nerve ligated rats. Pain 75:261-272
6. Jadad AR, Carroll D, Glynn CJ, Moore RA, McQuay HJ (1992) Morphine responsiveness

of chronic pain: a double-blind randomised cross-over study with patient controlled analgesia. Lancet I:1367-1371

7. Stein C, Yassouridis A (1997) Peripheral morphine analgesia. Pain 71:119-121
8. Kalso E, Tramer MR, Carroll D, McQuay HJ, Moore RA (1997) Pain relief from intra-articular morphine after knee surgery: a qualitative systematic review. Pain 71:127-134
9. Picard PR, Tramer MR, McQuay HJ, Moore RA (1997) Analgesic efficacy of peripheral opioids (all except intra-articular): a qualitative systematic review of randomised controlled trials Pain 72:309-318
10. McQuay HJ, Tramer MR, Nye BA, Carroll D, Wiffen PJ, Moore RA (1996) A systematic review of antidepressants in neuropathic pain. Pain 68:217-227
11. McQuay H, Carroll D, Jadad AR, Wiffen P, Moore A (1995) Anticonvulsant drugs for management of pain: a systematic review. BMJ 311:1047-1052
12 Webb J, Kamali F (1998) Analgesic effects of lamotrigine and phenytoin on cold-induced pain a crossover placebo-controlled study in healthy volunteers. Pain 76:357-363
13 Hannington-Kiff J (1974) Intravenous regional sympathetic block with guanethidine Lancet I:1019-1020
14 Toreborjk E, Wahren L, Wallin G, Koltzenburg M (1995) Noradrenaline-evoked pain in neuralgia. Pain 63:11-20
15. Campbell JN, Raja SN, Selig DK, Belzberg AJ, Meyer RA (1994) Diagnosis and management of sympathetically maintained pain In. Fields HL, Liebeskind JC (eds) Pharmacological approaches to the treatment of chronic pain. new concepts and critical issues. IASP Press, Seattle, pp 85-100
16. Davis KD, Treede RD, Raja SN, Meyer RA, Campbell JN (1991) Topical application of clonidine relieves hyperalgesia in patients with sympathetically maintained pain Pain 47 309-317
17. Glynn CJ, O'Sullivan K (1996) A double-blind randomised comparison of the effects of epidural clonidine, lignocaine and the combination of clonidine and lignocaine in patients with chronic pain Pain 64:337-343
18 Felsby S, Nielsen J, Arendt-Nielsen L, Jensen TS (1996) NMDA receptor blockade in chronic neuropathic pain: a comparison of ketamine with magnesium chloride Pain 64:283-291
19. Pud D, Eisenberg E, Spitzer A, Adler R, Fried G, Yarnitsky D (1998) The NMDA receptor antagonist amantadine reduces surgical neuropathic pain in cancer patients. a double-blind, randomised, placebo-controlled trial. Pain 75:349-354
20. Eide PK, Jorum E, Stubhaug A, Bremmes J, Brevik H (1994) Relief of post-herpetic neuralgia with N-methyl-D-aspartatic acid receptor antagonist ketamine: a double-blind, cross-over comparison with morhine and placebo. Pain 58:347-354

Chapter 5

Role of the central nervous system in processing pain stimuli and perspectives of pharmacological intervention

E. MASOERO, L. FAVALLI, S. GOVONI

Pain, perceivable through conscious integration of nociceptive stimuli, is classified into somatic pain, characterized by intense and localized sharp sensation, and visceral pain, characterized by diffuse, deep and slow-in-onset painful sensation. Based on the current knowledge, the proposal of the existence of a single central pain centre has to be rejected due to the complexity of the systems that modulate pain transmission. It is worth considering that each cerebral area perceives as pain signals received from alterations in the peripheral region on which it exerts its own control (objective sensation). Moreover, affective and emotional components play an important role in pain perception (subjective sensation).

Acute pain serves as a physiological warning to preserve the integrity of the organism. It is linked to known causes such as trauma and surgery, has limited duration and, normally, it improves to extinction when the triggering cause is removed.

On the other hand, signals for chronic pain have no apparent significance as a protective measure for the organism. Pain associated with extensive prolongued tissue damage tends to worsen with time, resulting in complex reactive changes of the nociceptive pathways. Frequently, the clinical situation is worsened by psychological components linked to fear and/or recollection of pain. Moreover, pain processes can be distinguished as being nociceptive or neuropathic. The first, caused by nociceptive receptor stimulation, is conducted through intact neuronal pathways, while the second is due to damage of neuronal structures and increased neuronal sensitivity.

Pain transmission pathways

Pain transmission pathways lead the nociceptive stimulus from the periphery to the brain through spinal cord and midbrain centres. Specific pain receptors (nociceptors) are located in different nervous fibres. C fibres, characterized by their small diameter, low conduction and lack of myelin, are activated by mechanical, chemical and thermal stimuli, whereas Aδ fibres have a high threshold, high conduction and are myelinated and activated by strong mechanical stimuli. These afferent fibres project to the spinal dorsal horn via a pathway through the dorsal roots of spinal nerves. Nociceptive primary fibres mostly terminate in the superficial laminae (laminae I, II, III and V) and then the deeper laminae are involved. Axonal extensions originate from neurones in the grey matter of the dorsal horn and project to different cerebral supraspinal structures (e.g., the spino-thalamic pathway whose axons project to the thalamus). The observation that the transection of the spino-thalamic pathway induces a strong but incomplete and short-lasting analgesia suggests the involvement of alternative pain pathways such as the spino-cervico-thalamic and the lemniscal pathway.

According to much evidence, the spinal cord cannot simply be considered as a passive bridge between the periphery and the brain. In fact, according to the gate control hypothesis, proposed by Melzack and Wall [1], spinal horn interneurones located in the substantia gelatinosa (lamina II) can modulate nociceptive transmission through inhibitory synapses on afferent primary fibres. As a consequence, the amount of nociceptive signal reaching the superior centres depends on the reciprocal activity of different inhibitory and excitatory fibres. The pain transmission system is further regulated through inhibitory and excitatory descending fibres originating from cortical and mesencephalic nuclei which project to the dorsal horn. Serotonergic and noradrenergic descending fibres have been demonstrated to project to neurones located in the laminae II of the spinal dorsal horn [2].

The periacqueductal grey (PAG) and several nuclei of the rostral ventral medulla (RVM), such as the nucleus raphe magnus (NRM) and the adjacent ventral reticular formation, are the most important areas from which descending fibres originate. The RVM receives afferent fibres from PAG and from the dorsolateral pontine tegumentum, another area implicated in nociceptive modulation [3]. Since intracerebral morphine injection either in the PAG or in the NRM induces naloxone-antagonized analgesia (as well as direct stimulation of both areas), a role for endogenous opioids has been postulated [4]. The excitatory actions of opioids on PAG neurones can stem from a local disinhibitory mechanism on a putative excitatory neurone [5]. Excitatory connections between PAG and NRM using transmitters such as glutamate, aspartate or neurotensin have been postulated [3, 6]. The NRM is the origin of the raphe-spinal pathway which, in turn, projects to the laminae I, II, V, VI of the dorsal horn. These descending axons are serotonergic and their activation induces antinociceptive effects on afferent fibres through a post-synaptic inhibition. Another important descending system originates in the dorsolateral pons and uses noradrenaline as a neurotransmitter. This system, if stimulated, also induces analgesia and inhibition of spinal nociceptive neurones.

The study of the regulatory mechanisms of nociceptive transmission is complicated by the involvement of a variety of neurotransmitters: besides serototonin and noradrenaline, γ-amino-butyric acid (GABA), excitatory aminoacids, enkephalins and neurotensin are involved both in descending and ascending pathways and their role is not yet fully understood. In the afferent fibres, putative candidate neurotransmitters are: somatostatin, cholecystokinin, calcitonin gene-related peptide and substance P, the latter being the most important [7, 8]. This peptide is detectable in approximately 20% of the spinal ganglionic neurones and is found in peripheral tissues, too. Since substance P is found in the superficial laminae of the spinal dorsal horn, in spinal intrinsic neurones and in terminals of descending fibres, a role as a nociceptive neurotransmitter can be postulated. In fact, capsaicin, the active constituent of red pepper, causes degeneration of small-diameter fibres and decreases their substance P content up to 50%, resulting in an increase of pain threshold and analgesia.

Enkephalins, endogenous peptides with opioid activity, are present in spinal interneurones and in propriospinal interneurones which project to the superficial laminae where the afferent substance P-containing fibres terminate. The distribution of enkephalins in the spinal dorsal horn parallels that of opioid receptors probably located on afferent substance P-containing fibres. This hypothesis is supported by the observation that the peripheral dissection of afferent fibres decreases the number of opiod receptors and the amount of substance P content. Moreover, local or systemic opiod administration inhibits substance P release from nervous terminals and induces naloxone-reversible analgesia [9]. Opiod receptors have both presynaptic and postsynaptic localizations. In fact, beyond the primary afferent nerves or dorsal rhizotomya, only 40% of receptor number is lost and spinal dorsal horn neurones can still be activated by opiods. Thus, the dorsal horn enkephalinergic system could be envisaged as the fine regulator of the afferent painful stimulus as hypothesized by the gate control theory. Increased met-enkephalin release by substance P has been demonstrated in rat spinal medulla in vivo [10]. During chronic pain the increase in met-enkephalin release potentiates the gate control activity to reduce the nociceptive information [11]. In the case of acute pain, where a strong pain avoidance reaction is required, gate control function is removed to reinforce the nociceptive afferent input.

As reported above, excitatory amino acids and GABA can play an important role in pain modulation. The excitatory amino acid glutamate is present either in the terminals of small-diameter primary fibres or in dorsal horn interneurones [12]. When glutamate is released, it activates n-methyl-D-aspartate (NMDA) receptors located in dorsal horn neurones which, in turn, induce the release of substance P [13]. This suggests that NMDA receptors are involved in the generation and maintenance of spinal hypersensitivity potentiating the transmission of nociceptive messages. This role is further supported by the fact that NMDA-antagonist administration can block or prevent enhanced pain states [14]. Recently it has been demonstrated that also alpha-amino-3-hydroxy-5-methyl-4-isoxazoleproprionate (AMPA) receptor activation may regulate nociceptive transmission in the spinal cord, particularly in the case of chronic pain [15].

Concerning the GABA-system, it is known that administration of the GABA-agonist muscimol in the PAG potentiates opioid-induced analgesia whereas the administration of the GABA-receptor antagonist bicucullin decreases the analgesic effect of enkephalin analogs. Moreover, administration of the opioid receptor antagonist naloxone blocks the action of muscimol [16]. Since the PAG contains a substantial number of GABA neurones, it can be postulated that the GABA system may modulate the activity in descending inhibitory pathways arising from this cerebral area. The relative balance between GABA and excitatory amino acid systems appears to be, in part, responsible for pain transmission.

Role of endogenous opioid peptides in pain transmission

Following the discovery in the mid-1970s of the existence of opiod receptors in every vertebrate and in some invertebrate species, many studies have been devoted to the search for endogenous ligands for these receptors [17].

To date, at least 18 active opiod peptides have been identified; the first identified pentapeptides met-enkephalin and leu-enkephalin were found in pig and ox brain [18]. The known peptides are now grouped in three different families: enkephalins, endorphins and dynorphins. Each family is derived from three large precursor proteins encoded by three different genes. The three precursors are pro-opiomelanocortin (POMC), proenkephalin and prodynorphin, from which lower-molecular-weight peptides are derived through enzymatic proteolytic cleavage at target sites.

POMC, detectable in the anterior and intermediate lobes of the pituitary gland and in the brain, is processed into melanocyte-stimulating hormone (γ-MSH), adrenocorticotropin (ACTH) and β-lipotropin (β-LPH) through proteolitic cleavage at the level of the basic amino acids arginine-lysine. β-LPH, in turn, gives origin to β-MSH and β-endorphin. Although β-endorphin contains the met-enkephalin sequence in its N-terminal end, this opiod peptide, as well as leu-enkephalin, is produced by a different precursor, proenkephalin, which was identified for the first time in the adrenal medulla.

Pro-dynorphin gives origin to different peptides containing the leu-enkephalin sequence, among them dynorphin A (1-17), dynorphin A (1-8), dynorphin B, α- and β-neoendorphin.

The anatomical distribution of opioid peptides varies for the different classes; in fact, peptides from POMC are present particularly in the arcuate nucleus, from which very long axons projections to amygdala, thalamus and PAG originate. Peptides derived from proenkephalin are found in areas related to the control of nociceptive transmission and in hippocampus, globus pallidus and median eminence, suggesting their involvement in controlling various physiological processes such as emotional, behavioural, motor, endocrine and immunological activities. Enkephalinergic pathways are mainly constituted by short axons and short neuronal circuits. Peptides from prodynorphin are co-localized with those originating from proenkephalin. Despite the fact that each family of peptides is usually present in different groups of neurones, occasionally some neurones can contain more than one family [19]. Opiod peptides have been found in peripheral tissues such as the gastroenteric tract (i.e., dynorphin 1-17 is found in duodenum), pancreatic islet cells and adrenal medulla. Detectable amounts of β-endorphins and met-enkephalins either in human or in animal plasma and liquor have been measured.

It is known that β-endorphin levels (such as ACTH) are circadian, with values higher in the first hours of the day when the pain sensitivity threshold is higher. In contrast, plasma levels of met-enkephalin are constant all day long, suggesting that the two peptides are regulated in an independent manner.

Opioid receptors

Using pharmacological criteria, opiod receptors have been divided in three major classes designated μ, κ and δ, which, in turn, are divided into subtypes.

These receptor proteins represent different molecules with distinct roles and are variously distributed in cerebral areas and peripheral tissues.

Using human cDNA, it has been possible to isolate genomic clones encoding μ, κ and δ opioid receptor genes. Each receptor class is encoded by a separate gene while within a given class subtypes originate from alternative splicing.

The class of μ receptors, subdivided into μ_1 and μ_2, have high affinity for morphine and endogenous peptides such as β-endorphin, enkephalins and dynorphin A. Some authors have also suggested that morphine may be naturally present in cerebral areas; accordingly, this alkaloid has been proposed as the natural ligand for this receptor. This hypothesis is, however, controversial. With in situ hybridization studies, mRNA (messenger RNA) for (receptor has been found in the cerebral areas and in the spinal cord involved in modulation of pain transmission, such as the PAG and *substantia gelatinosa*, and in nuclei involved in respiratory control and emesis. The human μ opioid receptor mRNA is highly expressed in the hypothalamus, thalamus and subthalamic nucleus, moderately expressed in the amygdala and caudate nucleus, while expression is low in hyppocampus, substantia nigra and corpus callosum (Table 1).

Activation of μ_1 and μ_2 receptor subtypes, characterized by means of selective antagonists, is responsible for supraspinal and spinal analgesia, respectively. It seems that morphine systemically administered in animal models, induces analgesia acting preferentially on μ_1 receptors whereas activation of μ_2 receptors is supposed to mainly mediate respiratory depression and decrease of gastric motility.

The class of κ receptors is divided into κ_1, κ_2 and κ_3 subtypes. The pharmacological properties have only been defined for κ_1 and κ_3 receptors. It is known that dynorphin A is a very potent endogenous ligand at κ_1 receptors that seem to be particularly involved in spinal analgesia, whereas κ_3 receptors are involved in supraspinal analgesia. Dysphoria and psychotomimetic effects are also due to activation of κ_1 receptors.

The last class of opioid receptors, largely present in the dorsal horn, is composed of δ receptors (δ_1 and δ_2) whose activation induces supraspinal and spinal analgesia, particularly in the case of pain due to thermal stimuli; their specific endogenous ligands are the enkephalins and deltorphine, a natural, highly selective peptide extracted from frog skin [17]. The human δ opioid receptor mRNA is found in cortical areas, in basal ganglia and hypothalamus, whereas in internal globus pallidus, thalamus and pituitary gland is not present. More information on opioid receptor classification and their ligands is reported in Table 1.

The role played by each receptor subtype in the nociceptive process is not fully understood and many studies have addressed this problem.

Knock-out mutant mice lacking μ receptor but endowed with regular popu-

Table 1. Opioid receptors. μ_1 receptors exhibit high affinity for several δ receptor agonists, except for DPDPE The μ, κ and δ receptors correspond to the μ_1, κ_1 and δ_2 subtypes [27–39]

Nomenclature	μ	κ	δ
Potency order	β-end> dynA> met=leu	β-end=leu=met> dynA	dynA>> β-end> leu> met
Selective agonists	DAMGO	Bremazocine Ethylketazocine	DSLET BUBU DPDPE (δ_1) Deltorphine II (δ_2)
Selective antagonists	β-FNA CTAP Naloxazine (μ_1)	norBNI	Naltrindole BNTX (δ_1) Naltrinbene (δ_2)
Effector	Gi/o	Gi/o	Gi/o
Gene/chromosomal localization	OPRM/ 6q24-25	OPRK/8q11 2	OPRD/1p34 3-36.1

DAMGO, Tyr-D-Ala-Gly-[NmePhe]-Gly-ol; *DPDPE*, [D-pen^2,D-pen^5]enkephalin; *BNTX*, 7-benzylidenenaltrexone; *BUBU*, Tyr-D-Ser(O-tert-butyl)-Gly-Phe-Leu-Thr(O-tert-butyl); *DSLET*, [D-Ser^2,Leu^5]enkephalin; *NorBNI*, norbinaltorphimine, *β-FNA*, β-funaltrexamine; *CTAP*, D-Phe-Cys-Tyr-D-Trp-Arg-Thr-Pen-T

lations of both κ and δ receptors were obtained by genetic engineering suppressing the specific μ receptor-expressing gene. In these mutant animals morphine failed to induce analgesia and physical dependence, suggesting that the μ receptor is the specific target of morphine in vivo. Moreover, κ and δ receptors seem not to be involved in mediating the major biological action of morphine when μ receptors are lacking [20]. It should be noted that antinociception and physical dependence are strongly correlated, making it impossible to separate the positive from the unwanted effect.

The role of κ receptor in opiod analgesia is not clear. Cooperativity between opioid receptors at molecular (allosteric interaction or second messenger production) or functional (separate neurones) level has been demonstrated. Recently, in vivo and in vitro studies have demonstrated that activation of κ receptors in the brainstem nucleus significantly reduces morphine-induced analgesia through hyperpolarization of neurones indirectly activated by μ receptors. This suggests a functional, opposing interaction between μ and κ receptors [21].

The first to be cloned were the δ receptors, obtained by expression cloning using cDNA libraries derived from NG-108 neuroblastoma-glioma cells, frequently used as a source of pure δ receptors [22].

To date, all the opiod receptors have been cloned using human cDNA, and the knowledge of their primary structures points out that they have very little similarity with all the other G protein-coupled receptors, except for somatostatin receptors which are approximately 65% identical [23].

All the opioid receptors are coupled to G proteins and their activation induces adenylate cyclase activity inhibition [24] (Fig. 1). It seems that all are also coupled to increase in K^+ conductance which, in turn, results in a decrease in calcium influx and that κ receptors inhibit directly the entry of calcium through voltage-dependent calcium channels. The consequent membrane hyperpolarization and the reduced calcium availability are both responsible for reduced presynaptic neurotransmitter release and blockade of pain transmission [17]. These mechanisms undergo adaptive changes during chronic treatment which underlie the process of tolerance and dependence development (Fig. 1).

Pharmacological treatment of pain

An adequate pain treatment implies individualization of pharmacological therapy, which requires different and appropriate strategies.

Acute pain is treated with non-steroid anti-inflammatory drugs (NSAIDs), regional anaesthesia and systemic administration of opioid drugs. The latter represents the first-choice analgesic treatment for severe chronic pain.

Opioid drugs have various classifications: weak and strong opioids (i.e. codeine and morphine, respectively); pure agonists (morphine), partial agonists (buprenorphine), agonist-antagonists (nalbuphine), antagonists (naloxone); and synthetic, semi-synthetic and natural derivatives (on the basis of their chemical structure). The characteristic of some common opioid analgesics available for pain treatment are summarized in Table 2. The most commonly used drugs in the treatment of pain are morphine and its analogs. The beneficial effects of these compounds are due to the stimulation of opioid receptors at the spinal and supraspinal levels. In fact, the simultaneous administration of opioids into spinal and supraspinal structures induces analgesia by means of synergistic effects: this allows lowering of the doses in order to obtain the same effect as achievable with independent administrations. It is known that opioid drugs are effective only in the presence of an active serotonergic tone. In fact, studies in animals and in humans demonstrated that a diet poor in tryptophan, the amino acid precursor of serotonin, induces a depletion of serotonin stores determining, eventually, opioid inefficacy. On the other hand, 5-hydroxytryptophan administration increases serotonin levels and opioid action. A likely explanation of these findings is that opiod drugs can stimulate the descending serotonergic inhibitory pathways.

Morphine and related compounds acting as full agonists, such as hydromorphone, levorphanol, oxicodone, petidine and fentanyl not only have an antinociceptive action but can relieve pain by improving the capacity to tolerate painful perceptions.

Agonist/antagonists (pentazocine, butorphanol) or partial agonists (buprenorphine) are endowed with moderately strong analgesic activity.

The main problem concerning opiod drugs is the presence of severe side effects which limit their use. Morphine at therapeutic doses induces respiratory

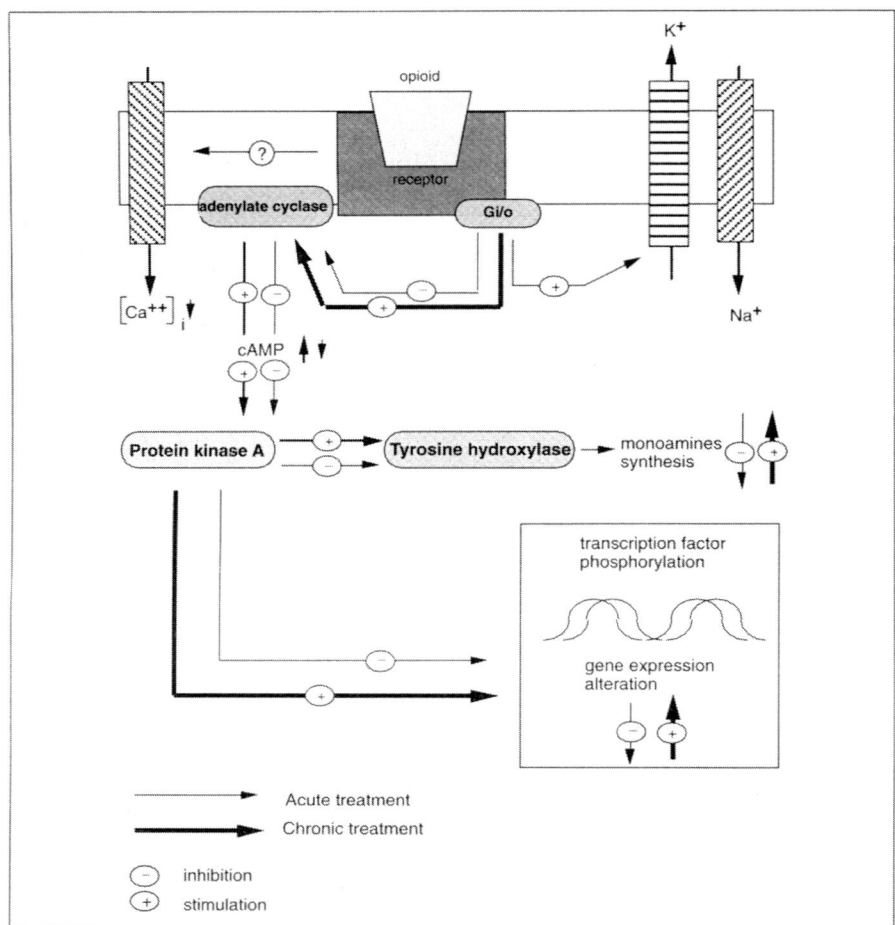

Fig. 1. Opioid mechanisms. Opioid receptors mediate their effects through pertussis toxin-sensitive G proteins. Opioid receptors agonists induce a reduction in the cyclic AMP synthesis and an increase in K$^+$ conductance. Following membrane hyperpolarization, Ca^{++} influx and Ca^{++} intracellular levels decrease. The activation of κ opioid receptors seems instead to directly inhibit calcium current trhough N-type calcium channels.

Acutely, the reduced phosphorylation of tyrosine hydroxylase and of transcription factors leads to a decrease in monoamine synthesis. During chronic treatment these transduction systems become hyperactive to contrast opioid action and contribute to opiate tolerance, dependence and withdrawal. The biochemical and cellular events responsible for the development of opioid tolerance and dependence remain unclear. Opioid tolerance seems to be associated with uncoupling of the opioid receptors from G proteins, resulting in a loss of the ability of these proteins to exchange GDP for GTP [25]. Moreover, following long-term administration, either down- or up- regulation of opioid receptors can occur, depending on the receptor type or subtype and on the CNS region examined. Since these changes appear after tolerance is established, it seems that they are not responsible for it. Further investigations using highly selective opioid agonists and antagonists are needed to understand the consequences of the chronic treatment at the level of a given receptor subtype. Also NMDA receptors and the NO system may play an important role in opioid tolerance [26]

Table 2. Comparison of the opioid agonists, agonist/antagonist and antagonists used in clinic therapy

Drug	Dose[a] (mg)	Therapeutics uses	Adverse effects
Agonists			
Morphine	10 (IM), 30-60 (O)	All these drugs are used for acute, post surgical and chronic pain treatment. They are not well recommended in parturients or in headhache and migraine therapy. Methadone is used in treatment of opioid abstinence syndrome and treatment of heroin users	Respiratory depression, constipation, nausea, vomiting, tolerance and physical dependence. Meperidine associated with MAO-inhibitors induces important side effects. Respiratory depression in newborns is lower than that induced by morphine. Constipation and urinary retention are less frequent
Hydromorphone	1.5 (IM), 7 5 (O)		
Oxymorphone	1 (IM)		
Levorphanol	2 (IM), 4 (O)		
Codeine[b]	130 (IM)		
Oxycodone	30 (O)		
Meperidine	100 (IM), 300 (O)		
Fentanyl	0.1 (IM)		
Sulfentanyl	0.02 (IM)		
Alfentanyl	0.4-0.8 (IM)		
Methadone	10 (IM), 10-20 (O)		
Propoxiphene	130-250 (O)		
Tramadol	100-400 (O, IM, EN,R)	Moderate, muscular/skeletal, postsurgical neurogenic and cancer pain, traumas and fractures	Dizziness, nausea, low incidence of cardiac and respiratory depression, low potential drug abuse
Agonist/Antagonists			
Pentazocine[c]	30-60 (IM, O, SC)	Obstetric postsurgical plain	Nausea, vomiting, sedation; respiratory depression
Butorphanol[c]	1-3 (IM)	Postsurgical pain	
Nalbuphine[c]	12 (IM)	Postsurgical and acute myocardialinfarction pain	
Dezocine	10 (IM)	Postsurgical pain	
Buprenorphine[c]	C.2-0 3 (IM)	Postsurgical and cancer pain	
Meptazinol	100 (IM)	Obstetric postsurgical and acute myocardial infarction pain	
Antagonists			
Naloxone	0.4-1.2 (EV)	Opioid overdose	
Levallorphan	1-2 (EV)		
Naltrexone	50 (O)		

[a] Dose is the amount that produces approximately the same analgesic effect as 10 mg of morphine administered intramuscularly or subcutaneously
[b] Antitussive dose is 10-20 mg (orally)
[c] Induces an abstinence syndrome in morphine-addicted subjects

depression in all respiratory activity phases by a direct action on the cerebral midbrain centre; moreover, nausea and vomiting (by direct stimulation of chemoreceptor trigger zone), constipation, sedation, neuroendocrine effects, euphoria and mood alterations are present. Although long-term treatment also induces physical dependence and tolerance in healthy subjects, it is nevertheless highly recommended in chronic pain such as cancer-related pain.

In chronic cancer pain, opioid drugs are often associated with other compounds acting with different mechanisms to potentiate analgesic activity or to reduce adverse effects by lowering opioid dose.

Adjuvant therapeutic approaches are NSAIDs, antidepressants, anti-epileptics and benzodiazepines [40]. Not only are NSAIDs a support in chronic pain treatment but also constitute the most common treatment in acute pain such as headache, neuralgia and rheumatic pathologies. Compounds such as aspirin and related drugs inhibit cyclo-oxygenase enzyme (COX), the enzyme-converting arachidonic acid, into intermediates among which the inflammatory mediators, prostaglandins, prostacyclin and leukotrienes are derived. The analgesic actions of NSAIDs are evident not only in peripheral tissues but also in the nervous system, where prostanoid release, following depolarization of C fibres in the spinal dorsal horn, is well documented. Furthermore, NSAIDs seem to reduce hyperalgesia induced by NMDA and substance P receptor activation, indicating that the analgesic effects can be dissociated from the anti-inflammatory actions [41]. However, it is necessary to consider that these drugs are also responsible for several side effects such as gastropathy, bleeding, renal failure and hepatic dysfunction.

Another class of drugs used in association with opioids includes antidepressants, particularly helpful for treating chronic pain with a neuropathic component. Antidepressants which act both on the noradrenergic and serotonergic systems (imipramine, clomipramine) have an intrinsic analgesic action and are preferable to the selective noradrenergic (desimipramine) or serotonergic (fluoxetine) antidepressants. The pain-relieving activity of these drugs is due both to an intrinsic analgesic effect, involving serotonergic, noradrenergic and endogenous opioid systems through unknown mechanisms, and to potentiation of the opioid effect by enhancement of serotonergic tone. It may be hypothesized that analgesia is not linked with the antidepressant activity since the former appears immediately and does not require 2-3 weeks from the beginning of treatment, and the effective doses are lower than those required to induce antidepressant effects.

A whole series of other drugs that may be used alone or in combination to control pain such as corticosteroids, anticonvulsivants, GABA-mimetics and others are briefly reported in Table 3.

New perspectives

The high incidence of side effects associated with the most commonly used drugs in the pharmacological therapy of pain has prompted the search for new molecules with fewer unwanted effects.

Table 3. Drugs used as adjuvants in pain therapy [40, 42–45]

Drug	Clinical use	Proposed analgesic mechanism
Corticosteroids	Acute nerve compression, visceral distension, rheumatic diseases, complex regional pain syndromes	Contribution to tumoral mass reduction through their anti-inflammatory and antiedema effects
Anticonvulsants (carbamazepine, valproate, phenytoin)	Neuropathic lancinating, tic-like pains (alone or in association with antidepressants), trigeminal nerve neuralgia	Interference with GABA transmission and ion channels
GABA-agonists (baclophen, benzodiazepines)	Neuropathic pain, trigeminal nerve neuralgia	Myorelaxants Interferences with GABA transmission
Capsaicin and its analogs (civamidine)	Neuropathic pain such as postherpetic neuralgia, diabetic neuropathy and osteroarthritis	They act through desensitization of sensory neurones by repeated administration
α_2 Adrenoreceptor-agonists (clonidine, dexmedetomidine)	Neuropathic pain	They activate α_2 adrenoreceptors located postsynaptically to noradrenergic terminals originating from brainstem and midbrain, inducing an inhibition of nociception and potentiating opioid-induced analgesia

Particularly in the case of opioid drugs several options are being explored. The knowledge of receptor sequence, following molecular cloning, and the quantitative analysis of structure action properties have led to the development of antisense or complementary sequences to receptors which can be used to regulate events mediated by receptor activation. To date, selective κ and δ agonists, which should have fewer effects on respiratory control and should induce less physical dependence (linked to μ-receptor activation), are being developed.

Another target of drug discovery concerns NMDA antagonists. It is worth remembering that a sustained activation of NMDA receptors induces central sensitization responsible for allodynia and hyperalgesia and reduces the magnitude and duration of opioid-induced analgesia. It has been shown that NMDA competitive/non-competitive antagonist administration in animals potentiates and prolongs opioid-induced antinociception. Moreover, coadministration of opioids with NMDA antagonists blocks or diminishes the development of long-term tolerance. Furthermore, NMDA antagonists re-established antinociceptive opioid effect in tolerant animals. Nevertheless, NMDA antagonists cannot be used in clinics since, acting at various sites of the receptor complex, they induce several side effects. Consequently, non-competitive antagonists are used, such as ketamine (general anaesthetic), dextromethorphan (antitussive) and memantine (anti-Parkinsonian), drugs which also induce adverse effects such as psychomimetic symptoms (ketamine) or are not effective in neuropathic pain (dextromethorphan). Additional clinical trials are needed to corroborate the results of the few clinical studies available up to now on the interactions between NMDA antagonists and opioid drugs [46].

A new drug, recently marketed in the USA for treatment of moderate pain, is tramadol, a synthetic analog of codeine. The analgesic effect of tramadol is only partially blocked by the opiod antagonist naloxone, suggesting an important non-opioid mechanism. In fact, this centrally acting drug acts through two different mechanisms: it binds weakly to μ-receptor (its affinity for μ-receptor being 6 000-fold lower than that of morphine) and inhibits serotonin and noradrenaline reuptake without interfering directly with monoamine metabolism. Tramadol is administered as a racemic mixture in which the two enantiomers seem to have complementary and synergic actions. In fact, the (−) enantiomer seems to have noradrenaline uptake-inhibiting ability, whereas the (+) enantiomer has modest opioid and serotonin uptake-inhibiting properties. Its major metabolite O-Desmethyl-tramadol (M1) may potentiate the antinociceptive action binding to μ-receptors with an about 200-fold higher affinity than the parent compound. In the treatment of postoperative pain its efficacy is comparable to that of meperidine and morphine and it is more effective than NSAIDs (comparative studies). Moreover, it is recommended in severe acute pain, in many types of severe and refractory cancer pain even if its efficacy is lower than that of morphine and in occlusive arterial pathology and postherpetic neurophaty. Low incidence of cardiac and respiratory depression and low potential drug dependence render tramadol an effective and alternative drug to other analgesics in different pain syndromes. Its co-administration with NSAIDs permits a reduction in close with potentiation of antinociceptive action and lower incidence of side effects such as dizziness, nausea, dry mouth and sedation [47-51].

Another line of research is concerned with the development of selective inhibitors of COX-2. In fact, NSAIDs inhibit the two isoforms of this enzyme, which is the common primary step in prostanoid synthesis. COX-1 isoform is a constitutive enzyme present in many tissues. It has an important role in production of prostanoids involved in intercellular communication and in local cellular modulation, whereas the COX-2 isoform, found in brain, kidney and testicles, is inducible by many stimuli such as proinflammatory agents (i.e., cytokinins and interleukins). In the central nervous system, COX-2 is localized in sensory and limbic neurones in particular and is induced in the dorsal horn following peripheral painful stimuli. New selective compounds for the COX-2 isoform could induce pain relief without the typical side effects of non-selective NSAID drugs (e.g., gastropathy), and it may be further hypothesized that blood-brain barrier-crossing compounds may be effective in chronic pain treatment.

Other targets of research are non-peptide antagonists of bradykinin receptors, substance P antagonists, calcium channel blockers, and inhibitors of enkephalin metabolism [52].

The use of new routes and new delivery systems of administration such as slow-release preparations, chronic infusions with indwelling catheters and transdermal system patches may also provide advancements in pain management.

Transdermal administration offers the advantages of simplicity and a non-invasive form of analgesic therapy which increase patient compliance. The use of transdermal opioids has been suggested for chronic pain therapy and for the treatment of postoperative pain. The transdermal morphine in patients with cancer relieves pain. In particular, transdermal fentanyl relieves pain in a way which is identical to sustained morphine release, decreasing constipation and the use of laxatives significantly [53].

Oral transmucosal delivery (OTM) may also be used for releasing peptides with analgesic properties and, furthermore, progress is being made in the development of an implantable opioid delivery device capable of releasing hydromorphone subcutaneously for the treatment of cancer pain [54].

Although the ideal analgesic drug to satisfactorily control different pain situations and without adverse effects is still lacking, significant advancement, as outlined above, has been made. The use of new and improved administration routes for old drugs (e.g., transdermal opioid administration) and the design of new compounds such as tramadol, acting synergistically by different action mechanisms (opioid and non-opioid) with fewer side effects, do represent attained goals. The drug treatment of pain in appropriate conditions following the current protocols should make it possible to safely treat most of patients even when long-term treatment is needed. Old taboos and fears about chronic pain treatment should be abated and a better quality of life guaranteed to all who suffer.

References

1. Melzack R, Wall PD (1965) Pain mechanism: a new theory. Science 150:971-979
2. Dubuisson D, Wall PD (1980) Descending influence of receptive fields and activity of single units in laminae I, II, III of cat spinal cord. Brain Res 199:283-298
3. Fields HL, Heinricher MM, Mason P (1991) Neurotransmitters in nociceptive modulatory circuits. Ann Rev Neurosci 14:219-245
4. Basbaum AI, Fields H (1984) Endogenous pain control systems: brainstem spinal pathways and endorphin circuitry. Ann Rev Neurosci 7:309-338
5. Gebhart GF (1982) Opiate and opiod effects on brain stem neurons: relevance to nociception and antinociception mechanism. Pain 12:93-140
6   Fields HL, Anderson SD (1978) Evidence that raphe-spinal neurons mediate opiate and midbrain stimulation produced analgesia. Pain 5:333-349
7. Jessel TM, Iversen LL (1977) Opiate analgesics inhibit substance P release from rat trigeminal nucleus Nature 268:549-551
8   Pernow B (1984) Substance P. Pharmacol Rev 35:86-114
9. Hosobuchi Y, Emson PC, Iversen LL (1982) Elevated cerebrospinal fluid substance P in arachnoiditis is reduced by systemic administration of morphine Biochem Psychopharmacol 33:497-500
10. Tang J, Chou J, Yang HYT, Costa E (1983) Substance P stimulates the release of met5-enkephalin-Arg6-Phe7 and met5-enkephalin from rat spinal cord. Neuropharmacology 22:1147-1150
11 Faccini E, Uzumaki H, Govoni S, Missale C, Spano PF, Covelli V, Trabucchi M (1984) Af-

ferent fibers medıate the ıncrease of met-enkephalın elıcıted ın rat spınal cord by local-ızed paın. Paın 18:25-31

12. Yamamoto T (1996) N-methyl-D-aspartate (NMDA) receptor and paın. Masuı 45:1312-1318

13. Lıu H, Mantyh PW, Basbaum AI (1997) NMDA-receptor regulatıon of substance P re-lease from prımary afferent nocıceptors. Nature 386.721-724

14. Dıckenson AH (1997) NMDA receptor antagonısts. ınteractıon wıth opıods. Acta Anaesthesıol Scan 41:112-115

15. Harrıs JA, Corsı M, Quartarolı M, Arban R, Bentıvoglıo M (1996) Upregulatıon of spınal glutamate receptors ın chronıc paın. Neuroscıence 74:7-12

16. Zakusov VV, Ostrovskaya RU, Bulayev VM (1983) GABA-opıates ınteractıons ın the ac-tıvıty of analgesıcs. Arch Int Pharmacodyn Ther 265:61-75

17. Sımon EJ (1991) Opıod receptors and endogenous opıod peptıdes. Med Res Rev 11:257-274

18. Hughes J (1975) Isolatıon of an endogenous compound from the braın wıth pharmaco-logıcal propertıes sımılar to morphıne. Braın Res 88:295

19. Weıhe E, Mıllan MJ, Leıbold A, Nohr D, Herz A (1988) Co-localızatıon of pro-enkephalın- and prodynorphın-derıved opıoid peptıdes ın lamınae IV/V spınal neu-rons revealed ın arthrıtıcs rats. Neuroscı Lett 29:187-192

20. Matthes HWD, Maldonado R, Sımonın F, Valverde O, Slowe S, Kıtchen I, Befort K, Dıerıch A, Le Meurs M, Dolle P, Tzavara E, Hanoune J, Roques BP, Kıeffer BL (1996) Loss of morphıne-ınduced analgesıa, reward effect and wıthdrawal symptoms ın mıce lackıng the mu-opıoid-receptor gene. Nature 383:819-823

21. Panz ZZ, Tershner SA, Fıelds HL (1997) Cellular mechanısm for antı-analgesıc actıon of agonısts of the kappa-opıod receptor. Nature 389:382-385

22. Evans C, Keıth D, Morrıson H, Magendzo K, Edwards R (1992) Clonıng of delta opıod receptor by functıonal expressıon. Scıence 258:1952-1955

23. Reısıne T, Brownsteın MJ (1994) Opıod and cannabınoid receptors. Curr opın ın Neu-robıol 4:406-412

24. Herz A (1993) Opıoıds I. Handbook of experımental pharmacology. Sprınger-Verlag, Berlın Heıdelberg New York, p 104

25. Collın E, Cesselın F (1991) Neurobıologıcal mechanısms of opıoid tolerance and de-pendence. Clın Neuropharmacol 14.465-488

26. Lıaw WJ, Ho ST, Wang JJ, Wong CS, Lee HK (1996) Cellular mechanısm of opıoid toler-ance. Acta Anaesthesıol Sın 34:221-234

27 Aceto MD, Dewey WL, Portoghese PS, Takemorı AE (1986) Effects of β-funaltrexamıne on morphıne dependence ın rats and monkeys. Eur J Pharmacol 123:387-393

28. Alexander SPH, Peters JA (1998) Receptor and ıon channel nomenclature. Trends Phar-macol Scı (Suppl 9):58-59

29. Baamonde A, Dauge V, Gacel G, Roques BP (1991) Systemıc admınıstratıon of Tyr-D-Ser(O-tert-butyl)-Gly-Phe-Leu-Thr(O-tert-butyl), a hıghly selectıve delta opıoid ago-nıst, ınduces mu receptor-medıated analgesıa ın mıce. J Pharmacol Exp Ther 257:767-773

30. Eısenberg RM (1993) DAMGO stımulates the hypothalamo-pıtuıtary-adrenal axıs through a mu_2 opıod receptor. J Pharmacol Exp Ther 266:985-991

31. Ho J, Mannes AJ, Dubner R, Caudle RM (1997) Putatıve $kappa_2$ opıoid agonısts are an-tıhyperalgesıc ın a rat model of ınflammatıon. J Pharmacol Exp Ther 281.136-141

32. Maldonado R, Negus S, Koob GF (1992) Precıpıtatıon of morphıne wıthdrawal syn-drome ın rats by admınıstratıon of mu-, delta- and kappa-selectıve opıoid antagonısts. Neuropharmacology 31.1231-1241

33. Menkens K, Bilsky EJ, Wild KD, Portoghese PS, Reid LD, Porreca F (1992) Cocaine place preference is blocked by the delta-opioid receptor antagonist, naltrindole. Eur J Pharmacol 219:345-346

34. Noble F, Cox BM (1996) Differences among mouse strains in the regulation by mu, delta$_1$ and delta$_2$ opioid receptors of striatal adenylyl cyclases activated by dopamine D$_1$ or adenosine A$_{2A}$ receptors. Brain Res 716:107-117

35. Raynor K, Kong H, Mestek A, Bye LS, Tian M, Liu J, Yu L, Reisine T (1995) Characterization of the cloned human μ opioid receptor. J Pharmacol Exp Ther 272:423-428

36. Simonin F, Befort K, Gaveriaux-Ruff C, Matthes H, Nappey V, Lannes B, Micheletti G, Kieffer B (1994) The human delta opiod receptor: genomic organization, cDNA cloning, functional expression, and distribution in human brain. Mol Pharmacol 46:1015-1021

37. Sofuoglu M, Portoghese PS, Takemori AE (1992) Maintenance of acute morphine tolerance in mice by selective blockage of kappa opioid receptors with norbinaltorphimine. Eur J Pharmacol 210:159-162

38. Takemory AE, Portoghese PS (1993) Enkephalin antinociception in mice is mediated by delta 1- and delta 2-opioid receptors in the brain and in spinal cord, respectively. Eur J Pharmacol 242:145-150

39. Ward SJ, Portoghese PS, Takemori AE (1982) Improved assays for the assessment of kappa- and delta-properties of opioid ligands. Eur J Pharmacol 85:163-170

40. Levy MH (1996) Pharmacologic treatment of cancer pain. New Engl J Med 335:1124-1132

41. Malmberg AB, Yaksh TL (1992) Hyperalgesia mediated by spinal glutamate or Substance P receptor blocked by spinal cyclooxygenase inhibition. Science 257:1276-1279

42. Brasseur L (1997) Revue des thérapeutiques pharmacologiques actuelles de la doleur. Drugs 53 (Suppl 2):10-17

43. Dray A, Urban L, Dickenson A (1994) Pharmacology of chronic pain. Trends Pharmacol Sci 15:190-197

44. Fusco BM, Giacovazzo M (1997) Peppers and pain, the promise of capsaicin. Drugs 53:909-914

45. Hua HY, Chen P, Hwang J, Yaksh TL (1997) Antinociception induced by civamidine, an orally active capsaicin analogue. Pain 71:313-322

46. Wiesenfeld-Hallin Z (1998) Combined opioid-NMDA antagonist therapies. Drugs 55:1-4

47 Lehmann KA (1997) Tramadol in acute pain. Drugs 53 (Suppl 2):25-33

48. Lewis KS, Han NH (1997) Tramadol: a new centrally acting analgesic. Am J Health Sys Pharm 54:643-652

49. Raffa RB, Nayak RK, Liao S, Minn FL (1995) The mechanism(s) of action and pharmacokinetics of tramadol hydrochloride. Rev Contemp Pharmacother 6:485-497

50 Raffa RB, Friderichs E (1996) The basic science aspect of tramadol hydrochloride. Pain Rev 3:249-271

51. Raffa RB (1996) A novel approach to the pharmacology of analgesics. Am J Med 101:40S-46S

52. Dray A, Urban L (1996) New pharmacological strategies for pain relief. Ann Rev Pharmacol Toxicol 36.253-280

53. Donner B, Zenz M, Tryba M, Strumpf M (1996) Direct conversion from oral morphine to transdermal fentanyl: a multicenter study in patients with cancer pain Pain 64:527-534

54 Lesser GJ, Grossman SA, Leong KW, Lo H, Eller S (1996) In vitro and in vivo studies of subcutaneous hydromorphone implants designed for treatment of cancer pain. Pain 65.265-272

Chapter 6

Pain and the genome

M.E. Ferrero, A. Fulgenzi, M. Tiengo

There is increasing evidence that genotype affects pain sensitivity and pain modulation. As an example in humans, 10% of a Caucasian population studied only poorly metabolized the liver isozyme P450IID6 (required for the O-demethylation of the widely used opiate drug codeine to morphine) [1]. So, for such people codeine is an inefficient analgesic. The enzymatic defect is related to a mutation in the CYP2D6 gene [2]. As an experimental example, a recent study in rats demonstrated that a form of stress-induced analgesia was naloxone-insensitive, but attenuated by dizocilpine in male C57BL/6J mice. The same type of analgesia in male DBA/2J mice was significantly attenuated by naloxone but was insensitive to dizocilpine antagonism, indicating the role exerted by the different rat strain (i.e., genetic factors) in determining the selective recruitment of alternative central mechanisms of pain inhibition [3].

Many useful genetic models to study pain-related phenomena have been identified in laboratory animals [4]. The use of transgenic technology to "knock out" a pain-relevant gene was employed to generate targeted mutant mice in which the tyrosine codon at position 179 of the propiomelanocortin gene was converted to a premature translational stop codon [5]. The resultant transgenic mice produced normal corticotropin and melanocyte-stimulating hormone, but presented deficient β endorphin generation. They exhibited unchanged morphine analgesic sensitivity, but lacked the opioid analgesia induced by mild swim stress; the same mice displayed significantly greater nonopioid analgesia than controls and also displayed paradoxical naloxone-induced analgesia. The data indicate that the mutant animals have upregulation of alternative pain inhibitory mechanisms; such upregulation is a compensatory response to the absence of β endorphin. By using different inbred mouse strains, it is evident that different types of nociception are mediated by various physiological mechanisms. In fact, D2 mice have a lower sensitivity than B6 mice as shown by hot-plate and tail-flick tests of nociception. However, the strains show no differences in sensitivity to intraperitoneal injection of acetic acid [6].

Sensory neurons

The activation of peripheral neurons in response to tissue damage plays an important role in pain regulation. Such neurons (nociceptors) are activated by many mediators such as ATP, bradykinin, serotonin, prostaglandins, inter-leukins, and nerve growth factor (NGF). Sensory neurons secrete some neu-ropeptides, including substance P and the calcitonin-gene-regulated peptide, which have the following functions: transmission of pain signals, stimulation of secretion by diverse types of cells such as endocrine and immune cells. The reg-ulation of peripheral neurogenesis requires the presence of genes which are proneural, neuronal, or neuron-specific (the latter for the generation of neu-ronal subtypes) [7]. In humans and mice, the neuronal gene C promoter binding factor-I encodes the expression of a DNA-binding protein involved in differenti-ation of peripheral nerve tissue. The regulation of neuronal fate is determined by many transcription factors: the transcript P_{2x3}, which encodes a functional ATP-gated cation channel and is similar to the P_{2x} receptor for ATP, is restricted to cell types with a predominantly nociceptive modality; its expression might be physiologically significant as a response to ATP released from damaged tissues.

Another transcript which has a restricted expression in small-diameter sen-sory neurons encodes an unusual tetrodotoxin-insensitive, voltage-gated Na^+ channel useful in the transmission of nociceptive information to the spinal cord. The tetrodotoxin is a toxin which reduces the current but does not block the channel. Such a transcript, expressed by small sensory neurons and also named SNS, is reduced by capsaicin, which ablates substance P-producing neurons. Transcription factors are differentially expressed in the two populations of small-diameter unmyelinated C fibers and in myelinated A fibers. The extent of noxious input to the spinal cord may thus be explained by this sequence of events: chemical mediators (released following tissue damage) activate C fibers through the binding of mediators to their receptors. Some signals regulate re-ceptor activation, possibly by involving protein kinase activation. Such signals also regulate the sensitivity of nociceptors to the propagation of the action po-tential, in which the tetrodotoxin-insensitive Na^+ channels are involved. Noxious input into the spinal cord occurs in superficial laminae through the release of glutamate and neuropeptides by sensory cells [7].

Nerve growth factor

NGF is a hyperalgesic mediator (i.e., induces an increased sensitivity to pain) re-leased during inflammation. Another hyperalgesic mediator is tumor necrosis factor (TNF), which leads to increased levels of NGF. NGF is able in upregulat-ing the ion flux carried by the tetrodotoxin-insensitive Na^+ channels on sensory neurons, thus favoring the transmission of nociceptive information.

NGF influences the differentiation and survival of neurons in the developing nervous system [8, 9], at the level of sympathetic and sensory ganglia (peripher-al nervous system) and in the brain (central nervous system) at the level of the basal forebrain cholinergic system (which is atrophied in Alzheimer's disease) [10]. The effect of NGF depletion on central and peripheral neurons has been studied in mice [11]. To inactivate NGF expression, a targeting vector was constructed by deleting some sequences and replacing them with a neoresistance gene cassette. The targeting vector was introduced into AB1 embryonic stem cells by electroporation. Eleven clones that had a disrupted NGF allele were identified and injected into blastocytes derived from C57 BL/6 female mice. Heterozygous NGF-targeted mice were then isolated and bred to obtain mice with both alleles disrupted: 24% were found to be homozygous (−/−), 44% heterozygous (+/−), and 29% wild type (+/+) for the disrupted gene (3% died). Many (−/−) mice appeared smaller at birth than (+/−) or (+/+) mice. Following the first week of life, some (−/−) mice did not ingest normal food, failed to gain weight, and died. Some animals surviving past the first week developed a tremor, which was more evident during locomotion. All mice surviving until 4 weeks displayed marked ptosis (drooping of the upper eyelid) as a consequence of lack of sympathetic innervation to the eye.

Superior cervical ganglia from (−/−) animals were smaller than those obtained from (+/+) mice, and dorsal root ganglia from (−/−) mice revealed selective cell loss. In addition, homozygous NGF null mutant mice had a significantly decreased response to a noxious stimulus (pinch applied to the tail) with respect to (+/+) and (+/−) mice. However, (−/−) mice developed basal forebrain cholinergic neurons (whose life possibly is independent of NGF).

NGF binds, other than the low-affinity p75 receptor Trk, a receptor tyrosine kinase encoded by the trk proto-oncogene. The effect of ablation of the Trk gene in embryonic stem cells by homologous recombination was studied [12] in mice. The homozygous mutant animals, normal at birth, were smaller than controls on successive days, many had died by the 20th day, and none of them has survived more than 55 days. Since the Trk gene is expressed in the trigeminal and dorsal roots and sympathetic ganglia of the peripheral nervous system, dorsal root ganglia of mutant mice were examined. There was extensive neuron loss: small neurons were preferentially lost. In addition, mice lacking Trk had a decrease in the cholinergic basal forebrain projections to the hippocampus and cortex. The data showed the role of Trk as a mediator of the trophic activity of NGF in vivo.

Hereditary sensory neuropathies

Analogous to mice, mutations in the TRKA (a high-affinity receptor for NGF in humans) gene are responsible for four unrelated cases of congenital insensitivity to pain with anhidrosis (CIPA) [13], which is an autosomal recessive disorder known to be one of the five hereditary sensory neuropathies. They are: dominant hereditary sensory neuropathy (characterized by degeneration of dorsal root ganglia), recessive congenital sensory neuropathy (characterized by loss of unmyelinated A fibers and consequent deficits in mechanosensitivity), dysautonomia or Riley-Day syndrome (characterized by loss of unmyelinated C fibers), CIPA (characterized by loss of small diameter unmyelinated C fibers), and congenital insensitivity to pain without anhidrosis (characterized by the absence of small myelinated A delta fibers) [14]. Patients with CIPA have recurrent episodes of unexplained fever, absence of reaction to noxious stimuli, anhydrosis (absence of sweating and thus of thermoregulation), self-mutilating behavior, and mental retardation. The defects in pain and temperature sensations are related to complete absence of small myelinated and unmyelinated fibers and to the absence of eccrine sweat gland innervation (which is due to sympathetic cholinergic fibers originating from the paravertebral ganglia). Indeed, the NGF/TRKA system plays a role in the development and function of the nociceptive regulation in humans as well as in animals.

Pain and the immune system

TRKA and NGF have also been demonstrated to be expressed by cells of the immune system, i.e., lymphocytes [15]. NGF exerts its role in inflammatory disorders by activating the nociceptors. The immune response of each patient is genetically determined, for example, for the predominance of the Th1-type response or the Th2-type response. The Th2-type response is related to an increase in opioid peptide β endorphin synthesis (in the arcuate nucleus in the central nervous system, in the intermediate pituitary in the periphery, and in peripheral blood lymphocytes and monocytes). The Th1-type response is related to a decrease of β endorphin synthesis and occurs in many autoimmune diseases (multiple sclerosis, rheumatoid arthritis, and Crohn's disease). The inhibitory effect of β endorphin on immune functions could be corrected by therapeutic modulation of β endorphin production [16].

The effect of mediators (such as cytokines produced by immune cells) on nociceptive modulation has been previously studied.

In fact, peripheral administration of IL-1β was found to produce hyperalgesia, whereas the neutralization of IL-1, IL-6, and TNFα action reduced inflammatory hyperalgesia [16, 17].

Moreover, IL-6$^{-/-}$ mice displayed a significantly lower response threshold than IL-6$^{+/+}$ controls to mechanical and thermal stimulation. After localized carrageenan injection, the magnitude of hyperalgesia and plasma extravasation was lower in IL-6$^{-/-}$ than in control mice [18]. Furthermore, autotomy (see later), a sign of neuropathic pain, was significantly higher in IL-6 deficient females than in IL-6$^{-/-}$ male mice following peripheral nerve injury.

Such results indicate that cytokines could modulate the nociceptive response. In contrast, a recent study indicated that a mediator produced by sensory neurons, substance P, provokes IL-12 production by murine macrophages [19]. The latter data suggest the possible role of substance P in modulating cellular immunity.

Genetic predisposition to neuropathic pain

The severity of neuropathic pain symptoms varies among different individuals with similar nerve injury. A rat model of human deafferentation pain (self-injury to a denervated limb is called "autotomy") suggested that the variability of responses in animals was genetically determined [20]. In fact, two lines of rats were selected which showed high autotomy or low autotomy. Phenotypes of F1 heterozygotes and backcrosses were then studied, and autotomy appeared to be inherited as a single-gene autosomal recessive trait. In humans, some conditions, such as diabetic neuropathy, carpal tunnel syndrome and trigeminal neuralgia, seem to have a heritable component. However, is the susceptibility to the disease (for example, to diabetes) or the response to the nerve injury primarily inherited?

Further considerations

The neural adhesion molecule L1, a member of the immunoglobulin superfamily with binding domains similar to those of fibronectin [21], is involved in processes of the nervous system. Mutations in the human L1 gene are related to anomalous development of the nervous system, known as "CRASH" (corpus callosum hypoplasia, retardation, adducted thumbs, spastic paraplegia, and hydrocephalus). The mutant mice obtained by disruption of the L1 gene presented some malformations of the nervous system (reduced size of the corticospinal tract, enlarged lateral ventricles, and limited association with axons of the non-myelinating Schwann cells), were smaller than controls, and were less sensitive to touch and pain [22]. Studies on the function of L1 (in the nervous system) could clarfy whether it is dependent on genetic influences.

Conclusions

Many studies have given evidence of the influence of genetic factors on nociception activation. Knowledge of genetic mediation in pain response may be useful to understand some clinical conditions. Moreover, genetic investigation might allow us to improve analgesic therapy and immune responsiveness, which in turn would be useful to better address the issue of pain inhibition. In the future, gene therapy might be used in patients affected by chronic pain and insensitive to drugs such as morphine and opiate analogues.

References

1. Alvan G, Bechtel P, Iselius L et al (1990) Hydroxylation polymorphisms of debrisoquine and mephenytoin in European populations. Eur J Clin Pharmacol 39:533-537
2   Dayer P, Desmeules J, Leemann T et al (1988) Bioactivation of the narcotic drug codeine in human liver is mediated by the polymorphic monooxygenase catalyzing debrisoquine 4-hydroxylation (cytochrome P-450 dbl/bufl). Biochem Biophys Res Commun 152:411-416

3. Mogil JS, Belknap JK (1997) Sex and genotype determine the selective activation of neu-rochemically-distinct mechanisms of swin stress-induced analgesia. Pharmacol Biochem Behav 56(1):61-66

4. Mogil JS, Sternberg WF, Marek P et al (1996) The genetics of pain and pain inhibition. Proc Natl Acad Sci USA 93:3048-3055

5. Rubinstein M, Mogil JS, Japon M et al (1996) Absence of opioid stress-induced analge-sia in mice lacking beta-endorphin by site-directed mutagenesis. Proc Natl Acad Sci 93(9):3995-4000

6. Mogil JS, Kest B, Sadowski B, Belknap PK (1996) Differential genetic mediation of sen-sitivity to morphine in genetic models of opiate antinociception: influence of nocicep-tive assay. J Pharmacol Exp Ther 276:532-544

7   Akopian AN, Abson NC, Wood JN (1996) Molecular genetic approaches to nociceptor development and function. Trends Neurosci 19(6):240-246

8. Levi Montalcini R (1987) The nerve growth factor: thiry five years later EMBO J 6.1145-1154

9. Thoenen H (1991) The changing scene of neurotrophic factors. Trends Neurosci 14:165-170

10. Hefti F, Hartikka J, Knusel B (1989) Function of neurotrophic factors in the adult and agin brain and their possible use in the treatment of neurodegenerative diseases Neu-robiol Aging 10:515-533

11. Crowley C, Spencer SD, Nishimura MC et al (1994) Mice lacking nerve growth factor display perinatal loss of sensory and sympathetic neurons yet develop basal forebrain cholinergic neurons. Cell 76:1001-1011

12. Smeyne RJ, Klein R, Schnapp A et al (1994) Severe sensory and sympathetic neu-ropathies in mice carrying a disrupted Trk/NGF receptor gene. Nature 368:246-249

13. Indo Y, Tsuruta M, Hayashida Y et al (1996) Mutations in the TRKA/NGF receptor gene in patients with congenital insensitivity to pain with anhidrosis. Nature Genet 13:485-488

14. Wood JN (1996) No pain, some gain. Nature Genet 13:382-383

15. Ehrhard PB, Erb P, Graumann U et al (1993) Expression of nerve growth factor and re-ceptor tyrosine kinase Trk in activated CD4-positive T-cell clones. Proc Natl Acad Sci USA 90:10984-10998

16. Ferreira SH, Lorenzetti BB, Bristow AF et al (1988) Interleukin 1β as a potent hyperal-gesic agent antagonized by a tripeptide analogue. Nature 334:698-700

17. Watkins LR, Wiertelak E, Goehler LE et al (1994) Characterization of cytokine-induced hyperalgesia. Brain Res 654:15-26

18. Xu XJ, Hao JX, Jonsson SV et al (1997) Nociceptive responses in interleukin-6-deficient mice to peripheral inflammation and peripheral nerve section. Cytokine 9(12):1028-1033

19. Kincy-Cain T, Bost KL (1997) Substance P-Induced IL-12 production by murine macrophages. J Immunol 158:2334-2339

20. Devor M, Raber P (1991) Experimental evidence of a genetic predisposition to neuro-pathic pain. Eur J Pain 12(3):65-68

21. Moos M et al (1988) Neural adhesion molecule L1 as a member of the immunoglobulin superfamily with binding domains similar to fibronectin. Nature 334:701-703

22. Dahme M, Bartsch U, Martini R et al (1997) Disruption of the mouse L1 gene leads to malformations of the nervous system. Nature Genet 17:346-349

PHARMACOLOGY

Chapter 7

Clinical pharmacology of local anaesthetic agents

L.E. MATHER, D.H.-T. CHANG

Local anaesthetic agents (LAAs) are defined as those agents which, when applied in the region of a neuronal structure, reversibly prevent its conduction, thereby producing an absence of sensation in the region innervated. Substances that are irreversible or otherwise neurolytic or act by systemic mechanisms clearly do not fit the definition. It may be reasonably added that they should do this predictably and with an acceptable difference between therapeutic and toxic doses but, for these agents, tissue toxicity is evaluated as foremost. Hence evaluation of the therapeutic index (defined in traditional pharmacological terms as the ratio of lethal to therapeutic doses) is not the primary question although it is the secondary question for agents passing the test of tissue toxicity. Only those LAAs that do not cause tissue toxicity can be further considered for their other pharmacological properties.

A multitude of LAAs have been used since the introduction of cocaine just over a century ago. However, the contemporary pharmacopoeia contains a relatively small list of drugs retaining the "classical" chemical structures defined for LAAs more than half a century ago. The requirements for a new local anaesthetic agent have not changed since they were written nearly 100 years ago (Table 1) [1], except for the choice of the standard agent by which a new agent should be compared, for an extended duration of action and for the ability to produce a useful differential neural blockade. A contemporary list is based upon retaining only those agents that are predictably anaesthetically active and minimally toxic. Unfortunately, these two properties do not sit well together [2].

Relevance of chemical structure

Chemical classifications for local anaesthetic structures

It is helpful to use a system for classifying drugs within pharmacological classes to make it easier to understand the relationships between drugs in the class: this also applies to LAAs. The contemporary viewpoint allows at least two ways of classifying LAAs based upon structural modifications to the molecules – by functional groups and by physicochemical properties. These classifications allow easy demonstration of the relationship between the chemistry and neural block-

Table 1. Requirements that a new local anaesthetic agent must fulfill according to Braun [1]

Besides producing local anaesthesia, any drug in this very numerous abundant class of agents must also have the following properties

- It must be less toxic relative to potency than. . (current standard[a])
- It must not cause irritation or damage to tissues .
- The substance must be soluble in water and be stable in solution ..
- The substance must be miscible with adrenaline
- The anaesthetic must be rapidly absorbed into the membrane. .

[a] Cocaine in the original

ade – side effect profiles as well as the pharmacokinetic properties of these agents.

Functional groups

The chemical structures of LAAs determine the ways in which the agents are formulated and interact pharmacologically with their intended ion channel targets in spinal and peripheral neurons, with unintended ion channel targets for side effects in the brain and heart, and with enzymic targets for metabolism in the liver and maybe elsewhere. The functional groups contained in "classical" LAAs were described in detail by Lofgren [3] as being an amino group which conveys hydrophilicity through its charged form (conjugate acid), an aromatic residue which conveys lipophilicity, and an intermediate or linking chain. This view was developed from the study during the first half of the twentieth century of hundreds of substances from the original local anaesthetic agent lead compound cocaine.

The phasing out of cocaine began soon after its introduction because of its toxicity and misuse potential. Indeed, its first successor, procaine, which was introduced in 1905, some 20 years before the structure of cocaine was completely elucidated in 1924, was based on improving upon these properties. Because cocaine and procaine have an ester group in the linking chain, ester groups were included in most LAAs and this presented a problem of chemical stability with

Table 2. Chemical characteristics of classical local anesthetic agents having general structures according to Lofgren [3] of an "amine group – intermediate chain – aromatic residue"

Ester-caines: i.e., procaine, amethocaine, benzocaine, butamben
- Lead compound of cocaine
- Unstable chemically, especially to heat sterilization
- Widely distributed esterase metabolism
- Potentially allergenic metabolites

Amide-caines: i.e., lignocaine, prilocaine, mepivacaine-bupivacaine homologues
- Synthesized logically
- Stable chemically – promoted by steric factors
- Principally (solely?) hepatic metabolism
- Rarely allergenic metabolites

pharmacological implications (Table 2). The ester group is usually of an (aromatic) amine substituted benzoic acid: the aromatic amino group may be primary as in procaine or secondary as in amethocaine (tetracaine) and is always a very weak amine that is unionized at neural pH. The ester group in these aminoacylesters is subject to time-related hydrolysis that is promoted by increased temperature (as in heat sterilization) and increased pH (hence, the need to maintain acidic solutions). Experience in the 1930s showed that this group could be replaced with an isosteric but more chemically stable amide group. At first the amide group was of benzoic acid derivatives and these were reported to be "excellent local anaesthetics" giving the agents related to cinchocaine (dibucaine). Lofgren's research in the 1930s arose from studies of the structure of the indoleamine alkaloid gramine and its congeners, one of which had local anaesthetic action. In further investigations in 1943 he synthesized diethylaminoaceto-2.6-xylidine, i.e. lignocaine (lidocaine), with a local anaesthetic activity greater and a toxicity considerably smaller than that of analogous substances [3]. The 2.6-dimethyl aniline (= 2.6-xylidine) structure or its isostere is found in every new clinically successful LAA since lignocaine. The para-amino benzoic acid (or its derivative) aromatic head that formed part of the ester group has been replaced, usually by a sterically hindered aniline derivative. Changes to the aromatic head are connected to changes in the intermediate acyl bridge that also enhance stability. Modern amide-caines are derived from 2.6-dimethyl aniline, except for prilocaine which is derived from 2-methyl aniline. The aromatic methyl substitutions have the impact of forcing the amide-link out of the plane of the aromatic ring, thus hindering its chemical and enzymic hydrolysis. In prilocaine there is far less hindrance than with the dimethyl substituted molecules but it is supplemented somewhat by alkyl (methyl) substitution on the intermediate chain. These aminoacylanilines thus have the dual benefits of the chemically sturdier amide-link that allows the agents to be repeatedly heat sterilized without loss of potency as well as having the lower potential for causing allergy.

The amino group does not differ materially between the ester- and amidecaines. Although the group is a tertiary amine in most LAAs and is a secondary amine in prilocaine, a variety of substituents, usually aliphatic (methyl, butyl, etc) or less commonly alicyclic (piperidine, etc) but even aryl (aromatic) groups have been used in both types. The importance of the amino group lies in the fact that, as a weak base with a pK_a ca 8-9, it can attract a proton (hydrogen ion) at physiological pH to become an ionized water-soluble conjugate acid and thus be suitable for injection. The amino group is not essential for local anaesthetic activity. At the same time such an aqueous solution contains 1 mol of strong acid (usually HCl) for every mol of local anaesthetic and thus has an acidic pH, typically 4-6. Amino pK_a values of p-amino benzoic acid esters are much weaker bases (typical values ~4) and are thus unionized at extracellular fluid pH.

Ester-caines are now used so relatively infrequently that this classification has more historical than pharmacological importance for contemporary anaesthesiologists. Of the many hundreds of ester-caines found in the experimental and clinical literature over the past 100 years, few survive in current clinical practice.

Cocaine, procaine, 2-chloroprocaine and possibly benzocaine are still part of the contemporary international pharmacopoeia and continued research and development have seen the reincarnation of old agents in new biopharmaceutical forms, e.g., as novel, long-acting preparations of amethocaine and butamben, but current international clinical practice has favoured the amide-caines, lignocaine, prilocaine, mepivacaine, bupivacaine and, recently, ropivacaine. Indeed, many younger anaesthesiologists will know of the ester LAAs only from the literature rather than first-hand experience.

A third type of LAA derives from the guanidine-type biotoxins represented by tetrodotoxin and saxitoxin. These are not in clinical use and are not considered further in this review.

Physicochemical properties

A more useful classification, also developed by Lofgren, based upon physicochemical properties, concerns the relative lipophilicity and fraction ionized, and this applies across ester-amide classifications. Bupivacaine (amide), amethocaine and butamben (esters) have high lipophilicity; lignocaine (amide) and procaine (ester) have moderate lipophilicity. Excepting benzocaine and butamben which have no amino group to ionize (and thus make hydrophilic), the ester caines are stronger bases (higher pK_a) and thus have higher fractions in the ionized state at body pH than amide caines [4].

Classification based upon physicochemical properties is especially helpful because it facilitates analysis of the interaction of the chemical and physiological factors involved in drugs crossing membranes for distribution and for elimination. These properties directly influence the rates at which the drugs reach their intended targets in spinal and peripheral neuronal tissues (as well as their unintended targets from which they elicit their side effects, particularly the brain and heart). Although LAAs are usually administered in a water solution at a slightly acidic pH, i.e. the equilibrium favours the ionized conjugate acids, the pH of the tissue region injected resets the equilibrium of concentrations between conjugate acid and base. Both are believed to be necessary for optimal local anaesthetic action.

Bulk flow of LAA solution and diffusion of LAA solute determine the relative rates of effective (producing neural blockade) and ineffective distribution (dilution or loss of dose). Of the LAA base forms, agents with moderate lipophilicity have moderate durations of action and those with higher lipophilicity have longer durations of action. Bupivacaine and ropivacaine have slightly higher ionized fractions than lignocaine, prilocaine and mepivacaine – perhaps giving slightly longer onset times. Local anaesthetic agents work by blocking the transient rise in Na^+ permeability in the neural membrane that accompanies the propagation of an action potential, i.e. they prevent depolarization of the nerve and spread of the neural impulse (see below). This is achieved by the conjugate acid form of the LAA molecule binding to the Na^+ channel protein on the axoplasmic side (inside) of the neural membrane and temporarily inactivating it.

To work from the inside, the drug must have sufficient lipid solubility for a rapid rate of transfer across the neural membrane and a pK_a value between approximately 7.5 and 8.5 to allow sufficient concentrations of the conjugate acid to cause neural blockade.

The relative lipophilicity of LAAs is commonly represented by organic solvent to buffer distribution coefficients. There is a good rank order correlation between the organic solvent (typically *n*-octanol) distribution coefficients and the distribution of LAAs into fat and nerve tissue homogenates and with plasma protein binding [5] but these in vitro model systems can grossly overestimate the actual tissue: blood distribution coefficient found in vivo [6]. In general, binding is more hydrophobic than ionic, as shown by the increase of binding of LAAs with increase of pH [4].

Structural changes, principally in the aromatic head and in the amine group, markedly modify the important physicochemical properties of lipophilicity and hydrophilicity. These result in alterations to lipid/aqueous partition coefficients and to plasma and tissue protein binding and have, in turn, significant effects on potency, onset time, and duration of anaesthesia. The aqueous solubility of a local anaesthetic is directly related to its extent of ionization and inversely related to its lipid solubility. Despite large differences in lipid solubility of the LAA bases, differences in aqueous solubility of their conjugate acids are not remarkably different [4, 7].

Lipophilicity has implications for potency, onset time, and duration of anaesthesia. While such relationships may be intuitive, they have been more often assumed than measured. Net lipophilicity is independent of ester or amide links. Study of intrathecal injection of LAAs in mice showed a very strong correlation between lipophilicity and potency [8]. It is well known that lipophilicity has direct bearing upon duration of anaesthesia. This has often been explained in terms of drug partitioned into perineural fat acting as a depot but a drug interaction with hydrophobic components of receptors may also be important. The relationship to onset time, however, is more complex. The permeability coefficient of a series of drugs in an in vitro monkey spinal meninges preparation was found to have a "bell-shaped" relationship with lipophilicity [9]. This is not unexpected as passage of chemically similar molecules through lipoidal membranes generally has an optimal value. Within these limits, permeability is a simple diffusion process, independent of molecular weight, driven by the concentration gradient of solute [10].

Chirality

A great deal of recent attention has been accorded to the "chiral caines": these have one chiral centre (asymmetric carbon atom) which generates one pair of enantiomers. Enantiomers are stereoisomers bearing a mirror image relationship (also referred to as optical isomers). Racemates are drugs equi-molar mixtures of enantiomers (thus having with null optical rotation). Chiral drugs found in nature (i.e., tubocurarine, morphine, atropine) usually single enan-

Table 3. Considerations for racemic vs single enantiomer local anaesthetic agents

---

Racemates: i.e., bupivacaine, prilocaine, mepivacaine
• 50% chance of formation of each enantiomer
• Pharmacodynamically misleading to treat a mixture as a single substance
• Based upon pharmacological "sophisticated nonsense"
• Good science or commercial gain (?)

Single enantiomers: i.e., cocaine, ropivacaine, levobupivacaine
• Enzymic or chiral synthesis produces a single enantiomer
• Successful outcome depends on getting/choosing the "right one"
• Enantioselectivity in pharmacokinetics and pharmacodynamics is real
• Cost-effective or user pays (?)

---

tiomers because they are synthesized enzymatically and such reactions are usually produce one enantiomer only. Most synthetic chiral drugs are racemates because chemical reactions usually have an equal probability of producing both enantiomers. Lignocaine does not contain a chiral centre. Cocaine, a natural product, is a single enantiomer; mepivacaine, bupivacaine, prilocaine, etidocaine are made and used racemates. This has pharmacological and potentially economic implications (Table 3).

Many racemic drugs are used clinically; however, the time-course of their pharmacodynamic effects derives from the relevant biofluid concentrations of its enantiomers, thereby being subject to any differences in the pharmacokinetics of the enantiomers. The clinical complication caused by racemates is that the component enantiomers usually have different pharmacodynamic effects and different pharmacokinetic properties. Moreover, the body itself is a chiral environment due to its structures being made of numerous chiral components (e.g., natural amino acids and carbohydrates). Thus, although a racemate is injected as "a pure drug", the body recognizes the racemate as two drugs and allows the drugs to behave as reasonably independent entities with respect to their rates of distribution and elimination. Hence, the effect – side effect profile depends upon the dominating local concentration of the dominating enantiomer, i.e. both pharmacokinetic and pharmacodynamic properties of both enantiomers need to considered [11].

Enantiomers do not differ in an achiral environment, apart from their direction of rotation of plane-polarized light. However, physicochemical differences between the racemates and the separate enantiomers often occur, e.g., the aqueous solubility of *rac*-bupivacaine is nearly half that of its component enantiomers over the range of pH 3 to 5 but it is more soluble from pH 6 to 7.4 [7]. In the markedly chiral environment of the body, pharmacologically significant differences between enantiomers may occur in their interactions with biomembranes, enzymes and other biological systems.

Take the example of bupivacaine. Although $R(+)$-bupivacaine was found to be more potent in producing neural blockade in frog sciatic nerve in vitro, $S(-)$-bupivacaine exhibits a longer duration of intradermal anaesthesia in vivo [12, 13]. The latter is thought to be due to differences in effects on local vasculature

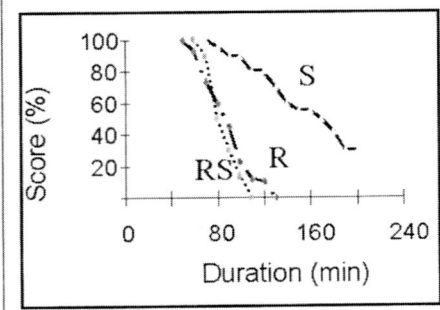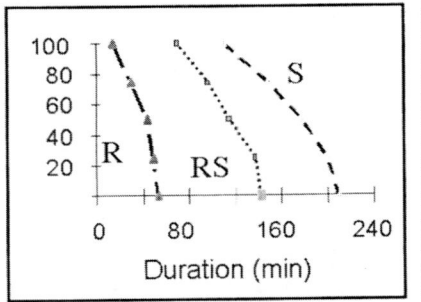

Fig.1. Importance of chirality in experimental neural blockade: intradermal skin wheal in the guinea pig. Left: data for bupivacaine from [2]; right: data for ropivacaine from [22]

rather than in intrinsic nerve-blocking potency, thereby maximizing the efficiency of their contact with neural structures. Enantio-selectivity for neural blockade as well as side effects has also been shown for mepivacaine and prilocaine [14, 15]. In general the S-enantiomers of chiral caines tend to have greater duration of neural blockade (Fig. 1) and generally lower toxicity than the R-enantiomers [16-18]. After direct administration, S(–)-bupivacaine is less toxic to the CNS and cardiovascular system in experimental animals than either racemic or S(–)-bupivacaine [16-18]; R(+)-bupivacaine has a greater mean total body clearance than S(–)-bupivacaine in experimental animals and humans due to its greater hepatic extraction [19-21].

Ropivacaine, which was introduced into trials during the 1980s, stands alone amongst LAAs in being designed de novo as a single enantiomer (the S(–)-enantiomer of the propyl homologue of bupivacaine) and, not surprisingly, it produces a similar neural blockade to bupivacaine although of slightly less potency [22, 23]. Most literature on LAAs, however, does not yet include discussion based upon the chirality of the "chiral caines", despite the pharmacodynamic and pharmacokinetic differences between enantiomers of bupivacaine, mepivacaine and prilocaine being known. It should be remembered that the same chemical properties that make bupivacaine longer acting than lignocaine also make it more toxic. Ropivacaine has been introduced with the aim of retaining the long action of bupivacaine and regaining more of the safety of lignocaine. Trials in experimental animals and humans of tolerability of ropivacaine indicate that this aim has been achieved [23]. Recently, the S(–)-enantiomer of bupivacaine (levobupivacaine) has entered trials [24, 25].

Biopharmaceutical implications

Ionization is relevant to the stability, solubility, activity and the equilibrium distribution of LAAs in various body compartments. Because their ionized forms are more water soluble than their free bases, the drugs are dispensed as their hydrochloride salts and the resultant solutions are acidic (typically pH 3-6). The low pH also stabilizes metabisulphite which is sometimes added to adrenaline-containing solutions to prevent oxidation of adrenaline. Whereas the chemical stability of the ester caines is greatest at pH 3.7, the amide caines are stable over a wide range of pH. Based upon the example of ropivacaine, there is no evidence of significant enantiomeric inversion of chiral caines even at strongly basic pH [26]. The aqueous solubility of a LAA is directly related to its extent of ionization and inversely related to its lipid solubility. Despite quite large differences in lipid solubility of the amide-caine bases, the differences in aqueous solubility of the conjugate acids are insignificant at clinically used dose concentrations. The long lag time after the introduction of bupivacaine before its clinical use in spinal anaesthesia resulted from concerns that its low aqueous solubility would result in its precipitation in CSF, with consequent neurotoxicity.

Activity is related to both drug distribution and intrinsic potency. The union-ized fraction is essential for drug passage through lipoidal barriers to the site of action on the nerve membrane. In principle, decreasing ionization by alkalin-ization of the solution for injection will effectively raise the initial concentration gradient of diffusible drug base, thereby increasing the rate of drug transfer; once at the nerve membrane, ionization is again necessary for complete anaes-thetic activity. This manoeuvre has not been found uniformly successful. A recent study attempted to clarify the effectiveness of alkalinization [27]. The results indicated that the latent period was usefully shortened for epidural block with lignocaine and bupivacaine, for sciatic/femoral block with mepivacaine and for brachial plexus block with lignocaine. However, the method of alkalin-ization was empirical by volume of bicarbonate such that the pH adjustment and the resultant CO_2 content was not uniform, so that the results of this com-monly used manoeuvre are still somewhat uncertain. Recent manoeuvres to ex-tend the duration of blockade with conventional long-acting LAAs include the incorporation of the more lipophilic agents into a lipoidal matrix [28], into li-posomes [29] and into polymer microspheres [30]. The principles of each of these is the same – of sustained release into the region of the nerve.

Although there is the potential for all drugs to undergo adsorptive losses into medical plastics such as polyvinyl chloride catheters and polypropylene syringes, this has not been found to be a problem [31]. Similarly, there is no evidence of instability or of precipitation when solutions of the amide LAAs are premixed with other organic bases such as opioids as long as pH of the solution is no higher than neutral.

Mechanisms of local anaesthetic actions

Basic concepts of neurophysiology

Neurons, nerve cells that are the basic units of the nervous system, are associat-ed with generating and conducting nerve impulses. They have four functional distinct components: a cell body, dendrites, axon, and axon terminal. Neurons can be classified by function as sensory neurons (afferent neurons) which carry signals (i.e., pain) from sensory receptors to the central nervous system, motor neurons (efferent neurons) which are responsible for conducting impulse to muscle from central nervous system, and interneurons which connect the sensory and motor neurons and integrate their function. The sensory neurons are the major targets for the LAAs action.

Like most cells, the membrane of nerve cells contains a double layer of lipids with integral membrane proteins penetrating it. The lipid layer forms the primary barrier to diffusion, while proteins perform most of the specific membrane functions. For example, these proteins can form protein pores (ion channels), which regulate the movement of ions, such as sodium ions (Na^+) and potassium ions (K^+) across the membrane.

In the resting state, a membrane potential exists in nerve cells, whereby the inside is negative (–60 to –90 mV) compared to the outside. Membrane potential is primarily due to the differences in distribution and membrane permeability of Na^+, K^+ and intracellular anions, which are the large, negatively charged intracellular proteins. The intracellular fluid concentration of K^+ is much greater than that in the extracellular fluid and vice versa for Na^+, with the concentration differences being maintained by the Na^+-K^+ pump using ATP as the source of energy [32]. Both Na^+ and K^+ passively diffuse across cell membranes along the concentration gradient via protein ion channels. K^+ diffuses 50-75 times more readily through the membrane than Na^+, because more potassium channels are available for diffusion. Intracellularly, the large negatively charged anions, which cannot diffuse through cell membranes, tend to hold the positively charged K^+ inside the cell. When these two opposing forces on K^+ balance each other, there would be an equilibrium potential for K^+ of –90mV. A similar equilibrium potential for Na^+ of +60 mV can be achieved from the balance between Na^+ and Cl^-, both being the predominant ions extracellularly. K^+ exerts a greater effect on resting membrane potential than Na^+ because of its greater membrane permeability.

The nerve cell membranes are called excitable membranes because they are capable of generating and conducting electrical signals, action potential, when excited. Initiation and propagation of an action potential depends on the concentration gradients and membrane permeability to different ions, particularly Na^+ and K^+. It starts with a sudden change from the negative resting membrane potential to pass through a value of zero to a slight positive overshoot before reversing rapidly back to the negative membrane potential. To conduct a nerve impulse, an action potential moves along the nerve fibre until it comes to the fibre's end.

Action potential can be divided into three different stages: resting, depolarization and repolarization. The resting stage is resting membrane potential before the action potential occurs. In depolarization stage, voltage-gated sodium channels open to allow increases of membrane permeability to Na^+ which move across the membranes into nerve cells along the concentration gradient. Initially, a slow phase of depolarization occurs as the cell becomes progressively less negative. When the threshold potential is reached, there is rapid and transient depolarization. In the repolarization stage, the sodium channels start to close, accompanied by opening of potassium channels, which allow rapid diffusion of K^+ into the extracellular fluid. As a result, the resting membrane potential is re-established. The disrupted ion concentration gradient by action potential is restored gradually by the Na^+-K^+ pump, but not necessarily after each action potential.

Molecular mechanism of LAA action

LAAs inhibit nerve impulse by interfering with the function of sodium channels to block Na^+ movement across the membrane of nerve cells. In the presence of local anaesthetic molecules, the threshold for electrical excitability increases, the rate of rise of the action potential decreases and the impulse conduction slows down. When the dose of LAAs is high enough, sufficient sodium channels are impaired and nerve conduction fails.

Na^+ channels of the mammalian brain consist of $\beta 1$ (33 kDa), $\beta 2$ (33 kDa) and α (260 kDa) subunits [33]. The large α-subunit is composed of four homologous domains (I-IV), each with six transmembrane domains or spans in a helical conformation (S1-S6). These four domains form the Na^+ selective transmembrane pore of the channels. In response to membrane depolarization, each of these domains in turn undergoes a conformational change. As a result, the Na^+ channel opens and Na^+ ions diffuse rapidly across the axonal membrane into the nerve cells. Within a few milliseconds after the opening, the inactivation gate between the domain III an IV shuts down and the transmembrane Na^+ conduction stops. This process can be divided into four different conformational stages, beginning with resting form, activating through closed intermediate form to reach an open form and then returning to an inactivated form.

LAAs block Na^+ channels in a complex voltage- and frequency-dependent manner [34]. Tertiary and quaternary amine LAAs, as well as neutral LAAs homologues produce the so-called tonic nerve block at low frequencies of impulse firing (<0.5 Hz). Increases in frequencies of firing result in a greater degree of nerve block, called phasic or use-dependent nerve block. It has been shown that LAAs have a higher affinity for the channels in open or inactivated form than for those in the resting state [35]. Tonic inhibition results from the binding of local anaesthetic molecules to nonactivated or resting Na^+ channels with relatively lower affinity. In phasic inhibition, local anaesthetic molecules bind more tightly to the sodium channels, which are opened or inactivated during the nerve stimulation, and stabilize the channels towards the resting equilibrium to achieve more potent anaesthetic effect.

More recently, it has been hypothesized that the molecules of tertiary amine LAAs can reach the sodium channels by two different pathways, both of them participating in nerve impulse blockade [36]. The charged form of the molecules may diffuse through the membrane and bind to a site close to the pores, blocking Na^+ channels from inside (hydrophilic route). Binding and dissociating of the molecules from this site, which is the binding site for phasic inhibition, are slow reactions with rates similar to those of the channel-gating processes. In the second pathway (hydrophobic route), the base form of LAAs binds to the other site, which is in a hydrophobic milieu, and interfere with the channel conformational changes which underlie the channel opening. This is the binding site for the tonic inhibition, since the drug molecules can reach and leave this site relatively rapidly and easily, even when the channels are closed. This is depicted in Figure 2.

The possible interaction of LAAs with other ion channels such as K^+ and Ca^{2+} channels may also contribute to the mechanism of their anaesthetic activity. It has been reported that delayed rectifier potassium currents are inhibited by LAAs [37]. However, since higher concentrations of LAAs are required to block this current, the contribution of this channel inhibition to the conduction block of nerve fibre is of minor importance. Recent studies showed that LAAs can also affect voltage-insensitive K^+ channels, i.e., flicker K^+ channels in peripheral nerve axons [38]. This inhibition may contribute to the mechanism of anaesthesia. The flicker K^+ channels are found mostly in the small nerve fibres, which in general conduct pain. Blockade of these channels by LAAs depolarizes the membrane and consequently reduces excitability of nerve conduction by increasing the portion of Na^+ channels in the inactivated state. Among the drugs studied, bupivacaine is the most potent agent and has a three times higher affinity to the channels than it has to the $\alpha 1$-acid glycoprotein in human serum, the protein with the highest affinity to LAAs known so far [39].

It has been shown that clinically relevant concentrations of LAAs also inhibit voltage-sensitive Ca^{2+} channels, although the interaction may be weaker than that with Na^+ channels. In cerebrocortical membranes of rats, LAAs dose-dependently inhibited [^{3}H]PN200-100, the channel antagonist, binding to L-type volt-

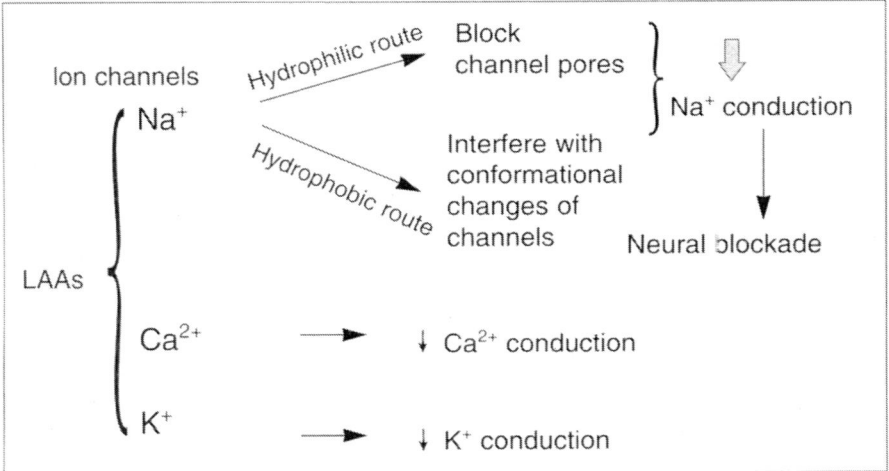

Fig. 2. A depiction of the molecular mechanisms of local anaesthetic agent actions at ion channels in neurons

age-sensitive Ca^{2+} channels [40]. Several electrophysiological studies also indicate that LAAs depress high voltage-activated Ca^{2+} currents with the rank order similar to their clinical rank order of potency [41-43]. Moreover, the L-type voltage-sensitive Ca^{2+} channel blocker verapamil potentiated spinal anaesthesia induced by LAAs [44]. The modulation of Ca^{2+} channels by LAAs may not only play a role in the mechanism of local anaesthetic action, but also contribute to the LAA-induced cardiac toxicity, although depression of myocardial contractility by the drugs has been suggested to be the result of intracellular Ca^{2+} release from the sarcoplasmic reticulum rather than Ca^{2+} conduction [45]. The relative actions of LAAs at neuronal and cardiac ion channels are depicted in Figure 2 and 3.

Accumulated evidence shows the enantiomer selectivity for LAA effect on voltage-gated Na^+ channels. In a study using the sucrose-gap method on desheathed nerves, $R(+)$-bupivacaine was shown to be more potent than $S(-)$-bupivacaine in both tonic and phasic inhibition of action potentials [12]. In general, enantiomers with relatively long, planar molecules slide more easily into the phasic blocking site and exert a greater anaesthetic effect, while their less potent enantiomers, which have an acutely angled conformation, have a higher affinity for the tonic blocking site [35, 46]. The enantioselectivity of LAAs has also been observed for Ca^{2+} channels. For example, the binding affinity of high Ca^{2+}-channel antagonist, dihydropyridines, to Ca^{2+} channels in rat brain membrane was antagonized by LAAs with a selectivity similar to that of Na^+ channels [47]. No enantioselectivity in the inhibitory effect of LAAs on delayed rectifier or transient outward K^+ channels has been observed.

Ion channel inhibition (especially Na^+ channel inhibition) by LAAs is the major contributor to their peripheral nerve block. In epidural and intrathecal

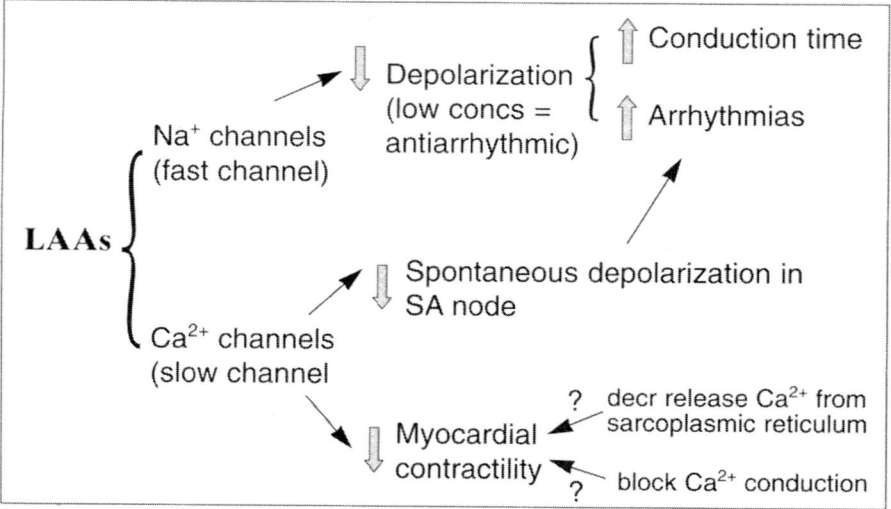

Fig. 3. A depiction of the molecular mechanisms of local anesthetic agent actions at ion channels in the heart

anaesthesia, however, the mechanism underlying LAA action is more complex. Besides ion channels, other membrane targets, including adenylate cyclase, guanylate cyclase, calmodulin-sensitive proteins, the ion-pumping enzymes Na^+/K^+-ATPase and Ca^{2+}/Mg^{2+}-ATPase, phospholipase A2 and phospholipase C, are affected by LAAs [34, 46]. At the neuromuscular junction, synaptic transmission can be inhibited directly by LAAs via modification of postsynaptic receptors such as nicotinic acetylcholine receptors, consequently inhibiting the chemical signal transmission across the synapse [35]. In presynaptic membrane within the spinal cord, several types of calcium channels, which facilitate the release of neurotransmitters, can also be inhibited by LAAs [47-49]. In general, epidural and spinal anaesthesia by LAAs may be the result of both Na^+ channel inhibition along the axons and blockade of other membrane-related activities mentioned above in spinal cord [34].

Pharmacokinetics

Local and systemic disposition

The dynamics of neural blockade are the result of complex pharmacokinetics involving the competition of LAA molecules moving in different directions – diffusion into and through neural and non-neural barriers, of exceeding a critical concentration in neural tissue to produce neural blockade and within a group of nerves to produce a differential blockade, and of uptake into vascular tissue to remove the drug irreversibly from the sphere of action. Although LAAs act at or near the site of injection, all of the drug will eventually be absorbed systemically with the potential for causing systemic effects (Table 4). Whether they do rests with the balance between the rates of drug absorption and of systemic distribution and elimination. The rate at which the drug is absorbed systemically depends principally upon the vascularity of the injection site, the drug and the addition of vasoconstrictor. Thus, the systemic effects of LAAs depend on whether they arrive in the blood rapidly or slowly. The well-known progression of LAA

Table 4. General principles of local anaesthetic agent pharmacokinetics after perineural injection

- Principles elucidated with intravenous regional and epidural anaesthesia in the 1970s [4]
- Data constantly being refined with more sophisticated techniques such as dual route-stable isotope label methodology — but confirm general principles
- Biphasic absorption is usual due to uptake in hydrophilic and lipophilic matrices in the body
- Typically biexponential absorption
- Fast rate: 50% of the dose with half life in minutes giving a C_{max} at 10-20 min
- Slow rate: remainder of dose with half life in hours giving absorption over 24 h
- Essentially same pattern for the different amide local anaesthetic agents
- Essentially same for all other nerve blocks

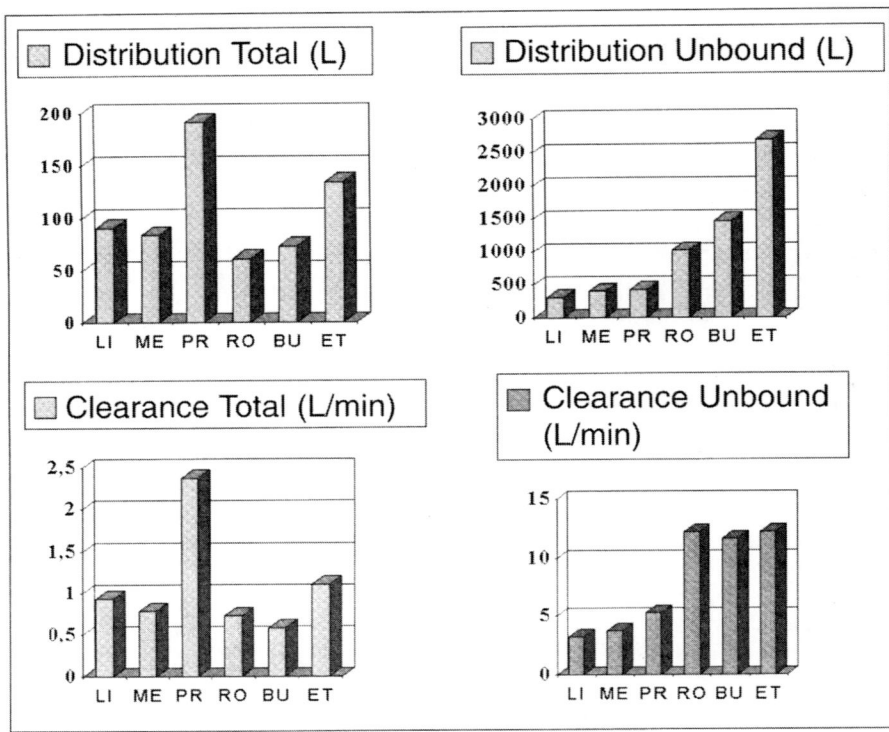

Fig. 4. A composite of the apparent volumes of distribution (Vss) and mean total body clearances for commonly used local anaesthetic agents calculated with respect to the drug total plasma concentration and with respect to the unbound concentration. While the apparent volumes of distribution and clearances calculated from total plasma concentrations do not follow a particular relationship to chemical properties, there is a gradation of clearance calculated from unbound concentrations, suggesting that the binding restricts the clearance. The agents are arranged in order of increasing lipophilicity from lignocaine to etidocaine. *LI,* lignocaine; *ME,* RS-mepivacaine; *PR,* RS-prilocaine; *RO,* ropivacaine; *BU,* RS-bupivacaine; *ET,* RS-etidocaine

toxicity from "early warning signs" of circumoral numbness, tinnitus, etc., to CNS excitation to CVS depression is the consequence of accumulation after perineural injection with increasing severity of effects. If the effects are due to accumulation, they should be expected to dissipate slowly. On the other hand, should the agent be injected intravascularly or be absorbed very rapidly then the progression may well be in the reverse order but will dissipate more rapidly [4]. Despite the pharmacokinetic complexity of neural blockade, the systemic and regional pharmacokinetics of LAAs are quite predictable and not very remarkable. By-and-large, they distribute into an apparent volume equal to about one to three times body mass, have a total body clearance from 1/3 to 2/3 of hepatic blood flow and a slow half-life of 2-3 h. They bind to plasma proteins in a concentration dependent manner from about 50% to 90% at non-toxic plasma concentrations but much less at toxic plasma concentrations, especially if the dose has been injected quickly into a vein [4].

After intravenous administration the pharmacokinetics of LAAs are characterized by simultaneous distribution and clearance [50-52] – some typical values are depicted in Figure 4. Less than a few per cent of the dose for all LAAs is excreted unmetabolized in urine and so their clearance is attributed to hepatic metabolism. Prilocaine is an exception and the metabolic clearance is greater than can be accounted for by hepatic metabolism alone [53]: metabolism in the lungs in vivo has been speculated but not proven. Both distribution and clearance are affected by plasma binding. Better appreciation of the differences between agents and of the relationship with lipohilicity can be gained by comparing drugs on the basis of unbound plasma concentrations, especially when comparing between enantiomers of racemic LAAs. Examples of differences between enantiomers is shown in Table 5.

After successful perineural injection, maximum arterial blood drug concentrations occur within 5-15 min: this is the time of maximum risk of side effects under most circumstances [4, 54, 55]. The more vascular the site the earlier and the higher the peak arterial blood drug concentration and the greater the potential risk [4]. The more lipid soluble the drug (i.e., bupivacaine more than lignocaine), the more it will be retained in fatty tissue and the slower it will be absorbed systemically. However, the peak arterial blood drug concentration still occurs at about the same time. Adrenaline acts as a vasoconstrictor to lower and delay the peak arterial blood concentrations of lignocaine more efficiently than those of bupivacaine. Pharmacokinetically, adrenaline decreases the fraction of dose absorbed rapidly [4].

The total body clearance should be the same after perineural and intravenous administration. Comparative pharmacokinetic studies have indicated that the

Table 5. Comparison of chiral-caine pharmacokinetics after i.v. administration to healthy adult volunteer subjects (mean (and SD) are given). (Ropivacaine data from [55], mepivacaine data from [52] and bupivacaine data from [51])

	Ropivacaine	S(–)-bupivacaine	R(+)-bupivacaine	S(+)-mepivacaine	R(–)-mepivacaine
CL (ml/min)	402 (108)	317 (67)	395 (76)*	350 (60)	790 (120)*
CLu (l/min)	8.0 (2.1)	8.71 (4 27)	7.26 (3.60)	1.43 (0 24)	2.24 (0 30)*
V^{ss} (l)	38 (8)	54 (20)	84 (29)*	57 (7)	103 (14)*
$V^{ss}u$ (l)	813 (274)	1498 (892)	1576 (934)	232 (30)	290 (32)*
T (min)	1.6 (0.4)	157 (77)	210 (95)*	123 (20)	113 (17)*
MRT (min)	100**	172 (55)	215 (74)*	165 (24)	131 (15)*
fu (%)	5.1 (2.0)	4.5 (2 1)	6.6 (3.0)*	25.1 (4.6)	35 6 (4.5)*

CL, mean total body clearance; CLu, mean total body clearance of unbound drug, V^{ss}, volume of distribution at steady state; $V^{ss}u$, volume of distribution at steady state of unbound drug; T, slow washout half-life; MRT, mean residence time in body
* Significant enantiomeric difference
** Estimated

slow or terminal half-life of LAAs tends to be slightly greater after perineural administration than after intravenous infusion. This may be attributed to the prolongation of absorption actually regulating the plasma half-life. Although there are small differences between LAAs in pharmacokinetics after perineural administration, the broad pharmacokinetic profiles of the agents are similar for the same type of injection.

Lung uptake is a particular aspect of the pharmacokinetics of LAAs to have received attention. The lungs provide the first region containing drug-metabolizing cytochromes that are encountered by drug collecting in the right side of the heart. It is well recognized that the lungs can exert a modulatory effect on the time course of arterial drug concentrations. By their vast capillary network, the lungs impose a transit delay in drug movement from the right to the left side of the circulation; drug bases may have some additional degree of prolonged residence due to ion-trapping in relatively acidic lung water. The lung uptake of LAAs (and of other basic drugs such as opioids) has been described extensively using the method of "first pass" drug uptake, i.e. relative to an intravascular marker dye, or by direct determination of the non-steady-state extraction ratio between pulmonary artery and artery. The results indicate that the pulmonary extraction can be substantial but time dependent and not, as appears for opioids, directly related to lipophilicity but to the unbound fraction in plasma [55-58]. Thus, this extraction should not be confused with pulmonary drug clearance, which is irreversible drug loss from the circulation under steady-state conditions. The first pass drug uptake described is reversible loss down a concentration gradient and is recovered when the gradient is reversed. This also applies to prilocaine. No direct evidence of their substantially metabolizing LAAs (or opioids) in vivo has yet been found. Moreover, no differences have been found between enantiomers of racemic LAAs with respect to their disposition in the lungs [57].

Metabolism

Metabolites of LAAs may possess pharmacological activity but are not considered to be important mediators of either local anaesthetic actions or toxic side effects. It was pointed out above that ester-caines are metabolized by widely distributed esterases and this gives very high total body clearances along with small distribution volumes because drug does not get sufficient time for equilibration with tissues. However, the hydrolytic acid end p-aminobenzoate metabolites are more likely to be allergenic. The amino-alcohol end metabolites of ester-caines are pharmacologically interesting. Diethylaminoethanol from procaine and chloroprocaine is active as a local anaesthetic agent [59] and may have CNS actions [60], being a chemical homologue of the choline precursor dimethylaminoethanol. Amino acid end metabolites of amide-caines also have potential activity. Pipecolic acid metabolites from the mepivacaine/bupivacaine [61] may be involved with central lysine pathways [62].

Amide-caines are principally metabolized in the liver and much has been written about the impact of hepatic pathophysiology on the clearance of ligno-

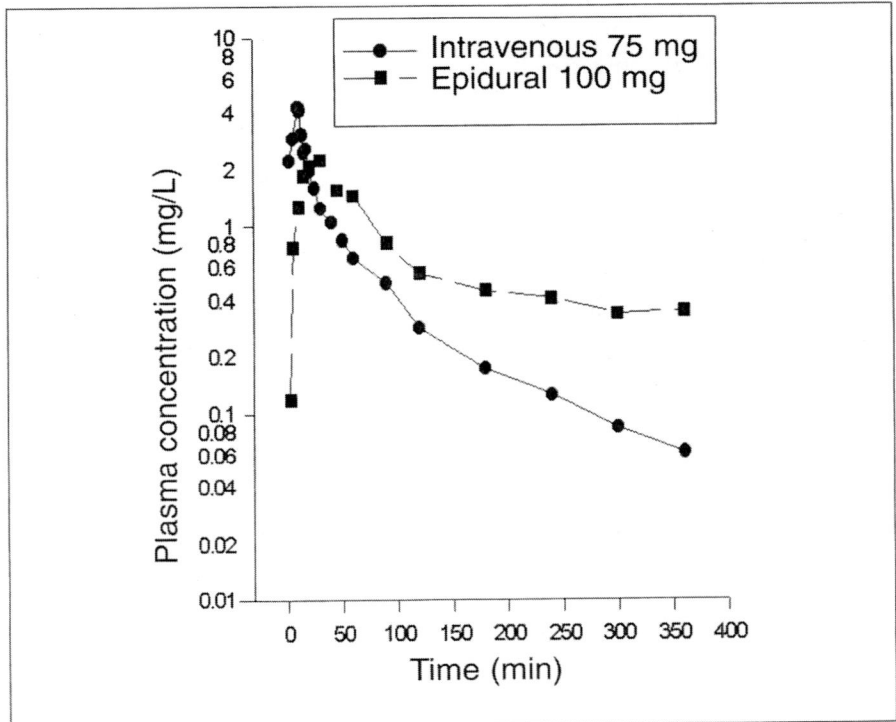

Fig. 5. A composite of the total arterial plasma rac-bupivacaine concentrations after intravenous administration of 75 mg over 10 min and epidural administration of 100 mg in a healthy volunteer subject on separate occasions. The washout half-life is longer after epidural administration because of continued slow absorption being the dominant feature

caine. Less is known about the impact of pathophysiology on the clearance of other amide-caines. Lignocaine has been most studied since its N-dealkylated metabolites that can be found in the circulation after neural blockade have been found to be antidysrhythmic. Bupivacaine and its congeners produce measurable quantities of N-dealkylated metabolites. However, varying extents of amide hydrolysis and aromatic hydroxylation produce the dominant metabolites in urine [4]. Metabolites of the racemic LAAs, all of which retain chirality, have not been subjected to a quantitative mass balance. As implied by the time course of effects, none of the metabolites are implicated in the toxicity resulting from accidental i.v. injection or rapid drug absorption although they may contribute to toxicity or other pharmacological effects upon prolonged administration.

Ropivacaine has been the most extensively studied of the LAAs [63, 64] since it was introduced only recently when sophisticated techniques for structural determination had become available. Like the other amide local anaesthetics, very little (ca 1%) ropivacaine is excreted unmetabolized into urine; most of the dose is metabolized oxidatively by hepatic enzymes and excreted into urine as N-dealkylated 2', 6'-pipecoloxylidide (PPX), aromatic hydroxylated 3'-hydroxyropiva-caine (3OHR) and 4'-hydroxyropivacaine (4OHR) [64]. Conjugated 3OHR is the main metabolite, accounting for 37% (average) of the dose with the total recovery of all metabolites at 86% (average) in urine and 9% (average) in faeces.

Conclusions

The history of local anaesthetic agents has been dominated by chemical attempts to decrease their toxicity and/or increase their duration of action. Overall, these have not materially improved the therapeutic index because the same chemical changes affect potency, duration and toxicity in parallel.

Neural blockade provides excellent surgical and/or emergency operating conditions and offers the possibility of the continuation of pain relief into the postoperative period. It is, however, an invasive procedure and the drugs used do have the potential for serious consequences should they be mistakenly injected intravascularly or be absorbed unexpectedly or too rapidly. Thus, a sound knowledge of the toxicological and pharmacokinetic characteristics of the drugs used is critical to minimizing the potential for morbidity. Although the newer agents such as ropivacaine and levobupivacaine provide a long duration with greater safety than their predecessors, this should not lead the anaesthesiologist into thinking that now we have safe long-acting LAAs. They are safer, not safe.

References

1   Braun H (1905) Uber einiger neue ortliche Anaesthetica (Stovain, Alypin, Novocain). Dtsch Klin Wochenschr 31·1667-1671
2.   Luduena FP (1969) Duration of local anaesthesia. Annu Rev Pharmacol 9:503-520
3.   Lofgren N (1948) Studies on local anaesthetics. Xylocaine: a new synthetic drug. PhD Thesis, University of Stockholm
4.   Tucker GT, Mather LE (1998) Properties, absorption and pharmacokinetics of local anaesthetics. In: Cousins MJ, Bridenbaugh PO (eds) Neural blockade in clinical anaesthesia. Lippincott-Raven, Philadelphia, pp 55-95
5.   Rosenberg PH, Kytta J, Alila A (1986) Absorption of bupivacaine, etidocaine, lignocaine and ropivacaine into n-heptane, rat sciatic nerve and human extradural and subcutaneous fat Br J Anaesth 58:310-314
6   Rutten AJ, Mather LE, McLean CF, Nancarrow C (1993) Tissue distribution of bupivacaine enantiomers in sheep Chirality 5:485-491
7.   Friberger P, Aberg G (1971) Some physicochemical properties of the racemates and the optically active isomers of two local anaesthetic compounds. Acta Pharm Suec 8:361-364
8.   Langerman L, Basinath M, Grant GJ (1994) The partition coefficient as a predictor of local anaesthetic potency for spinal anaesthesia: evaluation of five local anaesthetics in a mouse model. Anaesth Analg 79:490-494
9.   Bernards CM, Hill HF (1992) Physical and chemical properties of drug molecules governing their diffusion through the spinal meninges. Anaesthesiology 77.750-756

10. McEllistrem RF, Bennington RG, Roth SH (1993) In vitro determination of human dura mater permeability to opioids and local anaesthetics. Can J Anaesth 40:165-169
11. Mather LE, Rutten AJ (1991) Stereochemistry and its relevance in anaesthesiology. Curr Opin Anaesth 4:473-479
12. Lee-Son S, Wang GK, Concus A et al (1992) Stereoselective inhibition of neuronal sodium channels by local anaesthetics. Anaesthesiology 77:324-335
13. Reynolds F (1997) Does the left hand know what the right hand is doing – an appraisal of single enantiomer local anaesthetics? Int J Obstet Anaesth 6:257-269
14. Åkerman B, Persson H, Tegner C (1967) Local anaesthetic properties of the optically active isomers of prilocaine (Citanest). Acta Pharmacol Toxicol 25:233-241
15. Åberg G (1972) Toxicological and local anaesthetic effects of optically active isomers of two local anaesthetic compounds. Acta Pharmacol Toxicol 31:273-286
16. Mazoit JX, Boico O, Samii K (1993) Myocardial uptake of bupivacaine: II. Pharmacokinetics and pharmacodynamics of bupivacaine enantiomers in the isolated perfused rabbit heart. Anaesth Analg 77:477-482
17. Valenzuela C, Delpon E, Tamkun MM et al (1995) Stereoselective block of a human cardiac potassium channel (Kv1.5) by bupivacaine enantiomers. Biophys J 69:418-427
18 Huang YF, Pryor ME, Veering BT, Mather LE (1998) Cardiovascular and central nervous system effects of bupivacaine and levobupivacaine in sheep. Anaesth Analg 86:797-804
19. Mather LE, McCall P, McNicol PL (1995) Bupivacaine enantiomer pharmacokinetics after intercostal neural blockade in liver transplant patients. Anaesth Analg 80:328-335
20 Mather LE (1991) Disposition of mepivacaine and bupivacaine enantiomers in sheep. Br J Anaesth 67:239-246
21. Rutten AJ, Mather LE, McLean CF (1991) Cardiovascular effects and regional clearances of intravenous bupivacaine in sheep: enantiomeric analysis. Br J Anaesth 67:247-256
22 Akerman B, Hellberg IB, Trossvik C (1988) Primary evaluation of the local anaesthetic properties of the amino amide agent ropivacaine (LEA 103). Acta Anaesthesiol Scand 32:571-578
23. Markham A, Faulds D (1996) Ropivacaine – a review of its pharmacology and therapeutic use in regional anaesthesia. Drugs 52:429-449
24. Gristwood R, Bardsley H, Baker H et al (1994) Reduced cardiotoxicity of levobupivacaine compared with racemic bupivacaine (Marcaine): new clinical evidence. Exp Opin Invest Drugs 3.1209-1212
25. Cox CR, Faccenda KA, Gilhooly C et al (1998) Extradural S(–)-bupivacaine – comparison with racemic RS-bupivacaine. Br J Anaesth 80:289-293
26. Fyhr P, Hogstrom C (1988) A preformulation study of the kinetics of the racemization of ropivacaine hydrochloride. Acta Pharm Suec 25:121-132
27. Capogna G, Celleno D, Laudano D et al (1995) Alkalinization of local anaesthetics: which block, which local anaesthetic. Reg Anaesth 20.369-377
28 Langerman L, Grant GJ, Zakowski M et al (1992) Prolongation of epidural anaesthesia using a lipid drug carrier with procaine, lidocaine and tetracaine. Anaesth Analg 75:900-905
29. Boogaerts J, Declercq A, Lafont N et al (1993) Toxicity of bupivacaine encapsulated into liposomes and injected intravenously. comparison with plain solutions Anaesth Analg 76:553-555
30. Malinkovsky J-M, Bernard J-M, Le Corre P et al (1995) Motor and blood pressure effects of epidural sustained release bupivacaine from polymer microspheres a dose-response study in rabbits. Anaesth Analg 81.519-524
31 Jones JW, Davis AT (1993) Stability of bupivacaine hydrochloride in polypropylene syringes Am J Hosp Pharm 50 2364-2365

32. Rang HP, Ritchie JM (1968) On the electrogenic sodium pump in mammalian non-myelinated nerve fibers and its activation by various cations. J Physiol 196:183-221
33. Catterall WA (1988) Structure and function of voltage-sensitive ion channels. Science 242:50-61
34. Butterworth JF, Strichartz GR (1990) Molecular mechanisms of local anaesthesia: a review. Anaesthesiology 72:711-734
35. Strichartz GR (1998) Neural physiology and local anaesthetic action. In: Cousins MJ, Bridenbaugh PO (eds) Neural blockade in clinical anaesthesia. Lippincott-Raven, Philadelphia, pp 35-54
36. Olschewski A, Hempelmann G, Vogel W, Safronov BV (1998) Blockade of Na$^+$ and K$^+$ currents by local anaesthetics in the dorsal horn neurons of the spinal cord. Anaesthesiology 88:172-179
37. Arhem P, Frankenhaeuser B (1974) Local anaesthetics: effects on permeability properties of nodal membrane in myelinated nerve fibres from Xenopus. Acta Physiol Scand 91:11-21
38. Brau ME, Nau C, Hempelmann G, Vogel W (1995) Local anaesthetics potently block a potential insensitive potassium channel in myelinated nerve. J Gen Physiol 105:485-505
39. Mazoit JX, Cao LS, Samii K (1996) Binding of bupivacaine to human serum proteins, isolated albumin and isolated alpha-1-acid glycoprotein. Differences between the two enantiomers are partly due to cooperativity. J Pharmacol Exp Ther 276:109-115
40 Hirota K, Browne T, Appadu BL, Lambert DG (1997) Do local anaesthetics interact with dihydropyridine binding sites on neuronal L-type Ca^{2+} channels? Br J Anaesth 78:185-188
41. Carmeliet E, Morad M, Van der Heyden G, Vereecke J (1986) Electrophysiological effects of tetracaine in single guinea-pig ventricular myocytes. J Physiol 376:143-161
42. Oyama Y, Sadoshima J, Tokutomi N, Akaike N (1988) Some properties of inhibitory action of lidocaine on the Ca^{2+} current of single isolated frog sensory neurons. Brain Res 442:223-228
43. Sugiyama K, Muteki T (1994) Local anaesthetics depress the calcium current rat sensory neurons in culture. Anaesthesiology 80:1369-1378
44. Omote K, Iwasaki H, Kawamata M et al (1995) Effect of verapamil on spinal anaesthesia with local aesthetics. Anaesth Analg 80:444-448
45. Lynch C (1986) Depression of myocardial contractility in vitro by bupivacaine, etidocaine, and lidocaine Anaesth Analg 65:551-559
46. Li Y-M, Wingrove DE, Too HP et al (1995) Local anaesthetics inhibit substance P binding and evoked increases in intracellular Ca^{2+}. Anaesthesiology 82:166-172
47. Bolger GT, Marcus KA, Daly JW (1987) Local anaesthetics differentiate dihydropyridine calcium antagonist binding sites in rat brain and cardiac membranes. J Pharmacol Exp Ther 240:922-930
48. Rane SG, Holz GGIV, Dunlap K (1987) Dihydropyridine inhibition of neuronal calcium current and substance P release. Pflugers Arch 409:361-366
49. For AP, Nowycky MC, Tsien RW (1987) Kinetic and pharmacological properties distinguishing three types of calcium currents in chick sensory neurons. J Physiol 394:149-172
50. Emanuelson BM, Persson J, Sandin S, Alm C, Gustafsson LL (1997) Intraindividual and interindividual variability in the disposition of the local anaesthetic ropivacaine in healthy subjects. Ther Drug Monit 19:126-131
51. Burm AG, van der Meer AD, van Kleef JW et al (1994) Pharmacokinetics of the enantiomers of bupivacaine following intravenous administration of the racemate. Br J Clin Pharmacol 38:125-129
52. Burm AGL, Cohen IMC, van Kleef JW et al (1997) Pharmacokinetics of the enantiomers

of mepivacaine after intravenous administration of the racemate in volunteers. Anaesth Analg 84:85-89

53.   Tucker GT, Mather LE, Lennard MS, Gregory A (1990) Plasma concentrations of the stereoisomers of prilocaine after administration of the racemate: implications for toxicity? Br J Anaesth 65:333

54.   Veering BT, Burm AG, Vletter AA et al (1992) The effect of age on the systemic absorption, disposition and pharmacodynamics of bupivacaine after epidural administration. Clin Pharmacokinet 22:75-84

55.   Emanuelsson BMK, Persson J, Alm C et al (1997) Systemic absorption and block after epidural injection of ropivacaine in healthy volunteers. Anaesthesiology 87:1309-1317

56.   Kietzmann D, Foth H, Geng WP et al (1995) Transpulmonary disposition of prilocaine, mepivacaine, and bupivacaine in humans in the course of epidural anaesthesia. Acta Anaesthesiol Scand 39:885-890

57.   Sharrock N, Mather LE, Go G, Sculco TP (1998) Arterial and pulmonary arterial concentrations of the enantiomers of bupivacaine following epidural injection in elderly patients. Anaesth Analg 86:812-817

58.   Mather LE, Huang YF, Pryor ME, Veering BT (1998) Systemic and regional pharmacokinetics of bupivacaine and levobupivacaine in sheep. Anaesth Analg 86:805-811

59.   Butterworth JF IV, Lief PA, Strichartz GR (1988) The pH-dependent local anaesthetic activity of diethylaminoethanol, a procaine metabolite. Anaesthesiology 68:501-506

60.   Butterworth JF IV, Cole LR (1990) Low concentrations of procaine and diethylaminoethanol reduce the excitability but not the action potential amplitude of hippocampal pyramidal cells. Anaesth Analg 71:404-410

61.   Bruguerolle B, Attolini L, Gantenbein M (1994) Acute toxicity of bupivacaine metabolites in mice. Clin Exp Pharmacol Physiol 21:997-999

62.   Chang YF, Charles AK (1995) Uptake and metabolism of delta 1-piperidine-2-carboxylic acid by synaptosomes from rat cerebral cortex. Biochim Biophys Acta 1238:29-33

63.   Ekstrom G, Gunnarsson UB (1996) Ropivacaine, a new amide-type local anaesthetic agent, is metabolized by cytochromes p450 1a and 3a in human liver microsomes. Drug Metab Dispos 24:955-961

64   Halldin MM, Bredberg E, Angelin B et al (1996) Metabolism and excretion of ropivacaine in humans. Drug Metab Dispos 24:962-968

Chapter 8

Drug interactions and systemic toxicity

H. Adriaensen

The title of this contribution covers a large field of the pharmacological literature, and it is not easy to treat all aspects of the subject. Therefore we have defined the scope.

1. The starting point for the discussion will be the pharmacology of local anaesthetics (LA). The oral, parenteral or locoregional use of opioids, non-steroidal anti-inflammatory drugs, NMDA-antagonists, a_2 agonists or any other analgesic substances in the absence of LA will not be the subject of this paper.
2. Established techniques such as the combined use of LA with opioids will only be treated as far as new insights or innovative applications are concerned.

Hence, it is not our intention to conduct a meta-analysis or present a comprehensive review. We have chosen to search for data in the recent literature (Medline 1995-1998) and to focus on publications that triggered our intrest.

Although we were very impressed by the editorial "The systematic review: a good guide rather than a guarantee" [1], we fear that our review will not meet the criteria specified in that editorial: it will not be based on a complete review of the published material; it will not only refer to randomized controlled trials; and it will in some way reflect a personal viewpoint.

To justify such an approach we forward the following arguments:
- the title of this manuscript covers not one, but two subjects: drug interactions and systemic toxicity;
- we already restricted the field to LA but there are several LA a agents and many routes of administration, each leading to different drug interaction patterns and systemic toxicity problems;
- when searching the Medline with the key words "drug interactions", "systemic toxicity" or "adverse events" in combination with "local anaesthetics" (or local anaesthetics), or with one of the specific agents i.e. "lidocaine", "bupivacaine", "prilocaine", hundreds of abstracts are generated.

The poorly delineated subject, the heterogenicity of the drugs and the large amount of retrieved material are the reasons why we opted for a more eclectic discussion of the subject and for reporting mainly on papers thought to be clinically relevant or innovative: our aim is to update background knowledge and to furnish some additional information to the interested reader.

We have divided the paper into two parts:

- one part dealing with drug interactions, and including also some reflections on drug combinations, especially the use of LA in combination with clonidine;
- a second part reports on systemic toxicity of LA, with some specific data on ropivacaine and levobupivacaine.

Drug interactions

Drug-Drug Interaction is one factor among many others that may affect the therapeutic outcome of drug administration [2].

A potential drug interaction refers to the possibility that one drug may alter the intensity of the pharmacological effect of another drug given concurrently. The net result may be enhanced or diminished effects of one or both drugs, or the appearance of a new effect that is not seen with either drug alone.

Interactions may be either pharmacokinetic (i.e., alterations of absorption, distribution, biotransformation or excretion of one drug by another) or pharmacodynamic (i.e., drugs that interact at a common receptor site or that have additive or inhibitory effects due to actions at different sites in an organ). An additive, synergestic, potentiating or antagonizing action may be the final result [3].

Pharmacokinetic interactions

Several pharmacokinetic interactions of LA with commonly used drugs have been documented. One of the drugs most commonly used in connection with LA is 1/200 000 adrenalin added to the LA solution in order to increase the intensity of neural blockade, to prolong the action of the LA, and to decrease its absorption. Mazoit et al. [4] were able to show that, when epidurally administered, clonidine can also alter the pharmacokinetics of lidocaine: like adrenaline it may decrease lidocaine plasma peak concentrations (C_{max}), thus leading to a decreased toxicity.

Protein binding can also be affected. The use of oral contraceptives decreases the $\alpha 1$-acid glycoprotein, the fraction of plasma proteins that binds LA of the amide group [5]. Particularly bupivacaine and ropivacaine have a high protein-bound fraction.

A competitive binding of diazepam vs bupivacaine to plasma proteins with a larger free fraction of bupivacaine available for metabolism and elimination could explain the shorter half-life of bupivacaine under conditions of co-administration [6].

Drugs that decrease hepatic blood flow or enzymatic activity can decrease the clearance of the amide-type LA. Such an interaction has been described for propanolol [7] and cimetidine [8], when used in combination with lidocaine.

LA of the ester type agents (procaine-chloroprocaine and tetracaine) undergo biotransformation via hydrolysis by plasma pseudocholinesterases. An interaction with succinylcholine, inactivated by the same enzymes, has been decribed by Foldes et al. [9].

An interaction between monoamino oxidase inhibitors (isocarboxazid) and LA (with or without vasoconstrictors) was reported as being characterized by excessive CNS depression and resistance to the LA effects on peripheral nerves [10].

Pharmacodynamic interactions

The mechanisms by which LA act are reviewed by Strichartz and Ritchie [11]. LA have an effect on cell membrane excitability, mainly by blocking inward Na+ current. The receptor for LA is located inside the Na^+ channel. Besides the effect of LA on nerve conduction, they have also an effect on central nervous and cardiovascular functions.

The toxic action on the central nervous system (CNS) is related to an interference with inhibitory systems and can be antagonized by benzodiazpines, which is why diazepam or thiopentone are the drugs of choice for the treatment of CNS toxicity.

The toxic effect of LA on the cardiovascular system (CVS) is reflected by a decrease in myocardial contractility (translated into a negative inotropic effect) and by a slowing of impulse propagation (translated by dysrythmias), therefore LA may interfere with cardiovascular drugs with a negative effect on myocardial contractility or on electrical conduction. Drugs with an action on the heart such as β-blockers, calcium channel blockers, anti-arrythmic drugs (disopyramide, cibenzoline) and tricyclic antidepressants have all been reported to enhance LA cardiotoxicity [12].

LA have also ganglion-blocking properties. At the level of the neuromuscular junction, it has been shown that procaine and lidocaine can significantly enhance the action of both depolarizing and non-depolarizing blockers [13, 14].

The co-administration of LA with opioids has been one of the most noticed advances in locoregional anaesthesia (LRA). Especially in obstetrics and in postoperative analgesia, this drug combination has gained widespread use. Spinally applied LA act by blockade of axonal transmission, while opioids exert their effect by pre- and postsynaptic inhibition of signal transduction at the level of the dorsal horn. Both drugs act at the spinal level but by different mechanisms.

The combination of LA with clonidine and/or opioids has also been studied in depth. Courteix and coworkers [15] have shown that the systemic administration of clonidine on its own exerted an analgesic action in an animal model of diabetic neuropathy. In humans, De Kock et al. [16] described the use of epidural clonidine (bolus 2, 4, and 8 µg/kg; infusion 0.5, 1, and 2 µg/kg/per hour) as the sole agent during abdominal surgery. Escape medication was available to supplement clonidine if necessary. They described a dose-dependent analgesic effect with a success rate of 95% with the highest dosage, and a prolonged postoperative pain relief for ±6 h.

Rockemann et al. [17] cautioned about haemodynamic instability with the higher clonidine dosage of 8 µg/kg, administered epidurally.

Although clonidine has intrinsic analgesic properties, it is most often used in combination with LA, either mixed with an opioid or not. Such mixtures are reported to increase the analgesic quality of either component (faster onset, prolonged block, less rescue medication).

Many papers have been published on the association of clonidine to LA (most frequently bupivacaine). The route of administration of clonidine in these trials was not always the same and varied from systemic to different types of loco-regional applications.

Niemi [18] described the effects of intrathecal clonidine (3 µg/kg) on the duration of spinal anaesthesia with 0.5% bupivacaine (15 mg) for knee arthroscopy. He described a prolongation of the spinal block, but sedation and haemodynamic instability were the drawbacks of the technique.

Gentili and Bonnet [19] compared the combination bupivacaine-clonidine versus bupivacaine-morphine for spinal anaesthesia in patients undergoing hip surgery. They studied the incidence of bladder dysfunction and concluded that outcome was better with the bupivacaine-clonidine combination.

The combination bupivacaine-clonidine was also used in obstetrics by Cigarini et al. [20]. Transfer of clonidine through the placenta was documented, so that an effect on the foetus has to be taken into account.

When sufentanil 10 µg was added to the combination, a high incidence of foetal heart tracing abnormalities were observed. The dose of clonidine used in this trial was 100 µg or 150 µg [21].

Apart from epidural and spinal applications, clonidine has been combined with LA and/or opioids for several other locoregional blocks: for instance, for retrobulbar block for cataract surgery, where 2 µg/kg clonidine was used in combination with 2% lidocaine [22]. When compared to the control group receiving 2% lidocaine with saline, the block was not only prolonged from 128 to 241 min, but also a large decrease in intraocular pressure (from 13.5 to 7.7 mmHg), a small decrease in blood pressure and some sedation were observed.

Intravenous regional anaesthesia with 30 ml prilocaine 1% and 150 µg clonidine was described by Hoffmann et al. [23]. They described some residual analgesia after deflation of the tourniquet.

The use of clonidine (30, 90, or 300 µg) in combination with lidocaine (400 mg) for brachial plexus block was described by Bernard and Marcaire [24]. With the largest dose of clonidine (300 µg) they had serious hypotensive responses and a drop in SaO_2 below 90%. With the lowest dose (30 µg) they had a faster onset and a prolonged postoperative analgesia when compared to the control group.

Singeljn et al. [25] used a continuous popliteal sciatic nerve block for postoperative analgesia after foot surgery. When 1 µg/ml clonidine was added to the anaesthetic solution (bupivacaine 0.125% and sufentanil 0.1 µg/ml) the request for rescue analgesic medication was reduced.

The use of clonidine in epidural and caudal blocks for paediatric surgery has also been reported to improve and prolong analgesia into the postoperative period. In cases where up to 5 μg/kg clonidine was used bradycardia was recorded as an unwanted side effect [26-29].

When clonidine (150 μg) was added to 0.25% bupivacaine in order to prolong analgesia after wound infiltration in surgery for inguinal hernia repair, no prolonged action could be documented when compared to plain 0.25% bupivacaine [30].

Systemic toxicity

The toxicity of LA can be divided into three categories:
1. contact toxicity, as seen whith continuous spinal anaesthesia through thin spinal catheters: prolonged contact of nerve roots with locally accumulated lidocaine in higher concentration is thought to be responsible for eventual neural damage;
2. allergic phenomena, more common with the ester-type than with the amide type LA, and in some cases more likely to be caused by the preservative added as a stabilizer to the LA solution than by the LA itself;
3. systemic toxicity, frequently due to accidental intravascular injection or to overdose.

Our focus of interest is systemic toxicity, which is characterized by alterations of CNS or CVS function caused by intrinsic action of LA on these systems.

CNS toxicity starts with restlessness, visual and auditory disturbances, numbness of the lips or the tongue, light-headedness or a metallic taste in the mouth. If further muscle twitching occurs, this may progress towards convulsions and coma. CNS toxicity generally precedes CVS toxicity, with an exception made for bupivacaine.

CVS toxicity has three aspects: an effect on myocardial contractility, an impact on conduction and an effect on vascular smooth muscle.

A relationship exists between anaesthetic potency and the dose of LA necessary to induce signs of toxicity. In this respect bupivacaine has a lower safety margin than lidocaine.

Most LA are a racemic mixture of R(−) and S(+) enantiomers with different pharmacokinetic properties and differences in systemic toxicity.

The introduction of ropivacaine and/of the S(+) enantiomer of bupivacaine, levobupivacaine has renewed interest in the toxicity issue.

Huang and coworkers [31] compared the CNS and CVS effects of levobupivacaine and bupivacaine enantiomers in sheep. The negative inotropic effect was simular for both drugs, while convulsions occurred at a lower dose with bupivacaine than with levobupivacaine.

These pharmacodynamic findings were matched by a pharmacokinetic study by the same group showing that mean brain concentrations of 0.2%-1% dose were reached earlier after administration of bupivacaine than after levobupivacaine [32]. They conclude that levobupivacaine may offer a greater safety margin than bupivacaine.

The toxicity profile of ropivacaine, which is also a S(+) enantiomer and chemically related to bupivacaine, has been studied in comparison to bupivacaine. An interesting review was presented by Cuvillon et al. [33] at the last meeting of the JEPU in Paris in 1998.

Several authors have studied the toxicity profile of ropivacaine in vitro and in animal experiments. Their results suggest a lower cardiotoxicity of ropivacaine. In the isolated and perfused heart, Moller and Covino [34] have shown that myocardial contractility as well as conduction of the Purkinje fibres were less depressed by ropivacaine than by bupivacaine.

Knudsen et al. [35] administered bupivacaine vs ropivacaine intravenously in progessively increasing doses in human volunteers. The doses at which CNS and CVS toxicity occurred were higher for ropivacaine than for bupivacaine.

This suggest that the safety margin of ropivacaine is larger than that of bupivacaine and explains why its obstetrical use is now being explored [36].

Conclusions

The expansion of locoregional techniques in anaesthesia has stimulated interest in the pharmacology of LA. Drug interactions and toxicity profiles have become better documented and add to the safety of daily practice.

References

1. Crombie IK, McQuay HJ (1998) The systematic review: a good guide rather than a guarantee. Pain 76:1-2
2. Nies AS, Spielberg SP (1996) Principles of therapeutics. In: Hardman JG, Limbird LE, Molinoff PB, Ruddon RW (eds) Goodman & Gilman's: the pharmacological basis of therapeutics, 9th edn. Mc Graw-Hill, New York, pp 43-62
3. Klaassen CD, (1996) Principles of toxicology and treatment of poisoning. In: Hardman JG, Limbird LE, Molinoff PB, Ruddon RW (eds) Goodman & Gilman's: the pharmacological basis of therapeutics, 9th edn. Mc Graw-Hill, New York, pp 63-76
4. Mazoit SX, Benhamou D, Veilette Y, Samii K (1996) Clonidine and/or adrenaline decrease lignocaine plasma peak concentrations after epidural administration. Br J Clin Pharmacol 42(2):242-245
5. Ferrante FM (1998) Pharmacology of local anaesthetics. In: Longnecker DE, Thinker JH, Morgan GE (eds) Principles and practise of anaesthesiology, 2nd ed. Mosby, St Louis, p 1342
6. Giasi RM, D'Agostino E, Covino BG (1980) Interaction of diazepam and epidurally administered local anaesthetic agents. Reg Anaesth 5:8-11
7. Ochs HR, Carstens G, Greenblatt DJ (1980) Reduction in lidocaine clearance during continuous infusion and co-administration of propanolol. N Engl J Med 303:373-377
8. Feely J, Wilkinson GR, Mc Allister CR et al (1982) Increased toxicity and reduced clearance of lidocaine by cimetidine. Am J Intern Med 96:592-594
9. Foldes FF, Foldes VM, Smith JC et al (1963) The realation between plasma cholinesterase and prolonged apnea caused by succinylcholine. Anaesthesiology 24:208-210

10. Mueller RA, Lundberg DBA (1992) Manual of drug interactions for anaesthesiology, 2nd edn. Churchill Livingstone, New York, p 202

11. Strichartz GR, Ritchie JM (1987) The action of local anaesthetics on ion channels of excitable tissues. In: Strichartz GR (ed) Local anaesthetics. Springer-Verlag, Berlin Heidelberg New York, pp 22-52

12 Bruelle P, Cuvillon P, Viel E, Eledjam JJ (1998) Quand et à qui ne faut-il pas proposer une anaesthésie locorégionale? Nouvelles Techniques en Anaesthésie Locorégionale JEPU. CRI St-Germain-en-Laye, pp 1-16

13. Katz, Gissen (1969) Effects of intravenous and intra-arterial procaine and lidocaine on neuromuscular transmission in man. Acta Anaesthesiol Scand Suppl 1(36):103-113

14. Hirst GDS, Wood D (1971) On the neuromuscular paralysis produced by procaine. Br J Pharmacol 41:94-104

15. Courteix C, Bardin M, Chantelauze C, Lavarenne J, Eschalier A (1994) Study of the sensitivity of the diabetes-induced pain model in rats to a range of analgesics. Pain 57(2):153-160

16. De Kock M, Wiederkher P, Laghmiche A, Scholtes JL (1997) Epidural clonidine used as the sole analgesic agent during and after abdominal surgery. A dose-response study. Anaesthesiology 86(2):285-292

17. Rockemann MG, Brinkmann A, Goertz A, Seeling W, Georgieff M (1994) Analgesia and hemodynamics under 8 μg/kg clonidine for pain therapy following major abdominal surgery. Anaesthesiol Intensiv Med Notfallmed Schmerz Ther 29(2):96-101

18. Niemi L (1994) Effects of intrathecal clonidine on duration of bupivacaine spinal anaesthesia, haemodynamics, and postoperative analgesia in patient undergoing knee arthroscopy. Acta Anaesthesiol Scand 38(7):724-728

19. Gentili M, Bonnet F (1996) Spinal clonidine produces less urinary retention than spinal morphine. Br J Anaesth 76(6):872-873

20. Cigarini I, Kaba A, Bonnet F, Brohon E, Dutz F, Damas F, Hans P (1995) Epidural clonidine combined with bupivacaine for analgesia in labor. Effects on mother and neonate. Reg Anaesth 20(2):113-120

21. Chassard D, Mathon L, Dailler F, Golfier F, Tournadre JP, Bouletreau P (1996) Extradural clonidine combined with sufentanil and 0.0625% bupivacaine for analgesia in labour. Br J Anaesth 77(4):458-462

22. Msahed K, El Harrar N, Hamdani M, Amraoui M, Benaguida M (1996) Lidocaine-clonidine retrobulbar block for cataract surgery in the eldery. Reg Anaesth 21(6):569-575

23. Hoffmann V, Vercauteren M, Van Steenberge A, Adriaensen H (1997) Intravenous regional anaesthesia. Evaluation of 4 different additives to prilocaine. Acta Anaesthesiol 48(2):71-76

24. Bernard SM, Marcaire P (1997) Dose-range effects of clonidine added to lidocaine for brachial plexus block. Anaesthesiology 87(2):277-284

25. Singelijn FJ, Ayr F, Gouverneur JM (1997) Continuous popliteal sciatic nerve block: an original technique to provide postoperative analgesia after foot surgery. Anaesth Analg 84(2):383-386

26 Motsch J, Bottiger BW, Bach A, Bohrer H, Skoberne T, Martin E (1997) Caudal clonidine and bupivacaine for combined epidural and general anaesthesia in children. Acta Anaesthesiol Scand 41(7):877-883

27. Jamali S, Monin S, Begon C, Dubousset AM, Ecoffey C (1994) Clonidine in pediatric caudal anaesthesia. Anaesth Analg 78(4):663-666

28. Lee JJ, Rubin AP (1994) Comparison of a bupivacaine-clonidine mixture with plain bupivacaine for caudal analgesia in children. Br J Anaesth 72(3):258-262

29. Cook B, Grubb DJ, Aldridge LA, Doyle E (1995) Comparison of the effects of adrenaline, clonidine and ketamine on the duration of caudal analgesia produced by bupivacaine in children Br J Anaesth 75:698-701
30. Elliott S, Eckersall S, Figelstone L, Jothilingam S (1997) Does the addition of clonidine affect duration of analgesia of bupivacaine wound infiltration in inguinal hernia repair? Br J Anaesth 79(4):446-449
31. Huang YF, Pryor ME, Mather LE, Veering BT (1998) Cardiovascular and central nervous system effects of intravenous levobupivacaine and bupivacaine in sheep Anaesth Analg 86(4):797-804
32. Mather LE, Huang YF, Veering B, Pryor ME (1998) Systemic and regional pharmacokinetics of levobupivacaine and bupivacaine enantiomers in sheep. Anaesth Analg 86(4):805-811
33. Cuvillon P, L'Hermite E, Viel E, De La Coussaye JE, Eledjam JJ (1998) Cardiotoxicité des anaesthésiques locaux: quoi de neuf? Nouvelles techniques en anaesthésie locorégionale (JEPU). CRI, St Germain-en Laye, pp 29-38
34 Muller RA, Covino BG (1990) Cardiac electrophysiologic properties of bupivacaine and lidocaine compared with those of ropivacaine, a new amide local anaesthetic Anaesthesiology 72:322-329
35. Knudsen K, Beckman SM, Blomberg SS, Edvardson N (1997) Central nervous and cardiovascular effects of i.v. infusion of ropivacaine, bupivacaine and placebo in volunteers. Br J Anaesth 78:507-514
36. Brichant JF, Hans P (1998) La ropivacaine pour l'anaesthésie et l'analgésie obstétricale· l'avenir? Nouvelles tecniques en anaesthésie locorégionale (JEPU). CRI, Saint Germain-en-Laye, pp 39-48

Chapter 9

Placental transfer of pharmacological agents

E. Margaria, I. Castelletti, P. Petruzzelli

The placenta acts as an interface between maternal and fetal circulations. It transmits biological substances essential for fetal growth and development. Drugs cross the placenta by diffusing at varying rates, depending on their physical and chemical properties. Nonionized particles cross more rapidly than ions and small molecules more rapidly than large ones.

Drugs administered to mothers have the potential to cross the placenta and reach the fetus. Under certain circumstances, the comparison of the drug concentration in the maternal and fetal plasma may give an idea of the exposure of the fetus to maternally administered drugs [2].

Several drugs rapidly cross the placenta and pharmacologically significant concentrations equilibrate in maternal and fetal plasma. Their transfer is termed "complete". Other drugs cross the placenta incompletely, and their concentrations are lower in fetal than in maternal plasma. The majority of drugs fit into one of these two groups. A limited number of drugs reach greater concentrations in fetal than maternal plasma. These drugs have an "exceeding" transfer.

However, a careful analysis of the literature suggests that all drugs cross the placenta, although the extent varies considerably.

The amount of a drug that actually reaches the fetus depends upon:

1. dose and route of administration to the mother;
2. amount of free drug in the mother's serum;
3. amount of protein binding – the extent of drug binding to plasma protein has limited influence on the type of drug transfer across the human placenta;
4. molecular weight – drugs with a molecular weight greater than 500 have an incomplete transfer;
5. hydrosolubility – the molecular weight limit of hydrophilic drugs is 100;
6. lipid solubility – for lipid-soluble drugs, transfer occurs easily up to a molecular weight of 600;
7. concentration of nonionized free drug – strongly dissociated acid drug molecules should have an incomplete transfer, but this does not seem to be an absolute rule. For example, ampicillin and methicillin transfer completely and they are strongly dissociated at physiological pH;
8. uterine blood flow;
9. hypoxia and hypercapnia;

10. the pKa (pH at which the drug is 50% ionized).

Placental transfer of glucose and some other carbohydrates occurs via facilitated diffusion, transfer via a membrane-bound carrier at rates significantly greater than would occur via simple diffusion. Transfer is still down a physicochemical gradient, so that fetal plasma glucose levels are lower than in the mother. It is important to note that with maternal/fetal exchange of nutrient molecules (i.e., carbohydrates, lipids, amino acids), the placenta does not function simply as an organ of transfer, but rather also is a significant consumer and/or converter of these compounds.

The term permeability is used to denote the number of molecules of a given solute that cross a defined area of a membrane during a defined time period under the conditions of a known concentration difference across the membrane [1]. Permeability coefficients have the dimensions of a velocity and if the concentration of the solute is given in moles per milliliter, the area of the membrane in square centimeters and the time of transfer in seconds, then the unit of permeability would be centimeters per second.

When dealing with a whole organ such as the placenta, the unit area available for transport is usually not known. Therefore, the term permeability is derived from the number of molecules that transfer per unit time per unit concentration difference, and it has the dimensions of milliliters per second.

In measurements of solute concentrations across complex organs such as the placenta, it is difficult to estimate the true concentration difference because only inflow (arterial) and outflow (venous) samples are available for measurement. The term placental clearance has been used to define the number of molecules that are transferred per unit of time divided by the concentration difference between the maternal uterine artery and the fetal umbilical artery. As for respiratory gas, instead of moles per milliliter, the concentration differences across the placental are expressed as partial pressure, with units of millimeters of mercury and the amount transferred per unit time, given as milliliters per minute.

Methodologies in the in vivo study of placental transport

The amount of solute transferred can be measured by application of the Fick's law of diffusion:

$$Q/t = K (A(Cm - Cf)/D)$$

where Q/t is the rate of diffusion (quantity per unit time), A is the surface area, Cm is the maternal and Cf the fetal concentration, D is the thickness of the membrane, and K the diffusion constant of the drug.

The major potential limitation of this approach is that not all uterine blood flow is placental blood flow. The Fick principle applied to placental transfer also assumes that the solute under study is not metabolized or otherwise sequestered in the placenta itself, as occurs for nutrients such as glucose. To determine the amount of metabolized solutes tranferred to the fetus, the Fick principle must be

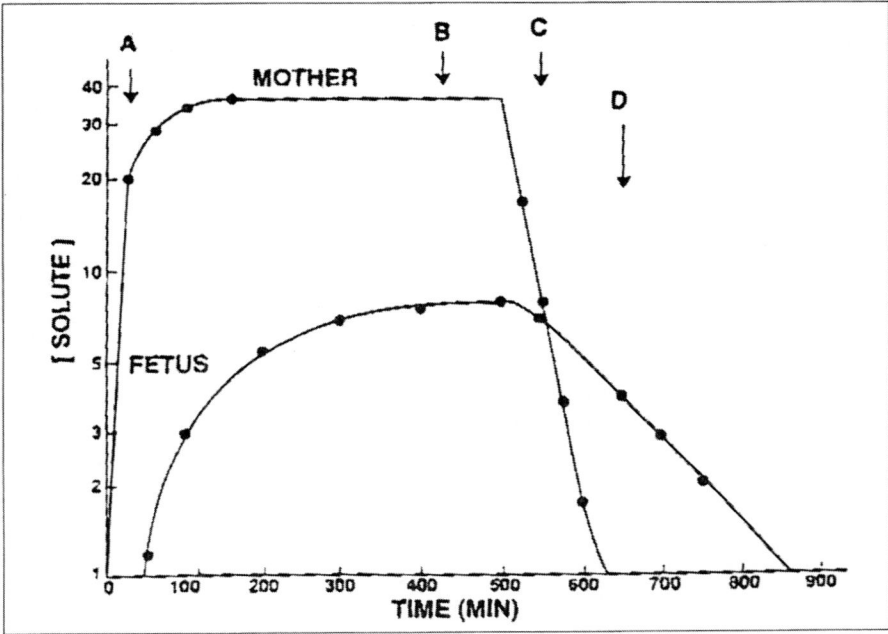

Fig. 1. Relationship of sampling time to interpretation or maternal-fetal transport across the placenta. Hypothetical data shown for a solute which in the steady state has a relatively low placental transport. Single samples at time A in maternal and fetal blood umbilical cord blood at delivery would lead to the conclusion that the placenta is impermeable to this solute. Sampling at point B would lead to the proper interpretation that the solute is relatively permeable and fetal levels are about one-fourth of those in the mother at steady state conditions (note log scale of the Y-axis). Blood obtained at point C would lead to the conclusion that the placenta is freely permeable to the solute, and sampling at point D would be interpreted as evidence for active transport from mother to fetus. (From [11])

applied to the concentration difference between the umbilical vein and artery and umbilical blood flow.

An attempt is often made to estimate placental transport from single samples taken from the mother and from cord blood. The results are then expressed as a percentage of the maternal level and inferences made concerning the effectiveness of transfer across the placenta. Substances in which the fetal concentration is a significant percentage of the maternal one are considered to be transferred efficiently (Fig. 1).

The four most prioritized organs for distribution are the brain, the heart, the kidney and the liver/placenta. Because the brain acts essentially as a lipid barrier, the drug entry rate is determined by its lipid solubility and unionization ratio; there is an increase in the blood – brain barrier permeability in neonates. Protein binding also decreases a drug's permeability to the blood – brain barrier because the large protein molecules do not pass readily; permeability to drugs is also increased with conditions of hypoxia and or hypercarbia.

Anaesthesiologic implications

The placenta transmits most anaesthetic drugs to the fetus, because most have low molecular weights, low ionization and high lipid solubility. According to the Fick equation, it is readily apparent that the primary determinant of the numerator, other than surface area of membrane for diffusion, is the concentration of the drug in the maternal compartment. This concentration is directly controlled by the anaesthesiologist, who determines both the amount of drug given and the rate at which that given amount is administered.

General anaesthesia

In *preanaesthesia* usually parasympaticolitic plus sedative drugs are given. Atropine can cross the placenta and induce fetal tachycardıa. Benzodiazepine reaches greater concentrations in fetal than maternal plasma, so, also due to their slow metabolism, they are rejected in obstetric anaesthesia until the fetus is in the uterus. The best drug that can be given is prometazina, which combines sedative and anthistaminic properties.

Induction

Both barbiturate and propofol cross the placenta within a different time. Finally, the definitive work of a clinical study confirmed that barbiturate transfer is almost instantaneous and, in fact, that barbiturate levels peak by 3-5 minutes and are low again by 6-8 minutes. Propofol is not allowed in Italy for obstetric anaesthesia; nevertheless its advantages, because of some questions, were raised about neonatal adaptive scores (NACS), due to its important placental passage.

Mainteinance

All inalation anaesthetics traverse the placental barrier with ease. The transfer is due to their diffusion capability, their high fat solubility, and their low molecular weight. It is still a common practice today to use N_2O/O_2 analgesia or anaesthesia at the time of delivery. It is known that N_2O transfer is about 90% (SD=6%) when the maternofetal flow ratio is 2 and about 75% (SD=13%) when the ratio is 1.

Both isoflurane and halothane (halogenated anaesthetics) are present in the earliest fetal blood samples, suggesting rapid placental passage [5]. The new methyl-ethyl ethers desflurane and sevoflurane presently not used in obstetrics could be especially beneficial agents.

Opioids

A drug that has gained enormous popularity is fentanyl. Its placental transfer is intermediate between meperidine and bupivacaine. Maternal levels remain 2.5 times greater than fetal levels and declined similarly during the degradation phase. Fentanyl is the drug used most in the obstetric management of the first stage of labor [5]. Sufentanil [6] crosses the placenta rapidly at a rate two-thirds that of the transfer marker antipyrine; it increases linearly with the maternal concentration (r=0.999).

Muscle-paralyzing drugs

Suxamethonium chloride does not cross the placenta. Pancuronium, vecuronium, atracurium, used for muscle relaxation in cesarean section, have an umbilical venous to maternal venous ratio of about 0.22, but this value increases with prolongation of the incision to delivery interval. Neonatal depression associated with this drug is rare.

Loco regional anaesthesia

All local anaesthetics readily cross the placenta. Thus, it becomes critically important to understand the factors that influence the amount and rate of drug transferred from the maternal circulation to the fetus. The transfer of the local anaesthetic from the mother to the fetus via the placenta is influenced by factors specific to each. Once the drug reaches the intervillous space, the quantity of local anaesthetic transferred per unit of time is given by this equation:

$$Q/t = A\ (C1\text{-}C2)\ k\ D\text{-}1$$

where the quantity diffusing per unit of time (Q/t) depends upon the thickness (D) and surface area (A) of the membrane, the concentration gradient of the substance (free, unbound drug in the case of local anaesthetic) from one side to the other (C1-C2), and a diffusion costant (k) for each substance that is related to the physicochemical properties of the drug, including molecular weight, extent of ionization, and lipid solubility.

Bupivacaine is confirmed to have fast systemic absorption and rapid elimination, and may be used without risk of acute toxicity both in mother and child, even at a 0.375% concentration [3].

The new drug ropivacaine [10], with less cardiocirculatory toxicity, is now at first place in obstetric anaesthesia at 0.1% for labor and 0.75% for cesarean section.

References

1   Bonica JJ, Mc Donald JS (1995) Principles and practice of obstetric analgesia and anaesthesia. Williams and Wilkins, Baltimore, pp 176-186
2   Pacifici GM, Nottoli R (1995) Placental transfer of drugs administered to the mother Clin Pharmacokinet 28 235-269

3   Decocq G, Brazier M, Hary L, Hubau C, Fortaine MR, Gondry J, Andrejak M (1997) Fundam Clin Pharmacol 11:365-370

4.   Kaneko T, Iwama H, Tobishima S, Watanabe K, Komatsu T, Tacheichi K, Tase C (1997) Placental transfer of vecuronium administered with priming principle regimen in patients undergoing Caesarian section JPEN J Anaesthesiol 46:750-754

5.   Fernando R, Bonello E, Gill P, Urquhart J, Reynolds F, Morgan B (1997) Neonatal welfare and placental transfer of fentanyl and bupivacaine during ambulatory combined spinal-epidural analgesia for labour. Anaesthesia 52:517-524

6.   Johnson RF, Herman N, Arney TL, Johnson HV, Paschall RL, Downing JW (1997) The placental transfer of sufentanil: effects of fetal pH, protein binding, and sufentanil concentration. Anaesth Analg 84:1262-1268

Chapter 10

Clinical perspectives of cholecystokinin antagonists in pain management

M. Amanzio, F. Benedetti

Cholecystokinin in the nervous system

Cholecystokinin (CCK) is a peptide widely distributed in the central nervous system. Since its characterization in the porcine intestine, evidence has accumulated that it plays an essential role in several brain functions such as nociception, anxiety, memory, sleep and dopamine modulation. In mammalian brain, CCK is mainly found as an octapeptide (CCK-8) and tetrapeptide (CCK-4) and its effects are mediated by two types of receptors: CCK-A and CCK-B [1, 2]. CCK-8 acts at both receptors whereas CCK-4 shows its main activity at the CCK-B receptors. The distribution of the type-A and type-B receptors shows species differences and this fact has important clinical implications [3]. For example, CCK-B binding sites are predominant in the spinal cord of rodents whereas CCK-A receptors prevail in the spinal cord of primates and humans. Therefore, the original nomenclature of peripheral alimentary (type A) and brain (type B) receptors no longer holds. It should be pointed out that, whereas the gene *cckA* encodes for the CCK-A receptor, the gene * cckB* encodes for both the CCK-B and gastrin receptor, thus indicating that the type-B binding site is better defined as CCK-B-gastrin receptor.

The distribution of CCK and its receptors in the brain matches that of the opioid peptides at the spinal and supraspinal level [4-6], and several lines of evidence indicate that CCK acts as an anti-opioid peptide. For example, CCK has been reported to inhibit analgesia induced by morphine [7] and β-endorphin [8]. In addition, it has been shown that, after peripheral nerve damage, an increase of spinal CCK is associated with a reduction in the analgesic effectiveness of morphine [9]. The mechanisms of the anti-opioid action of CCK have been unraveled only in part. The CCK receptors occupy both the pre- and post-synaptic regions of the primary afferent fibers (C fibers), mirroring the opioid receptor distribution in the spinal cord [10, 11]. Opioids probably interact with CCK at both the spinal and supraspinal levels [12]. At least two mechanisms appear to be involved. First, the presynaptic CCK receptors may induce the mobilization of Ca^{2+} from the intracellular stores [13] (Fig. 1a). This Ca^{2+} increase antagonizes the Ca^{2+} reduction caused by the opioid agonists, which represents the basis for opioid reduction of transmitter release [14]. Second, CCKergic neurons may antagonize opioidergic neurons (Fig. 1b), such that CCK has excitatory effects, whereas opioids have inhibitory effects [12]. Another possible

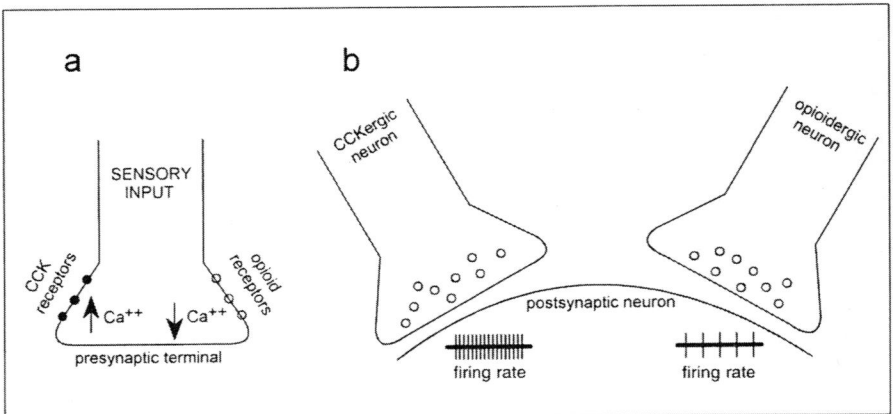

Fig. 1a,b. Mechanisms of the antagonism between endogenous opioids and endogenous cholecystokinin (CCK) at the presynaptic (a) and postsynaptic (b) level

mechanism is represented by the inhibition of enkephalin release by CCK [15, 16].

Taking all these considerations into account, the use of CCK antagonists in pain management has received particular attention. In fact, the blockade of CCK receptors by specific CCK antagonists results in the potentiation of opioid analgesia and thus in the reduction of opioid intake.

Cholecystokinin antagonists

Most of our knowledge about pain modulation by CCK comes from the use of CCK antagonists [1]. Several antagonists have been developed in past years, and, recently, highly specific receptor antagonists have been synthetized. Although Figure 2 shows four CCK antagonists widely used in pain research, it should be pointed out that numerous antagonists have been tested. Proglumide is a glutamic acid-based antagonist and was one of the first CCK antagonists used in pain research; however, its low specificity for type-A ($IC_{50}=6.3\times10^{-3}$ M) and type-B ($IC_{50}=1.1\times10^{-2}$ M) receptors poses some limitations. The binding affinity is expressed here as IC_{50}, that is, the concentration required to inhibit by 50% the specific binding of ^{125}I-Bolton-Hunter CCK-8. By contrast, the benzodiazepine-based antagonist devazepide (or L-364718) is highly specific for CCK-A receptors ($IC_{50}=0.08$ nM for CCK-A and 270 nM for CCK-B), whereas the benzodiazepine based antagonist L-365260 ($IC_{50}=2$ nM for CCK-B and 280 nM for CCK-A) and the peptoid antagonist CI-988 (also PD134308) ($IC_{50}=1.7$ nM for CCK-B and 4300 nM for CCK-A) are highly specific for CCK-B binding sites. In conclusion, several specific antagonists are available to block selectively CCK-A and CCK-B receptors.

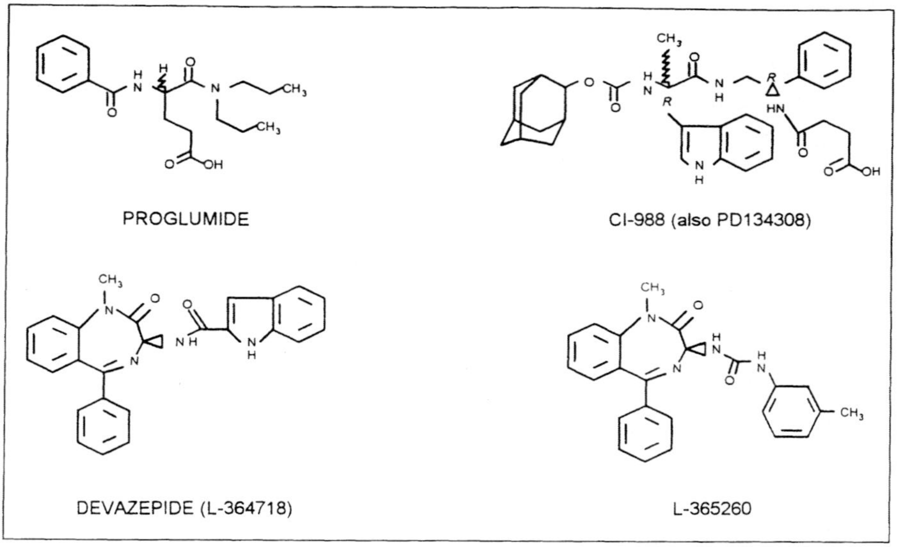

Fig. 2. Structural formula of 4 widely used CCK antagonists in pain research

Cholecystokinin antagonists potentiate endogenous opioids

Cholecystokinin antagonists per se are not analgesic drugs since their administration in some painful conditions does not relieve pain. However, CCK antagonists can potentiate analgesia induced by procedures that activate endogenous opioid systems [3]. In other words, CCK antagonists appear to produce their potentiating effects only when endogenous opioids are activated. This notion comes from several studies showing the antagonism between endogenous opioids and endogenous CCK. For example, early studies with proglumide and the CCK-A receptor antagonist devazepide showed a potentiation of endogenous opioid-induced antinociception. In the first case, proglumide was reported to enhance endogenous opioid analgesia induced by front-paw shock in the rat [17] (Fig. 3a), whereas in the second case, devazepide was found to enhance endogenous opioid-mediated analgesia induced in the rat by restraint stress [18]. However, recent studies with specific CCK-B antagonists indicate that potentiation of endogenous opioids occurs through the blockade of the CCK-B receptor in rodents. Figure 3b,c shows two examples. In the first case, the CCK-B antagonist CI-988 was administered to rats with chronic allodynia induced by spinal cord injury. This treatment produced an increase in pain thresholds, an effect that was reversed by naloxone [19]. In the second case, antinociceptive effects were induced by means of the inhibitor of the enkephalin-degrading enzyme RB-101. Such effects were potentiated by CCK-B antagonists such as CI-988 and L-365260 [20]. Further evidence of the antagonism between endogenous CCK and endogenous opioids comes from two recent studies. In the first study

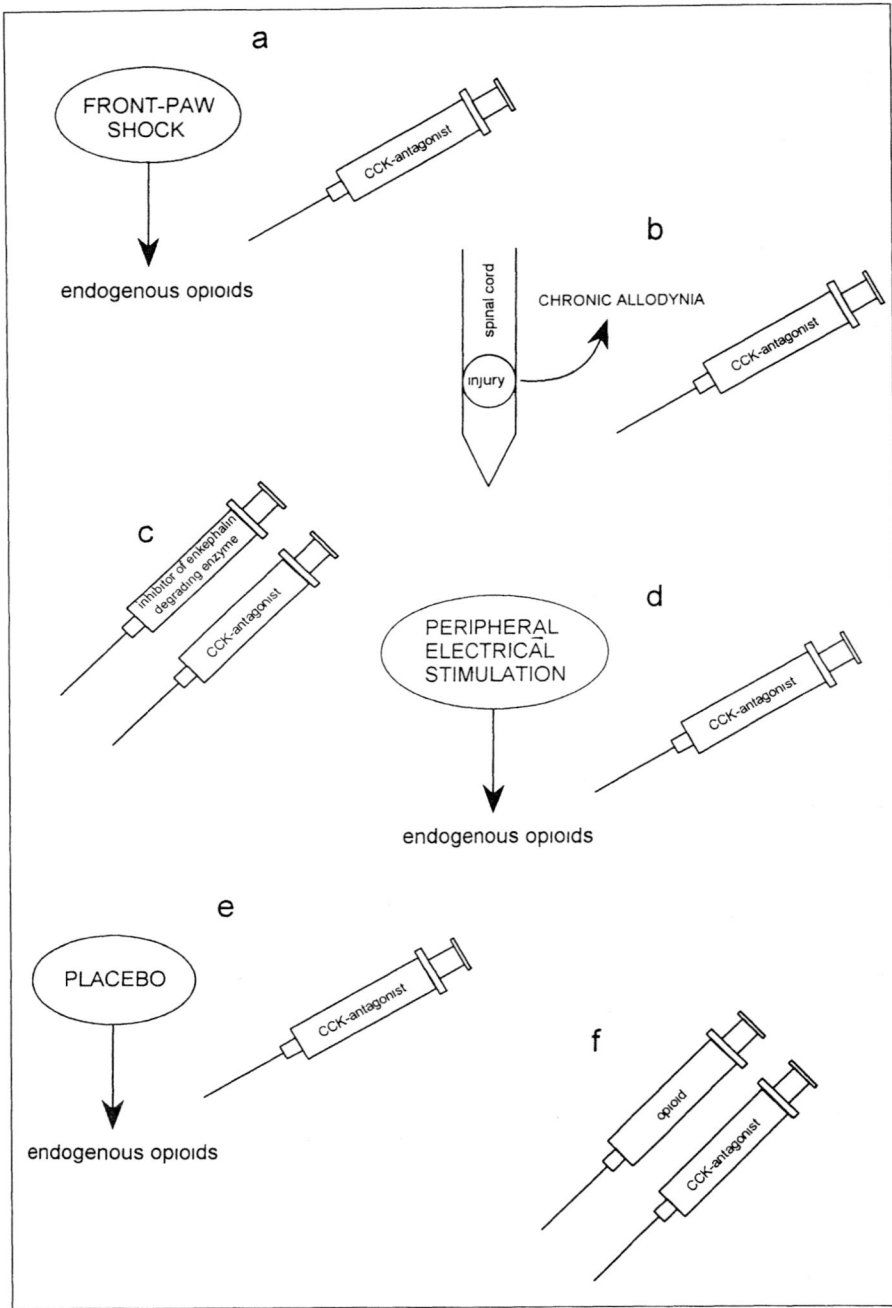

Fig. 3a-f. Different procedures to induce opioid potentiation by CCK antagonists Whereas in a-e CCK antagonists potentiate endogenous opioids, in (f) a CCK antagonist enhances a coadministered opioid (i.e., morphine)

(Fig. 3d), it was shown that the CCK-B antagonist L-365260 is capable of enhancing electrical stimulation-induced analgesia in the rat, which is known to be mediated by endogenous opioids [21]. In the second study (Fig. 3e), placebo-induced analgesia, which is mediated by endogenous opioids, was found to be potentiated by the CCK antagonist proglumide in humans, both in clinical [22] and experimental pain [23].

Enhancement of morphine analgesia by cholecystokinin antagonists

Whereas Figure 3a-e is concerned with the different possibilities to potentiate endogenous opioids by means of a CCK antagonist, Figure 3f shows that the coadministration of an opioid and a CCK antagonist results in an enhanced analgesic effect. Several studies performed in animals and humans showed that administration of morphine in combination with CCK antagonists results in a potentiation of morphine analgesia. For example, it was found that the selective CCK-B antagonist CI-988 produces a greater antinociceptive effect of morphine in rodents [24]. Similarly, another study in the monkey showed the morphine-enhancing effect of the selective CCK-A antagonist devazepide [25]. Interestingly, in this study only morphine analgesia was enhanced, while respiratory depression was not affected. Similar results have been obtained in humans in both experimental [26] and clinical pain [27] by using the CCK antagonist proglumide.

Taken together, all these findings indicate that CCK antagonists represent promising drugs for the management of pain, although the role of CCK-A and CCK-B receptors has yet to be clearly established. Therefore, the development of new specific CCK receptor antagonists will be of primary importance for clinical trials.

Acknowledgements. This work was supported by grants from MURST and CNR "Coordinate Project on Trigeminal Pain".

References

1   Woodruff GN, Hughes J (1991) Cholecystokinin antagonists. Ann Rev Pharmacol Toxicol 31:469-501

2. Crawley JN, Corwin RL (1994) Biological actions of cholecystokinin. Peptides 15:731-755

3. Benedetti F (1997) Cholecystokinin type A and type B receptors and their modulation of opioid analgesia. News Physiol Sci 12.263-268

4. Stengaard-Pedersen K, Larsson LI (1981) Localization and opiate receptor binding of enkephalin, CCK and ACTH/beta-endorphin in the rat central nervous system. Peptides 1.3-19

5. Gall C, Lauterborn J, Burks D, Seroogy K (1987) Co-localization of enkephalin and cholecystokinin in discrete areas of rat brain Brain Res 403.403-408

6   Gibbins IL, Furness JB, Costa M (1987) Pathway-specific patterns of coexistence of substance P, calcitonin gene-related peptide, cholecystokinin and dynorphin in neurons of the dorsal root ganglia of the guinea pig. Cell Tissue Res 248.417-437

7. Faris PL, Komisaruk BR, Watkins LR, Mayer DJ (1983) Evidence for the neuropeptide cholecystokinin as an antagonist of opiate analgesia. Science 219:310-312

8. Itoh S, Katsuura G, Maeda Y (1982) Caerulein and cholecystokinin suppress beta-endorphin-induced analgesia in the rat. Eur J Pharmacol 80·421-425

9. Xu X-J, Puke MJC, Verge VMK, Wiesenfeld-Hallin Z, Hughes J, Hokfelt T (1993) Upregulation of cholecystokinin in primary sensory neurons is associated with morphine insensitivity in experimental neuropathic pain in the rat Neurosci Lett 152.129-132

10 Ghilardi JR, Allen CJ, Vigna SR, McVey DC, Mantyh PW (1992) Trigeminal and dorsal root ganglion neurons express CCK receptor binding sites in the rat, rabbit, and monkey: possible site of opiate-CCK analgesic interactions. J Neurosci 12:4854-4866

11. Stanfa LC, Dickenson AH, Xu X-J, Wiesenfeld-Hallin Z (1994) Cholecystokinin and morphine analgesia. variations on a theme. Trends Pharmacol Sci 15:65-66

12. Baber NS, Dourish CT, Hill DR (1989) The role of CCK, caerulein, and CCK antagonists in nociception. Pain 39·307-328

13 Wang J, Ren M, Han J (1992) Mobilization of calcium from intracellular stores as one of the mechanisms underlying the antiopioid effects of cholecystokinin octapeptide. Peptides 13·947-951

14. North RA (1989) Drug receptors and the inhibition of nerve cells. Br J Pharmacol 98:13-28

15. Vanderah TW, Lai J, Yamamura HI, Porreca F (1994) Antisense oligonucleotide to the CCK-B receptor produces naltrindole- and (Leu5) enkephalin antiserum-sensitive enhancement of morphine antinociception. NeuroReport 5·2601-2605

16. Ossipov MH, Kovelowski CJ, Porreca F (1995) The increase in potency produced by carrageenan-induced inflammation is blocked by naltrindole, a selective delta opioid antagonist Neurosci Lett 184:173-176

17. Watkins LR, Kinscheck IB, Kaufman EFS, Miller J, Frenk H, Mayer DJ (1985) Cholecystokinin antagonists selectively potentiate analgesia induced by endogenous opioids. Brain Res 327:181-190

18. Dourish CT, Clark ML, Iversen SD (1988) Analgesia induced by restraint stress is attenuated by CCK and enhanced by the CCK antagonists MK-329, L-365260 and CR-1409. Soc Neurosci Abstr 14:120

19. Xu X-J, Hao J-X, Seiger A, Hughes J, Hokfelt T, Wiesenfeld-Hallin Z (1994) Chronic pain-related behaviors in spinally injured rats: evidence for functional alterations of the endogenous cholecystokinin and opioid systems. Pain 56·271-277

20. Valverde O, Maldonado R, Fournie-Zaluski MC, Roques BP (1994) Cholecystokinin B antagonists strongly potentiate antinociception mediated by endogenous enkephalins. J Pharmacol Exp Ther 270:77-88

21. Zhou Y, Sun YH, Han JS (1993) Increased release of immunoreactive CCK-8 by electroacupuncture and enhancement of electroacupuncture analgesia by CCK-8 antagonist in rat spinal cord. Neuropeptides 24:139-144

22. Benedetti F, Amanzio M, Maggi G (1995) Potentiation of placebo analgesia by proglumide Lancet 346.1231

23 Benedetti F (1996) The opposite effects of the opiate antagonist naloxone and the cholecystokinin antagonist proglumide on placebo analgesia Pain 64:535-543

24. Xu X-J, Hokfelt T, Hughes J, Wiesenfeld-Hallin Z (1994) The CCK-B antagonists CI988

enhances the reflex-depressive effect of morphine in axotomized rats. NeuroReport 5:718-720

25. Dourish CT, O'Neill MF, Schaeffer LW, Siegl PKS, Iversen SD (1990) The cholecystokinin receptor antagonist devazepide enhances morphine-induced analgesia but not morphine-induced respiratory depression in the squirrel monkey. J Pharmacol Exp Ther 255:1158-1165

26. Price DD, Von der Gruen A, Miller J, Rafii A, Price C (1985) Potentiation of systemic morphine analgesia in humans by proglumide, a cholecystokinin antagonist. Anaesth Analg 64:801-806

27. Lavigne GJ, Hargreaves KM, Schmidt EA, Dionne RA (1989) Proglumide potentiates morphine analgesia for acute postsurgical pain. Clin Pharmacol Ther 45:666-673

Chapter 11

Clinical pharmacology of non-steroidal anti-inflammatory drugs: novel acquisitions

A. Sala, R. Ballerio, S. Viappiani, S. Zarini

Arachidonic acid metabolism and non-steroidal anti-inflammatory drugs; overview and novel perspectives

Prostaglandins (PGs), thromboxanes (TXs), leukotrienes (LTs), and hydroxye-icosatetraenoic acids (HETEs) are collectively referred to as eicosanoids because they are derived from 20-carbon essential fatty acids that contain three, four or five double bonds (i.e. 8, 11, 14-eicosatrienoic acid, 5, 8, 11, 14-eicosatetraenoic acid or arachidonic acid and 5, 8, 11, 14, 17-eicosapentaenoic acid). In humans, arachidonic acid represents the most abundant percursor.

Since the concentration of unesterified arachidonate in the cell is very low, the biosynthesis of eicosanoids depends primarily upon its availability to the eicosanoid-synthesizing enzymes. The first step is the liberation of arachidonic acid from membrane phospholipids, tightly regulated by acylhydrolases as a consequence of the interaction of hormones, autacoids or other substances with their receptors (or physical stimuli) which induce an elevation in cytosolic Ca^{2+} [1].

Synthesis of PGs is accomplished in a stepwise manner by a ubiquitous complex of microsomal enzymes. The first enzyme, PGH synthase, possesses two distinct catalytic activities: it oxygenates and cyclizes unesterified arachidonic acid to form the cyclic endoperoxide PGG_2 (cyclo-oxygenase or COX activity) and it possesses peroxidase activity, reducing the –OOH group at position 15 of PGG2 to OH in PGH2 [2]. The endoperoxides are chemically unstable ($t_{1/2} = 5$ min) and are transformed enzymatically into various products, including PGD_2, PGE_2, PGF_{2a}, PGI_2, TXA_2. Whereas TX synthase and PGI synthase have been characterized, purified and cloned [3-6], the nature of the isomerases generating PGE_2, D_2 and $F_{2\alpha}$ is more elusive. The latter are relatively stable molecules, whereas TXA_2 ($t_{1/2} = 30$ s) and PGI_2 ($t_{1/2} = 3$ min) are chemically unstable and undergo non-enzymatic hydrolysis to TXB_2 and 6-keto-$PGF_{1\alpha}$, respectively. Although practically all tissues are capable of synthesizing the PGG_2/H_2 intermediates, their further metabolism varies in each tissue, depending on the specific enzymes that are present. For example, platelets contain TX synthase as the principal metabolizing enzyme of PGH_2 whereas endothelial cells contain primarily PGI synthase.

PGH Synthase-2 (PGHS-2, COX-2)

The oxygenation of arachidonic acid to PGH_2 is catalysed by two closely related enzymes, PGHS-1 and PGHS-2, also referred to as COX-1 and COX-2 [2]. Apart from red blood cells which do not make PGs or platelets that only contain COX-1, most nucleated cells have the gene for the inducible COX-2 which can be expressed in response to cell activation.

Human COX-2 has subsequently been cloned [7] and expressed. The primary sequence of the two isozymes presents approximately 60% homology between the deduced amino acid sequences within a given species. Mature COX-1 contains 576 residues compared to 587 for COX-2. COX-2 contains a C-terminal sequence of 18 amino acids, absent in COX-1; antibodies prepared against this peptide specifically identify COX-2 by western blotting.

The catalytic activities of the two COX isozymes are identical and all amino acids identified as important for catalysis in COX-1 are conserved in COX-2. The kinetic properties of the two isozymes are similar. However, the substrate binding sites exhibit subtle differences as COX-2 seems more permissive than COX-1 in its ability to transform 18-carbon polyunsaturated fatty acids [8] due to a somewhat larger, more accommodating, cyclo-oxygenase active site. Such differences may contribute to the development of highly selective inhibitors of the two isoforms [9].

PGH synthases are integral membrane proteins and they represent the first example of monotopic proteins (i.e. inserted only onto the inner membrane leaflet). The crystal structure of COX-1 suggests that three short amphipatic a-helices present in the amino-terminus of the enzyme interact with the membrane. Similar features have been found concerning the crystal structure of COX-2 [10]. COX-1 forms a dimer and these α-helices form two lipophilic poles which allow the protein to stand in the membrane. COX-1 appears to be located equally on the luminal side of the endoplasmatic reticulum and on the nuclear envelope, whereas COX-2 is slightly more abundant in the nuclear envelope.

Interactions of non-steroidal anti-inflammatory drugs with COX-1 and COX-2

Vane first demonstrated that aspirin inhibits the biosynthesis of prostaglandins [11]. A few months later, Smith and Lands reported that aspirin and indomethacin inhibited the oxygenation of arachidonic acid in a time-dependent manner [12]. Finally, in 1974, Roth and Majerus showed that ^{14}C-acetylsalicyclic acid selectively acetylated a platelet protein with a molecular weight of 70kDa [13]. This protein is now referred to as COX-1.

Aspirin

Aspirin is the only non-steroidal anti-inflammatory drug (NSAID) known to re-act covalently (and time dependently) with the cyclo-oxygenases by selective acetylation of a specific serine residue (Ser^{529} for human COX-1 and Ser^{516} for human COX-2). Although it can also acetylate other proteins, higher concentrations of aspirin are usually required. It should be noted that salicylic acid is a very weak inhibitor of PGH synthases and no firm data support a link between its anti-inflammatory action and an effect on arachidonic acid metabolism. A unique consequence of aspirin acetylation of COX-2 Ser^{516} is that the enzyme retains an oxygenase reaction, albeit modified in its capacity to transform arachidonic acid as its results in the formation of 15(R)-HETE. The biological significance of this stereoisomer of the 15(S)-metabolite of the corresponding lipoxygenase is largely unknown, although it has been suggested that aspirin-triggered formation of 15(R)-HETE may be involved in its alleged protection against colorectal cancer through transcellular conversion to novel bioactive eicosanoids.

Other NSAIDs

Based upon biochemical in vitro work, other NSAIDs can be divided into competitive (i.e. "instantaneous") or time-dependent competitive inhibitors of COX (i.e. after a certain time of binding with the enzyme, they will cause a conformational change leading to an irreversible loss of activity).

Measurement of TXB_2 production during whole blood clotting is used as an index of platelet COX-1 activity, while PGE_2 production in response to LPS added to heparinized blood samples reflects the time-dependent induction of COX-2 in circulating monocytes. Based on this methodological approach, a large number of currently available NSAIDs and new chemical entities have been screened and found that they can be grouped in three categories [14, 15]:

1. non-selective inhibitors: the vast majority of the NSAIDs examined have COX-1/COX-2 rations between 0.5 and 3.0;
2. relatively selective COX-2 inhibitors, such as meloxicam and nimesulide, with COX-1/COX-2 rations between 10-20;
3. highly selective COX-2 inhibitors, such as SC-58136, NS-398 and L-745,337, with COX-1/COX-2 rations >100.

It is unclear at this stage whether there is an optimal degree of biochemical selectivity to achieve comparable efficacy and improved safety with respect to conventional NSAIDs. However, on theoretical grounds it would seem desirable to have compounds with IC_{50} ratio >100 in order to adequately test the hypothesis underlying the development of selective COX-2 inhibitors. The two compounds currently in clinical development, i.e. MK966 and celecoxib, appear to meet this criterion.

Celecoxib

In a comparative phase I clinical study, 7-day treatment with celecoxib (100 and 200 mg p.o. b.i.d.) did not produce gastric erosions or ulcers; naproxen (500 mg b.i.d.) given over the same period caused ulcers and gastric erosions in 19% and 72% of the subjects tested, respectively.

A double-blind endoscopic study of the gastroduodenal effects of celecoxib was performed in 128 healthy volunteers with endoscopically proven normal upper gastrointestinal (UGI) mucosa. Subjects were randomized to receive celecoxib (100 or 200 mg b.i.d.), naproxen (500 mg b.i.d.) or placebo 7 days, at which point they underwent UGI endoscopy. In this study, celecoxib was well tolerated and had a side effect profile similar to that of placebo.

In another placebo-controlled, phase II trial, the analgesic and anti-inflammatory efficacy of celecoxib (40, 100 or 200 mg b.i.d. for 2 weeks) was compared to placebo in 293 patients with osteoarthritis of the knee that had flared following withdrawal of NSAIDs. Withdrawal from trial due to a lack of efficacy was 14% for patients on placebo; for patients on 40, 100 and 200 mg celecoxib it was 8%, 1% and 4%, respectively. Patient's assessment of pain and global assessments by patients and physicians were all significantly better in the celecoxib groups than in the placebo group. Adverse events were mild and were comparable for active drug and placebo; thus included headache, change in bowel habits, abdominal discomfort and dizziness.

References

1. Dennis EA (1994) Diversity of group types, regulation and function of phospholipase A2. J Biol Chem 269:13057-13060
2. Smith WL, Garavito RM, DeWitt DL (1996) Prostaglandin endoperoxide H synthases (cyclooxygenases)-1 and -2. J Biol Chem 271:33157-33160
3. Back SJ, Lee K-D, Shen R-F (1996) Genomic structure and polymorphism of the human thromboxane synthase-encoding gene. Gene 173:251-256
4. Wang L-H, Chen L (1996) Organization of the gene encoding human prostacyclin synthase. Biochem Biophys Res Commun 226:631-637
5. Nakayama T, Soma M, Izumi Y, Kanmatsuse K (1996) Organization of the human prostacyclin synthase gene. Biochem Biophys Res Commun 221:803-806
6. Yokoyama C, Yabuki T, Inoue H, Tone Y, Hara S, Hatae T, Nagata M, Takahashi E-I, Tanabe T (1996) Human gene encoding prostacyclin synthase (PTGIS): genomic organization, chromosomal localization, and promoter activity. Genomics 36:296-304
7. Jones DA, Carlton DP, Mc Intyre TM, Zimmerman GA, Prescott SM (1993) Molecular cloning of human prostaglandin endoperoxide synthase type II and demonstration of expression in response to cytokines. J Biol Chem 268:9049-9054
8. Laneuville O, Breuer DK, Xu N, Huang ZH, Gage DA, Watson JT, Lagarde M, De Witt DL, Smith WL (1995) Fatty acid substrate specificities of human prostaglandin endoperoxide H synthase-1 and -2. Formation of 12-hydroxy-(9Z,13 E/Z, 15Z)-octadecatrienoic acids from 8-linolenic acid. J Biol Chem 270:19330-19336
9. Kurumbail RG, Stevens AM, Gierse JK, McDonald JJ, Stegeman RA, Pak JY, Gildehaus D,

Miyashiro JM, Penning TD, Seibert K, Isakson PC, Stallings WC (1996) Structural basis for selective inhibition of ciclooxygenase-2 by antiinflammatory agents. Nature 384:644-648

10. Luong C, Miller A, Barnett J, Chow J, Ramesha C, Browner MF (1996) Flexibility of the NSAID binding site in the structure of human ciclooxygenase-2. Nature Struct Biol 3:927-933

11. Vane JR (1971) Inhibition of prostaglandin synthesis as a mechanism of action for aspirin-like drugs. Nature New Biol 231:232-235

12. Smith WL, Lands WE (1971) Stimulation and blockade of prostaglandin biosynthesis. J Biol Chem 246:6700-6702

13. Roth GJ, Majerus PW (1975) The mechanism of the effect of aspirin on human platelets. I. Acetylation of a particulate protein fraction. J Clin Invest 56:624-632

14. Patrignani P, Panara MR, Greco A, Fusco O, Natoli C, Iacobelli S, Cipollone F, Ganci A, Cremmon C, Maclouf J, Patrono C (1994) Biochemical and pharmacological characterization of the cyclo-oxygenase activity of human blood prostaglandin endoperoxide synthases. J Pharmacol Exp Ther 271:1705-1712

15. Panara MR, Greco A, Santini G, Sciulli MG, Rotonda MT, Padovano R, di Giamberardino M et al (1995) Effects of the novel anti-inflammatory compounds, N-[2-(cyclohexyloxy)-4-nitrophenyl] methanesulphonamide (NS-398) and 5-methanesulphonamido-6-(2,4-difluorothio-phenyl)-1-indanone (L-745,337), on the cyclo-oxygenase activity of human blood prostaglandin endoperoxide synthase. Br J Pharmacol 116:2429-2434

Chapter 12

Opioids

A.E. PANERAI, M. BIANCHI, P. FERRARIO, P. SACERDOTE

Opioid drugs have not changed dramatically in the last 10 years and any progress is limited to a better knowledge of the characteristics of opioids as a group and of single drugs for specific properties. In conclusion, we are being helped more and more in making a choice that can best join efficacy and safety in each single therapeutic challenge that requires opioid drugs. As a matter of fact, the improvement in our use of these drugs has also suggested that they can be used safely, if necessary, for pathological conditions, previously considered not amenable to treatment with opioids, e.g. non-oncologic chronic pain. However, in this case it is even more important than in the case of oncologic pain to have a deep knowledge of each of the particular characteristics of each drug. Most of all, it is important to know the receptor specificity of each drug and its pharmacodynamic effects, also those not directly amenable to an interaction with opioid receptors [1].

The knowledge of these characteristics can help to address therapies according to the different pathologies, the pain location, and the side effects that one can expect and/or accept.

Opioid receptors

It is well known that opioid receptors can be traced back to three main families: μ (mu), κ (kappa) and δ (delta). The μ receptors are mainly located in the brain and at a lower density in the spinal cord. These receptors mediate all the classical effects of opioid drugs: analgesia, nausea, emesis, respiratory depression, endocrine effects, depression of intestinal transit, immunosuppression, and a generally depressive effect on the cardiovascular system. Differently from μ receptors, κ receptors are mainly located at the spinal cord level and at a lower density in the brain, where they exert their typical disforic effect. The κ receptors do not seem to be involved in respiratory depression and in immunosuppression, as are μ receptors, while they exert a generally stimulatory effect on the cardiovascular system. κ receptors also seem to exert, at the spinal level, a role in the control of motor activity. Finally, δ receptors are present in both the brain and the spinal cord, and they practically mediate the same effects as μ receptors. Their peculiarity is their presence in interneurons, thus mediating a fine neuromodulatory effect, i.e., at the nigrostriatal level, not characteristic of μ receptors.

This brief analysis of opioid receptors offers interesting suggestions as to the possible effects exerted by drugs acting on the three receptors. For instance, for drugs acting on brain μ receptors might elicit a highly modulated analgesic response that is not typical of the κ effect that is limited to the spinal cord. On considering side effects, one can expect a decrease in cardiac work from μ agonists, while cardiac work is increased by κ agonists.

Opioid drugs

According to the literature the most used drugs are morphine, methadone, codeine, buprenorphine and tramadol for the oral route; morphine, meperidine, fentanyl and hydroxymorphone for the epidural and spinal route [2]; and morphine and tramadol for the intra-articular route [3, 4]. Interestingly, there is little evidence for the use of dextropropoxyphene, unless it is used in combination with non-steroid anti-inflammatory drugs (NSAIDs); this could be due to its low potency, although it has the advantage of a long half-life.

Most of the quoted drugs interact with the μ receptor, and morphine, probably more than the other opioids, also exerts a significant effect on κ and δ receptors. Drugs active on the κ receptor are under active investigation and could be very useful, for example because their effect is mainly limited to the spinal cord, or since they are devoid of the respiratory depressive effects of agonists. A drug that, although indirectly, acts on κ receptors is clonidine. It has been shown, in fact, that beyond its effects on the modulation of noradrenergic neurotransmission, this drug – better known as an agonist of the α2 adrenergic receptor – can induce the secretion of dynorphin, i.e., the endogenous ligand of κ receptors [5]. This indirect effect of clonidine on the κ receptor is proved by the blockade of its analgesic effect by antagonists of the κ opioid receptor.

In order to avoid misunderstandings, it is important to remember that all opioid drugs active on the same receptor class exert at equi-analgesic doses, independent of the administration route (with the exception of the intra-articular route), the same side effects and induce cross tolerance.

Beyond their receptor specificity, some opioid drugs or their derivatives are also characterized by their pharmacodynamic effects, which might be independent of the activation of these receptors. Four drugs are of main interest from this point of view: methadone, dextromethorphan, tramadol and sameridine.

Methadone, a classical μ opioid receptor agonist, and dextromethorphan, an opioid drug that, due to the structural changes, has lost its specific opioid receptor ligand characteristics, share an interesting effect as antagonists of the NMDA glutamate receptor, thus exerting an inhibitory effect on the neurotransmitter role of this excitatory amino acid [6, 7]. It is easy to understand how this characteristic might be interesting for the control of chronic oncologic and non-oncologic pain such as neuropathic pain. Tramadol, besides having a weak agonist effect on the μ opioid receptor, is a potent inhibitor (its potency is similar to that of imipramine) of serotonin and norepinephrine re-uptake [8]. The analgesic effect of amine re-uptake inhibitors such as imipramine or amitryptiline is well known, as is their efficacy in increasing the effect of opioid drugs and their efficacy in pain syndromes with a neuropathic component. Finally, sameridine [9] is an interesting drug since it exerts both an effect as a μ receptor agonist and as a local anaesthetic. If it can be confirmed clinically, sameridine may be a good candidate for the epidural and spinal administration routes. It is well known, in fact, that pain therapists often co-administer opioids and local anaesthetics, and this drug could substitute for the combination of the two drugs and avoid the pharmacokinetic problems that can arise from drug associations.

Opioid drugs and immune responses

It has been claimed for many years that opioid drugs exert an inhibitory effect on immune responses. However, this claim cannot be generalized to all opioid drugs, and for many of them it is possible to predict the degree of dissociation between their effects on immune responses and analgesia [10]. We know now that morphine is an imunosuppressive drug and that this effect of the opioid does not show tolerance. All morphine derivatives that had the –OH group in position 6 substituted, e.g., hydroxymorphone, are more potent analgesic drugs than the parent drug, but have lost the immunosuppressive effect. The same is true for codeine. This opioid maintains vs morphine the same potency ratio for both its effect on analgesia and immune responses. However, oxycodone, the codeine derivative with the substitution of the –OH in position 6, is a more potent analgesic than the parent drug, but does not exert any effect on immune responses.

Interestingly, antagonistic drugs that carry substitutions in both the 6 and 17 position, such as naloxone or naltrexone, behave as immunostimulatory drugs. In fact, they relieve the tonic immunosuppressive effect exerted by endogenous opioids, e.g., β-endorphin [11]. A peculiar drug is nalorphine. This drug maintains the same –OH group in positions 3 and 6 as in morphine, and it is substituted only in 17. This substitution results in a drug which has lost the analgesic effects, but preserves only the immunosuppressive effects of the parent drug morphine. Considering the immune effects of opioids, another peculiar drug is tramadol. This drug, probably due to its effect as an inhibitor of serotonin re-uptake, exerts both an analgesic and an immunostimulatory effect [12].

The knowledge of the immune effects of opioid drugs is probably one of the most important parameters to know when using and chosing one of them in oncologic and non-oncologic pain. Let us consider some examples. In oncologic pain, hydroxymorphone should be, at least theoretically, preferred to morphine. Morphine is in fact an immunosuppressor and could worsen the progression of the pathology, while hydroxymorphone exerts a more potent analgesic effect without immunosuppression. In rheumatic pain, hydroxymorphone is more potent than morphine, but morphine can exert both an analgesic and immunosuppressive effect and, therefore, it might also slow the progression of the immune disease. In post-operative pain, tramadol should be the opioid of choice because of its immunostimulatory effect that counterbalances the immunosuppression that is induced by the surgical stress and is worsened by morphine. Another type of pain in which, for totally different reasons, tramadol should exert a good therapeutic effect is neuropathic pain. Although it has been recently shown that both morphine and codeine can be effective in this type of pain, we know that the most effective drugs in neuropathic pain are tricyclic antidepressant drugs. Tramadol, which conjugates both the μ opioid receptor agonistic effect of morphine and codeine and the inhibition of serotonin and norepinephrine re-uptake that is typical of tricyclic antidepressants, should exert good effects in this pathology, although clinical data have not been presented yet.

Peripherally administered opioids

A chapter on its own is represented by the "topical" use of opioids drugs in oncologic and non-oncologic pain. It is easy to understand that such a treatment could drastically decrease the presence of the systemic side effects of these drugs. This approach has been attempted in extremely different situations: during surgery not accompanied by a relevant inflammatory component and in post-operative, arthritic, and oncologic pain with a substantial amount of inflammation. It became evident that the peripheral "topical" use of opioids, mainly morphine, was devoid of any substantial effect in the absence of inflammation. The effect was, in contrast, positive when inflammation was an important component of the pathology. The explanation of the different effects derives from findings, both in experimental animal studies and in tissues obtained from patients, that opioid receptors appear on the surface in inflamed tissues, whereas they are usually absent in non-inflamed "normal" tissues [3]. These receptors are specific and anatomically limited to the damaged tissues, therefore increasing the "topical" effect of the applied treatment [3]. The observation is even more important if one considers the intra-articular administration of morphine or other opioids. In fact, the impermeability of synovial tissue should drastically inhibit the systemic leakage of the drug and, hence, systemic side effects of hydrophilic drugs (such as morphine). Moreover, some opioids have also been shown to exert an anti-inflammatory and immunosuppressive effect. Both effects could contribute, beyond the analgesic effect, to their therapeutic efficacy in these pathologies.

Tolerance, dependence and addiction

The problems of tolerance, dependence and addiction are only relevant in the use of opioids for the therapy of chronic non-oncologic pain. Tolerance is not a real problem. It can even be turned to be an useful event, if its development implies the tolerance to the frightening side effects of opioids such as respiratory depression. In contrast, the lack of development of tolerance to effects such as stipsis represents one of the more important drawbacks of the use of opioids. Physical dependence develops similarly during both the chronic treatment of oncologic and non-oncologic pain. However, while it is highly improbable that an oncologic patient will interrupt treatment, this is a real possibility in non-oncologic patients. Therefore, there are two possible therapeutic behaviors: either the slow decreases in dosage toward "detoxification" or the use of drugs (e.g., clonidine) that can help in diminishing the withdrawal symptoms. This approach must be always kept in mind since it could be the only possible when treatment has to be suddenly interrupted, e.g., to treat the concomitant appearance of an acute disease not compatible with the use of opioids. Finally, the development of addiction seems not to be a problem in the therapeutic use of opioids in either oncologic or non-oncologic pain [2].

Conclusions

We have learned how to use opioids better and this knowledge contributes to a broader use of them, e.g., in non-oncologic pain. Opioids can be used to alleviate non-oncologic pain when patients are not responsive to other analgesic drugs. However, careful selection of the patient, the pathology and the opioid to be used in each individual case is mandatory, even more so than for the therapy of oncologic pain.

References

1. Reidine T, Pasternak G (1995) Opioid analgesics and antagonists. In: Hardman JG, Limbird LE (eds) The pharmacological basis of therapeutics. McGraw-Hill, New York, pp 521-555
2. Portenoy RK (1997) Current status of intrathecal therapy for nonmalignant pain management. J Pain Sympt Manag 14 (Suppl 3):1-48
3   Stein C (1995) The control of pain in peripheral tissues by opioids. N Engl J Med 332:1685-1690
4. Budd K (1996) The analgesic effect of tramadol hydrochloride when administered intraarticularly. 8th World Congress of Pain, Vancouver, 1(A41):229
5. Bianchi M, Brini A, Rovati L, De Giuli-Morghen C, Panerai AE (1989) Possible involvement of dynorphin in clonidine induced analgesia. Med Sci Res 17:351-352
6   Netzer R, Pflimlin P, Trube G (1993) Dextromethorphan blocks N-methyl-D-aspartate-induced currents and voltage-operated inward currents in cultured cortical neurons. Eur J Pharmacol 238:209-216
7   Shimoyama N, Shimoyama M, Elliott KJ, Inturrisi CE (1997) d-Methadone is antinociceptive in the rat formalin test. J Pharmacol Exp Ther 283:648-652
8. Wilder-Smith CH, Schimke J, Osterwalder B, Senn HJ (1994) Oral tramadol, a mu opioid agonist and monoamine reuptake blocker, and morphine in strong cancer related pain Ann Oncol 5:141-146

9. Swedberg MDB, Hellberg IB, Ask AL, Ericson AC (1997) Sameridine: assessment of physical dependence potential in mice of a novel type opioid with anaesthetic and analgesic effects. 27th Soc Neuroscience Meeting, New Orleans, 1(A58.13):126
10. Sacerdote P, Manfredi B, Mantegazza P, Panerai AE (1997) Antinociceptive and immunosuppressive effects of opiate drugs: a structure-related activity study. Br J Pharmacol 121:834-840
11. Manfredi B, Sacerdote P, Bianchi M, Locatelli L, Veljic-Radulovic J, Panerai AE (1993) Evidence for an opioid inhibitory effect on T cell proliferation. J Neuroimmunol 44:43-48
12. Sacerdote P, Bianchi M, Manfredi B, Panerai AE (1997) Effects of tramadol on immune responses and nociceptive thresholds in mice. Pain 72:325-330

Chapter 13

Psychoactive drugs and pain

K. KOUYANOU

We will present information on psychoactive drugs used for the management of pain. Opioids are the most potent pain-relieving drugs and are often the drugs of choice in the management of acute severe pain. Opioids are discussed elsewhere in this book. Psychoactive drugs other than opioids are mainly used in chronic pain as adjuvant treatment and have little or no place in the treatment of acute pain. They are mainly comprised by the classes of antidepressants, antipsychotics, anticonvulsants, and anxiolytics. We will briefly present the problem of chronic pain, the medication in chronic pain and the present status of psychoactive drug use.

The problem of chronic pain

Pain that persists beyond the expected course of an acute disease and lasting more than 6 months is defined as chronic. Chronic pain is a problem which is difficult to handle both for the patient and the health care system. The aetiology is complex and is undoubtedly multifactorial, involving differing combinations of physical, psychological, behavioural, social and cultural factors [1, 2]. It is now recognized that purely physical treatment for chronic pain based on the disease model has a low success rate. It has been suggested that the main strategy should now be to "de-medicalise" symptoms and to regard the problem as one of rehabilitation. Clinical management should place equal emphasis on both the physical and psychosocial aspects of chronic pain and disability [3-8]. The large number of therapeutic interventions available should not be regarded as treatments in themselves but rather as symptomatic measures – the focus should be on active exercise and rehabilitation.

A guiding principle in evaluating patients with chronic pain is to assess both emotional and organic factors before initiating therapy. Addressing these issues together rather than waiting to "rule out" organic causes of pain improves compliance, in part because it assures patients that a psychological evaluation does not mean that the physician is questioning the validity of their complaint. Even when an organic cause for a patient's pain can be found, it is still wise to look for other factors. For example, cancer patients with painful bony metastases also may have pain due to nerve damage and significant depression. Optimal therapy requires that each of these factors be looked for and treated.

Pharmacologic therapy is widely used to provide pain relief for most conditions. Nevertheless, successful outcomes are dependent on a comprehensive, multidisciplinary approach that may include patient education, pharmacologic intervention, minimally invasive procedures, i.e., acupuncture, transcutaneous electrical nerve stimulation TENS (transcutaneous electrical nerve stimulation), psychologic counselling, behaviour modification, physiotherapy and, in some instances, surgery and a variety of other non pharmacologic modalities [9].

Once the evaluation process has been completed and the likely causative and exacerbating factors identified, an explicit treatment plan should be developed. A multidisciplinary approach may require referral to a pain clinic. However this is not necessary for all chronic pain patients. For some, pharmacologic management alone can provide significant help.

Medication in chronic pain

Medication usually provides limited relief and side effects are common [10, 11]. It is possible that by treating pain complaints with acute pain relief interventions we indirectly contribute to the maintenance of disability among patients with chronic pain [12]. For example, the use of pro re nata medication schedules often results in drug-seeking behaviour in patients that mimic those seen in psychological dependence [13, 14]. In their widely publicised clinical guidelines, the Clinical Standards Advisory Group Report on back pain [3] recommends avoiding narcotics if possible and to never prescribe them for more than 2 weeks. Simple analgesics are adequate for most patients. Medication should be given on a regular basis for a fixed duration to control pain, and not intermittently ("prn").

Previous reports have shown that a significant percentage of chronic pain patients suffer from drug abuse/dependence [15, 16] which, in turn, may contribute to physical and psychological dysfunction. We have previously reported that 12% of a chronic pain population studied in two large teaching hospitals in South London met the DSM-III-R criteria for active drug abuse or dependence [17]. We also observed that a substantial percentage (17%) occasionally used medicines in doses well above the highest recommended dose (drug misuse) and that 9.6% met DSM-III-R criteria for drug abuse or dependence in remission. Furthermore, a number of patients were using medication in an inappropriate time schedule and were not aware or had inaccurate information about the possible side effects of such use.

Psychoactive drugs should be carefully considered as adjuvant treatment in chronic pain. Amitriptyline, nortriptyline and clomipramine have well-documented benefits but those benefits do not necessarily emerge immediately and are not thought as the first line of treatment. Anticonvulsants are used for the pain of trigeminal neuralgia and are widely employed to treat other stabbing pains. Antipsychotics are thought to be helpful for some chronic pain.

Psychoactive drugs

Antidepressants

Antidepressant drugs have been used for the treatment of chronic pain for over 30 years. Numerous studies have now been carried out which show that antidepressants have a clear benefit in reducing pain in patients with chronic pain. Although the relief of pain sometimes results because the antidepressant improves an associated depression, it is now well established that the beneficial effect of tricyclic antidepressants is distinct from the proper antidepressant activity. The analgesic effect of tricyclics has a more rapid onset of action and occurs at a lower dose than is typically required for the treatment of depression [18-20]. The possible explanations about the analgesic effect of antidepressants were presented by Feinmann in a review article [21]. Firstly, the antidepressant agent may alleviate depressive symptoms associated or consequent to chronic suffering [22-25]. However, if this is simply relief of an "overlay" of depression then it appears to be more susceptible to pharmacotherapeutic intervention than affective illness normally is [26]. Secondly, there may be a common biochemical mechanism underlying both depression and pain. Sternbach has suggested that the low brain serotonin turnover may cause hypersensitivity to pain and depression [27]. Pain perception can be reduced by giving serotonin precursors such as L-tryptophan which also potentiates endogenous opiates whereas reserpine, which lowers both noradrenaline and serotonin in the brain, increase pain awareness and accelerates tolerance to morphine. It is widely accepted that the tricyclics can inhibit neuronal uptake and increase synaptic serotonin, noradrenaline and dopamine. Also, monoamine oxidase inhibitors increase uptake and consequently increase release of serotonin, noradrenaline and possibly dopamine, which enhances the locally available concentration of these transmitters in the brain. This phenomenon is thought to be directly or indirectly responsible for their antidepressant activity and possibly responsible for pain relief [28, 29]. While controversy has continued as to whether the analgesic effect is separable from effect of the antidepressants on mood, many reports showed analgesic benefit without significant change on mood measurements [30, 26]. Watson et al. showed that amitriptyline was effective in patients with post-herpetic neuralgia who were free of depression when compared with inactive drug treatment [31]. Feinmann et al. found dothiepin to be an effective treatment in patients with facial pain [32]. Shara et al. had similar findings [33].

Finally, the close relationship between serotonin and the endorphins and enkephalins in nerves involved in the transmission of painful stimuli makes it likely that agents which reduce available serotonin are also likely to reduce endorphin release with concequent increase in the effect of substance P. The converse also holds true; increased activity in nerves where endorphins or enkephalins are the neurotransmitters will result in an increase in available serotonin [34].

Systematic reviews of randomised trials have provided strong evidence that tricyclic antidepressants are effective treatment in chronic pain [35-37]. In their systematic review of the effectiveness and safety of antidepressants in neuropathic pain, McQuay et al. showed that tricyclics are of particular value in the management of neuropathic pains such as painful diabetic neuropathy and postherpetic neuralgia, for which there are few other therapeutic options [35]. According to this review, antidepressants clearly have an effect when compared with placebo in neuropathic pain. This effect was apparent for several different pain syndromes and was of similar magnitude, despite the presumed differences in the underlying pain mechanisms. Of 100 patients with neuropathic pain who are given antidepressants, 30 will obtain more than 50% pain relief, 30 will have minor adverse reactions and four will have to stop treatment because of major adverse effects. In the same review it was noted that the adage that burning pain should be managed with antidepressant and shooting pain with anticonvulsant is not supported. If benefit was found, it occurred independently of the type of pain [38]. The only randomised comparison of antidepressant with anticonvulsant showed greater benefit at lower risk with antidepressants [39]. This is not supported by the systematic reviews, which show little to choose between antidepressants and anticonvulsants.

The commonest side effects are drowsiness, dry mouth, and constipation, which occur in one in three cases. About one in 30 patients has to stop taking the drug because of intolerable side effects. The tricyclics that have been shown to relieve pain have significant side effects. Unfortunately, some of the newer antidepressants (selective serotonin reuptake inhibitors-SSRIs) such as fluoxetine, paroxetine, and citalopram which have fewer and less serious side effects were also less effective [38, 40].

Antidepressants should be used in cases in which pain relief is inadequate with conventional analgesics or when pain relief is combined with unacceptable side effects. Antidepressants can also be used in addition to conventional analgesics. This can be particularly effective when conventional analgesics fail to control the variety of symptoms which may accompany terminal cancer.

When the decision for using antidepressants has been made, the first choice is amitriptyline. A starting dose of 25 mg would be reasonable although in frail patients only 10 mg should be used. Patients should take the medicine a few hours before bedtime and increase the dose by one tablet of 10 mg each evening until they either achieve pain relief or adverse effects become unacceptable. Many patients will continue to achieve pain relief for long periods of time but others will not.

Anticonvulsants

In 1962 Blom introduced carbamazepine for the treatment of trigeminal neuralgia. Since then anticonvulsants have been used in pain management. These drugs inhibit the firing of central or peripheral nerve impulse generators and so pain that is triggered by such a mechanism, for example stump and phantom limb pain, are often responsive to these drugs. They are also effective in diffuse burning such as pains often known by the term "causalgia".

The clinical impression is that anticonvulsants are useful for neuropathic pain. Carbamazepine is usually the drug of choice for trigeminal neuralgia [41]. Phenytoin is also used for trigeminal neuralgia if carbamazepine is ineffective or if the patient cannot tolerate effective doses. Sodium valproate is used as an adjuvant combined with other drugs because it is better tolerated than carbamazepine [42]. Anticonvulsants are also prescribed in combination with antidepressants as in the treatment of post-herpetic neuralgia [43]. Anticonvulsants can cause serious side effects, including deaths from haematological reactions [44]. The commonest side effects are impaired mental and motor function which may limit clinical use, particularly in elderly people [44, 45].

The present status of anticonvulsant drug use for the management of pain is illustrated in a systematic review by McQuay et al. [46]. In their study the authors included only randomised, controlled trials of the analgesic effects of anticonvulsant drugs from 1966 to February 1994. A total of 20 studies met the inclusion criteria. The pain conditions investigated were chronic non-malignant pain (in 17 trials), cancer pain (one trial), postoperative pain (one trial), and acute herpes zoster (one trial). Anticonvulsants were ineffective in the report of postoperative pain [47] and in the one of acute herpes zoster [48]. It seems, therefore, that there is no logic in using anticonvulsants to manage acute nociceptive pain when there are other effective remedies. Regarding trigeminal neuralgia, the statement that approximately 70% of patients will have significant pain relief would seem to be about right. The use of anticonvulsants in diabetic neuropathy is rather controversial and the use in migraine prophylaxis seems to be effective but recent advances in migraine management may reduce the impact of these results. The conclusions of the review were that anticonvulsants were effective for trigeminal neuralgia, diabetic neuropathy and migraine prophylaxis. Minor adverse effects occurred as often as benefits.

Carbamazepine can be given 100 mg b.d. initially. It can be then increased slowly up to a total daily maximum of 1 200 mg, if tolerated. Plasma concentration should be checked during the third week (5-10 mg/l=21-42 mmol/l). Phenytoin can be given 100 b.d. initially and then increased to a daily maximum of 600 mg. Plasma concentration should be checked during the second week (10-20 mg/l=40-80 mmol/l).

Anxiolytic drugs

Anxiolytics is a commonly used class of medications for chronic pain patients. The most commonly prescribed within the group are the benzodiazepines. These drugs are effective in relieving muscle spasm and are probably of some value in musculoskeletal strain. It has been reported that chronic pain patients in the United States are three to four times more likely to be using benzodiazepines as the general population [49-53].

In a study of benzodiazepine use by chronic pain patients, King and Strain found a prevalence of 38% [10]. In their study on medication misuse, abuse and dependence in chronic pain patients Kouyanou et al. reported that 18% of their sample used benzodiazepines [17]. This difference might in part reflect differences in both prescribing practice between US and UK as well as changes in the prescription of benzodiazepines over time. Relatively low rates of benzodiazepine misuse (4.8%), abuse (4%), and dependence (3.2%) were also noted. It has also been observed that once treatment with benzodiazepines is initiated, it is continued for longer periods than among non-pain patients [54, 10]. Because chronic pain patients often report difficulty in sleeping, it is not surprising that these medications are commonly prescribed to alleviate this problem [55, 56]. They are also often employed as muscle relaxants [54]. A major problem with these drugs is their tendency to cause dependence and their sudden discontinuation can result in serious withdrawal reactions [57]. They also can produce a variety of side effects, most notably sedation and impairments in cognition, all of which interfere with the common goal of chronic pain management programmes to increase the activity of the patient. Perhaps the issue of greatest concern is that not only do these medications offer minimal benefits, if any, to chronic pain patients, but in some patients they may exacerbate pain [58, 59].

Furthermore, those patients who are abusing other medications are most likely to be at risk for abusing and becoming dependent upon benzodiazepines [60]. Generally, it is not recommended that they are prescribed for longer than 2 weeks at a time in most patients. It is vital that physician education about prescription of these medications for this patient cohort should be enhanced.

Antipsychotics

The antipsychotic agents are used in the treatment of both acute and chronic pain although the evidence for their efficacy is limited. Methotrimeprazine has been shown to decrease cancer pain in well-controlled studies and can reduce the dose of opiate required to control pain. The mode of action is not well known. It seems that they alter the patient's emotional response to pain. There are some authors advocating the use of antidepressants in combination with phenothiazines [61-63] but these are case report studies. Droperidol has been used for the treatment of status migrainosus and refractory migraine [64].

Conclusions

Antidepressant, anticonvulsant, anxiolytic and antipsychotic drugs, alone or in combination, are used in the treatment of certain intractable pain conditions that have failed to respond to other drugs. Controlled clinical trials on the efficacy of psychotropic drugs for the relief of chronic pain are limited and related mainly to the use of antidepressants and anticonvulsants. The analgesic action of these drugs differs from their other actions. Psychotropic drugs can play an important role in the treatment of some types of chronic pain. Drug treatment, however, should be considered part of a multidisciplinary approach.

References

1. Bonica JJ (1990) Definitions and taxonomy of pain. In: Bonica JJ (ed) The management of pain, vol 1, 2nd edn. Lea and Febiger, Philadelphia
2. Flor H, Turk DC (1984) Etiological theories and treatment for chronic back pain. I. Somatic models and interventions. Pain 19:105-121
3. Clinical Standards Advisory Group (1994) Report of a CSAG Committee on Back Pain. HMSO, London, p 63
4. Flor H, Fydrich T, Turk DC (1992) Efficacy of multidisciplinary pain treatment centers: a meta-analytic review. Pain 49:221-230
5. Turner JA, Chapman CR (1982) Psychological interventions for chronic pain: a critical review. II. Operant conditioning, hypnosis, and cognitive-behavioural therapy. Pain 12:23-46
6. Aronoff GM, Evans WO, Enders PL (1983) A review of follow-up studies of multidisciplinary pain units. Pain 16:1-11
7. Linton SJ (1986) Behavioural remediation of chronic pain: a status report. Pain 24:125-141
8. Philips HC (1987) The effects of behavioural treatment on chronic pain. Behav Res Ther 25:365-377
9. Katz WA (1996) Approach to the management of nonmalignant pain. Am J Med 101(suppl 1A):54S-63S
10. King SA, Strain JJ (1990) Benzodiazepine use in chronic pain patients. Clin J Pain 6:143-147
11. Turner JA, Calsyn DA, Fordyce WE, Ready LB (1982) Drug utilization patterns in chronic pain patients. Pain 12:357-363
12. Riley J, Ahern D, Follick M (1988) Chronic pain and functional impairment: assessing beliefs about their relationship. Arch Phys Med Rehabil 69:579-582
13. Fordyce WE (1976) Behavioural methods for chronic pain and illness. Mosby, St Louis
14. Weissman D, Haddox D (1989) Opioid pseudoaddiction – an iatrogenic syndrome. Pain 36:363-366
15. Maruta T, Swanson DW, Finlayson RE (1979) Drug abuse and dependence in patients with chronic pain. Mayo Clin Proc 54:241-244
16. Ready LB, Sarkis E, Turner JA (1982) Self-reported vs actual use of medication in chronic pain patients. Pain 12:285-294
17. Kouyanou K, Pither CE, Wessely S (1997) Medication misuse, abuse, and dependence in chronic pain patients. J Psychos Res 43:497-504
18. Jenkins DG, Ebbutt AF, Evans CD (1976) Tofranil in the treatment of low back pain. J Int Med Res 4:28-40
19 Monks R, Merskey H (1989) Psychotropic drugs. In: Wall PD, Melzack R (eds) Textbook of pain, 2nd ed. Churchill Livingstone, London, pp 702-721
20 McQuay HJ, Carroll D, Glynn CJ (1992) Low dose amitriptyline in the treatment of chronic pain Anaesthesia 47:646-652
21 Feinmann C (1985) Pain relief by antidepressants: possible modes of action. Pain 23:1-8
22. Lascelles RG (1966) Atypical facial pain and depression. Br J Psychiatry 112:651-659
23. Okasha A, Ghalet HA, Sadek A (1973) A double blind trial for the clinical management of psychogenic headache. Br J Psychiatry 122:181-185
24 Gringas M (1973) A clinical trial of tofranil in rheumatic pain in general practice. J Med Res 4(Suppl 2):41-49
25 Hameroff SR, Cook RC, Scherer K, Crago BR, Newman C, Wombley JK, Davis TP (1982) Doxepin effects on chronic pain, depression and plasma opioids J Clin Psychiatry 43:22-26

26. Hughes A, Chauvergre J, Lisslour J, Lafgarde C (1963) L' imipramine, utilisée comme antalgique majeur en carcinologie. étude de 118 cas. Presse Med 71:1073-1074

27. Sternbach R (1976) The need for an animal model of chronic pain. Pain 2:2-4

28. Iversen LL (1974) Monoamines in the mammalian nervous system and the actions of antidepressant drugs. In: Iversen LL (ed) Biochemistry and mental illness. Plenum, New York, pp 57-83

29. Lee R, Spencer PSJ (1977) Antidepressants and pain. A review of the pharmacological data supporting the use of certain tricyclics in chronic pain. J Int Med Res 5.146-156

30. Lance JW, Curran DA (1963) Treatment of chronic tention headache. Lancet 1:1236-1239

31. Watson CPN, Evans RJ, Reed K, Merskey H, Goldsmith L, Warsh J (1982) Amitriptyline versus placebo in post-herpetic neuralgia. Neurology 32:671-673

32. Feinmann C, Harris M, Cawley R (1984) Psychogenic pain: presentation and treatment. Br Med J 228:436-438

33. Shara Y, Singer E, Schmidt E, Dionne RA, Dubner R (1987) The analgesic effect of amitriptyline on chronic facial pain. Pain 31:199-209

34. Basbaum AT, Fields HL (1984) Endogenous pain control mechanisms: review and hypothesis. Ann Neurol 4:451-462

35. McQuay HJ, Tramèr M, Nye BA, Carroll D, Wiffen PJ, Moore RA (1996) A systematic review of antidepressants in neuropathic pain. Pain 68:217-227

36. Onghena P, Van Houdenhove B (1992) Antidepressant-induced analgesia in chronic non-malignant pain· a meta-analysis of 39 placebo-controlled studies. Pain 49.205-219

37. Volmink J, Lancaster T, Gray S, Silagy C (1996) Treatments of postherpetic neuralgia: a systematic review of randomized controlled trials. Fam Pract 13:84-91

38. Max MB, Lynch SA, Muir J, Shoaf SF, Smoller B, Dubner R (1992) Effects of desipramine, amitriptyline, and fluoxetine on pain on diabetic neuropathy. N Engl J Med 326:1250-1256

39. Leijon G, Boivie J (1989) Central post-stroke pain: a controlled trial of amitriptyline and carbamazepine. Pain 36:27-36

40. Sindrup SH, Bjerre U, Dejgaard A, Brosen K, Aaes-Jorgensen T, Gram LF (1992b) The serotonin reuptake inhibitor citalopram relieves symptoms of diabetic neuropathy. Clin Pharmacol Ther 52:547-552

41. Loesser JD (1994) Tic douloureaux and atypical facial pain. In: Wall PD, Melzack R (eds) Textbook of pain, 3rd ed. Churchill Livingstone, London, pp 699-710

42. Twycross R (1994) The management of pain in cancer. In: Nimmo WS, Rowbotham DJ, Smith G (eds) Anaesthesia, 2nd ed. Blackwell, Oxford, pp 1635-1651

43. Monks R (1994) Psychotropic drugs. In: Wall PD, Melzack R (eds) Textbook of pain, 3rd ed. Churchill Livingstone, London, pp 963-989

44. Reynolds JEF (1993) Martindale: the extra pharmacopoeia, 30th ed. Pharmaceutical Press, London, pp 292-314

45. Graham-Smith DG, Aronson JK (1992) Oxford textbook of clinical pharmacology and drug therapy, 2nd ed. Oxford University Press, Oxford, pp 433-436, 529-717

46. McQuay H, Carroll D, Jada AR, Wiffen P, Moore A (1995) Anticonvulsant drugs for managementof pain: a systematic review. Br Med J 311:1047-1052

47. Martin C, Martin A, Rud C, Valli M (1988) Comparative study of sodium valporate and ketoprofen in the treatment of postoperative pain. Ann Fr Anaesth Reanim 7:387-392

48. Keczkes K, Basheer AM (1980) Do corticosteroids prevent post-herpetic neuralgia? Br J Dermatol 102:551-555

49. Hendler N, Cimini C, Ma T, Long D (1980) A comparison of cognitive impairment due to benzodiazepines and to narcotics. Am J Psychiatry 137:828-830

50. King SA, Strain JJ (1990) Benzodiazepine use by chronic pain patients. Clin Pain 6:143-147

51. Mellinger GD, Balter MB, Uhlenbuth EH (1984) Prevalence and correlates of long-term regular use of anxiolytics. JAMA 251:375-379

52. Turner JA, Calsyn DA, Fordyce WE, Ready LB (1982) Drug utilization patterns in chronic pain patients. Pain 12:357-363

53. Ziesat HA, Angle HV, Gentry WD, Ellinwood EH (1979) Drug use and misuse in operant pain patients. Addict Beh 4:263-266

54. Hollister LE, Conley FK, Britt RH, Shuer L (1981) Long-term use of diazepam. JAMA 246:1568-1570

55. Atkinson JH, Ancoli-Israel S, Slater MA, Garfin SR, Gillin JC (1988) Subjective sleep disturbance in chronic back pain. Clin J Pain 4:225-232

56. Pilowsky I, Crettenden I, Townley M (1985) Sleep disturbance in pain clinic patients. Pain 23:27-33

57. Greenblat DJ, Shader RJ, Abernethy DR (1983) Current status of benzodiazepines. New Engl J Med 309:410-416

58. Haefely W (1985) The biological basis of benzodiazepine actions. In: Smith DE, Wesson DR (eds) The benzodiazepines: current standards for medical practice. MTP Press, Lancaster, pp 7-41

59. Mantegazza D, Tammiso R, Vincentini L, Zambotti F, Zonta N (1980) The effects of GABAergic agents on opiate analgesia. Pharmacol Res Commun 12:239-247

60. Adams JE (1989) News from the council on research: task force on benzodiazepine dependency. Psychiatry Res Rep 4:3

61. Kocher R (1976) The use of psychotropic drugs in the treatment of chronic severe pains. Eur Neurol 14:458-464

62. Sherwin D (1979) New method for treating "headaches". Am J Psychiatry 136:1181-1183

63. Clarke IM (1981) Amitriptyline and perphenazine in chronic pain. Anaesthesia 36:210-212

64. Wang SJ, Silberstein SD, Young WB (1997) Droperidol treatment of status migrainosus and refractory migraine. Headache 37:377-382

REGIONAL TECHNIQUES

Chapter 14

Trigeminal neuralgia and atypical facial pain: current concepts on etiopathogenesis and diagnosis

G. Broggi, I. Dones, P. Ferroli, D. Servello

Facial pain can be related to a dysfunction of the nervous system or to diseases affecting the various anatomical structures of the face. Physicians tend sometimes to see only those aspects of the patient's problem that fit their notions of pathogenesis or therapeutic repertoire. Understanding and treating facial pain requires concepts derived from neuroscience, physiology, anatomy, oral and maxillo-facial surgery, general dentistry, neurosurgery, neurology, internal medicine, clinical psychology, psychiatry, otorhinolaryngology, orthopaedic surgery, physiatry and anaesthesiology. Thus, a multidisciplinary approach to this problem is strongly warranted for a correct diagnosis. If the medical literature in the past two decades has demonstrated major improvement in the diagnosis and treatment of typical facial pain or "tic douloureux", atypical facial pain remains a waste-basket diagnosis that contains several distinct pain syndromes with no widely accepted etiology, categorization and treatment. In these chapter we attempt to clarify current concepts of etiopathogenesis and diagnosis of trigeminal neuralgia (TN) and atypical facial pain.

Typical facial pain or typical TN or trigeminal "tic douloureux"

Although the classification of facial pain is often unclear, classical features of "tic douloureux" are well known and separate typical TN from other painful syndromes of the face. They can be summarized as follows:
- electric shock-like, brief, stabbing pains;
- pain-free intervals between attacks when the patient is completely asymptomatic;
- unilateral pain during any one attack;
- pain of abrupt onset and equally abrupt termination;
- pain restricted to the trigeminal nerve distribution;
- no gross sensory alterations in the trigeminal distribution;
- non-nociceptive triggering of pain, almost always ipsilateral to the pain and usually from the perioral region.
    Deviations from these criteria can occur and complicate differential diagnosis. The most common variant is the patient who has electric shock-like pain superimposed upon a background of burning, continuous discomfort. A small

amount of burning immediately after a jab of pain is not uncommon, either. If the patient has been previously submitted to a nerve-damaging procedure, a burning or dysesthetic component of neuropathic origin is common and it is important to ascertain that this kind of constant pain was not part of the original symptom complex. Careful questioning may reveal that the patient is actually describing a flurry of brief attacks recurring at rapid rate and that between each jab a pain-free interval does exist. Some patients initially may describe a dull, aching, continuous pain, responsive to carbamazepine, named by Fromm [1] "pre-trigeminal neuralgia". Approximately 3% of patients with tic douloureux have pain on both sides of their face, but never simultaneous bilateral pain. Generally an interval of years separates the pains on the two sides of the face. Although the early literature on TN suggested that women are afflicted more than men and that the right side of the face was a more common site of pain than the left, recent studies have not upheld these findings: dextral predominance is minimal and over 45% of patients are male. All ages can be affected, but the majority of patients with tic douloureux are in the 50- to 70-year age group.

Although the overwhelming majority of patients have pain restricted to the trigeminal nerve distribution, a small number may have pain in the glossopharyngeal or nervus intermedius or a combination of two or three of these sensory cranial nerves. Nervus intermedius involvement is suggested by pain localized in the external ear or external auditory meatus, vagoglossopharyngeal involvement by pain in the posterior tongue, tonsillar fossa or larynx. On rare occasions, in these cases tic is associated with syncopal attacks, presumably due to involvement of branches from the carotid sinus. When vagoglossopharyngeal or nervus intermedius pain is present, the third division is the most likely site of associated trigeminal pain. Tic pain most commonly involves the third division of the trigeminal nerve, least commonly the ophthalmic division. The maxillary division is involved less often than the mandibular one; the combination of second and third divisions is the most frequent in many reported series. Every combination of pain sites in the trigeminal distribution can and does occur. The triggering stimulus for tic pain is tactile stimulation, almost always of the perioral or nasal region. The triggering sites bears no necessary relation to the painful areas; they may be in the same division of the trigeminal nerve or may be widely separated. Many patients do not recognize a specific trigger but state that the pain is brought on by chewing, talking, swallowing, smiling, or exposure to temperature change, usually cold air. An occasional patient may describe a trigger area outside the trigeminal distribution; upper cervical segments are the most common sites. The trigger zone is always ipsilateral to the pain. Patients with triggering from the scalp will often refuse to brush their hair; shaving may be impossible for the man with a trigger zone in the upper lip or chin; triggering from the teeth or gingivae may preclude oral hygiene. Patients with pain triggered by chewing may have insufficient oral intake to maintain caloric requirements adequately. TN can be an intermittent disease. Many patients report intervals of months or years between episodes of pain, but it is common for the intervals to become shorter over time. Recurrences are usually in the same area of the face, but it is characteristic for the regions of pain to spread to involve a wider area over time. Some patients never enter remission once their pain begins. Others will have episodes lasting days to months, only to have the pain stop completely; a recurrence is likely but by no means certain. In the patient with tic douloureux, emotional or physical stress usually increases the frequency of attacks and their severity. Even with these individual variants, the clinical picture of tic douloureux is so unique that it should not be confused with any other pain state.

Etiology of tic douloureux

Although many theories try to explain mechanisms of typical trigeminal tic douloureux, its causes and physiopathology are not completely understood, yet. Classically, a distinction between the symptomatic and "so-called" idiopathic form is made.

Symptomatic TN

It can be related to central or peripheral causes.

Central causes

Multiple sclerosis. TN is 300 times more common among multiple sclerosis patients than among general population: 1% of patients with multiple sclerosis have TN, 2% of patients affected by TN have multiple sclerosis [2] and 18% of patients with bilateral TN have multiple sclerosis [3]. Sometimes a neuropathic component is present, but very often a typical tic douloureux is found. Generally tic douloureux developes in the late course of multiple sclerosis, but in about 1% of cases [4] TN is the first and only symptom. Althoug the causal relationship between plaques and tic douloureux is not completely understood, multiple sclerosis patients with TN has been seen to have a demyelinating plaque in the trigeminal root both under the surgical microscope and in surgical specimens [5]. However, plaques have also been found in the descending trigeminal tract and nucleus and throughout the lemniscal system; it is not possible to state that a plaque in the root is either sufficient or necessary to cause tic douloureux. Recently, we have observed patients affected by multiple sclerosis with an artery compressing the trigeminal nerve [6].

Other central causes. A case of syringobulbia [7] and a case of neurinoma invading the descending trigeminal tract at C1-C2 [8] have been reported accompanied by severe paroxysmal provocable facial pain.

Peripheral causes

Tumors. It is proven and generally accepted that, although very rarely, the typical clinical picture of tic douloureux could be due to a small "irritative" lesion in the cerebellopontine angle such as acoustic neuromas, meningiomas, epidermoids, or osteomas [9, 10]. Exceptionally, lesions affecting the gasserian ganglion or distal divisions elicit the typical syndrome; more commonly, tumors cause an atypical form with a neuropathic character. The more slowly the mass evolves, the more likely it is that the accompanying pain will mimic TN. Furthermore, some exceptional cases in which a typical TN was due to a contralateral cerebellopontine angle tumor are reported [11].

Vascular malformations. A typical tic douloureux is due to a dolichomegabasilar/vertebral artery in about 2% of cases [12], exceptionally to cerebellopontine angle arteriovenous malformations, aneurysms, or persistent primitive trigeminal artery [13, 14].

Other peripheral causes. Arachnoidal cysts [15], arachnoidal adhesions binding the rootlets together or against the side of the brain stem [16], basilar impression or the congenital origin or that associated to Paget's disease [17] are also reported associated with pain similar to TN .

So called "idiopathic TN"

The observations of Dandy previously [16] and Jannetta [9] and many other neurosurgeons more recently, have shown that the great majority (85%) of patients with the so-called idiopathic trigeminal typical tic douloureux have compression of the trigeminal root adjacent to the pons, usually by an artery, occasionally by a vein. When the pain is in the second or third trigeminal division, the usual finding is compression of the rostral and anterior portion of the root by the superior cerebellar artery. When first division pain is present, the most frequent finding is cross-compression of the caudal and posterior portion of the trigeminal nerve by the anterior inferior cerebellar artery. Other vessels may occasionally be responsible for compression of the nerve [18, 19]. Some still doubt the causal relationship between a compressive artery and trigeminal root. A small number of autopsy studies have been performed on patients who had tic douloureux; the findings have not been clearcut. A recent clinical and autopsy study [20] clarifies some of the ambiguities and, in conjunction with magnetic resonance imaging (MRI) studies, confirms the concept that vascular compression of the trigeminal root is the principal cause of tic douloureux. These authors not only carefully observed the site of compression by the vessel in their surgical patients, but also found no such indentation of the trigeminal nerve in autopsies on patients who did not have tic. When they perfused the vessels in cadavers, they could observe vessels adjacent to the nerve in 40% of their 50 specimens. This fits with the MRI observation of vessels adjacent to the nerve in about one third of patients who have had MRI studies for reasons other than face pain. The evidence of cross compression of the trigeminal nerve adjacent to the root entry zone in patients with tic douloureux is overwhelming; the causal relation to tic is less clear. In neurosurgical series of patients affected by TN who underwent cerebellopontine angle exploration a neurovascular conflict is reported in 60%-100% of cases. The question of adequate exposure or interpretation of the findings can always be raised, but it seems to be true that not every patient with tic has an important vascular groove on the trigeminal root and that sometimes the neurovascular conflict is very subtle.

There are many theories (central hypothesis, peripheral hypothesis and more recently a hypothesis trying to reconcile central and peripheral hypothesis) which try to explain the mechanisms of typical pain paroxysms of TN: nevertheless, they remain a mystery. The lack of a good animal model hampers research on this topic.

Central hypothesis

Since the last century many authors have posited seizure-like activity in trigeminal pathways in the central nervous system [21, 22], usually leaving open the precise epileptogenic process. Clinical features suggesting a hyperactive epileptic-like central nervous system dysfunction are: spontaneous fluctuations in the frequency of attacks; triggering of pain paroxysms by innocuous gentle stimulations to the discrete trigger zone; increase in pain intensity during the attack both with repeated stimulations and increase in size of the area of stimulation; persistence of pain after stimulation is ceased; absolute and relative refractory periods after each attack; spontaneous remission of paroxysms and/or progress of disease, in spite of certain treatments with increase of frequency and severity of the attacks up to an epileptic-like status; and control of pain paroxysms with anti-epileptic drugs.

Peripheral hypothesis

The unequivocal observation that TN could be related to space-occupying lesions or vascular malformations led some authors to look for a peripheral mechanism explaining pain paroxysms. Demyelination of the posterior root [23], ectopic electrogenesis and ephapses in the trigeminal nerve root fibers demyelinated by trauma [24], high sensitivity of dorsal root ganglion neurons to mechanical distortion [25], after discharge phenomena [24] have been invoked. All these mechanisms have been generally considered, but do not completely explain such clinical features of TN as long periods of spontaneous remission, paroxysmal pain, presence of mechanical compression of the root without TN, and presence of a trigger zone outside the trigeminal territory. Recently, a novel peripheral hypothesis, more comprehensive than previous theories, but already criticized [26], the so-called "trigeminal ganglion ignition hypothesis" was proposed by Rappaport and Devor [27]. They believe that trigger stimuli set off bursts of activity in small clusters of trigeminal ganglion neurons rendered hyperexcitable as a result of trigeminal ganglion or root damage, thus spreading from this ignition focus to involve wide portions of the ganglion. After a brief period of firing, refractoriness to further spontaneous activities ensues, with cessation of TN attacks.

Mixed central-peripheral hypothesis

Clinical data suggesting a central hypotesis and pathological observations pointing to a peripheral origin led to the more commonly accepted and current mixed hypothesis: epileptogenic activity in the central nervous system could be triggered by partial deafferentation [28] or by ectopic neural discharge in the peripheral nervous system [29, 30].

In our experience based on more than 300 explorations of the cerebellopontine angle (including 12 patients in which trigeminal neuralgia was thought to be due to multiple sclerosis) we found a vascular contact in all cases, even in patients with multiple sclerosis. Although there are some obvious and evident deformities of the trigeminal root, sometimes involved vessels are more subtle and the root does not appear grossly compressed. In reoperated cases a missed vessel, a new compressing vessel (an intratrigeminal vein in a case of ours with sigmoid sinus thrombosis at preoperative MRI) or a teflon-mediated compression can be seen, but sometimes only an arachnoiditis is found. A similar arachnoiditis can be observed when reoperating on patients previously operated in the cerebellopontine angle, without TN, and in the unlikelihood that we were to explore a pain-free patient previously submitted to neurovascular decompression we might observe similar findings. This apparent contradiction and many others (different rate of neurovascular conflicts in different series, patients having TN with little or no vascular compression, evidence of neurovascular conflict without neuralgia, vascular compression of the motor branch without hemimasticatory spasm, patients certainly well decompressed with persistent pain and so on) [30-32] can be partially explained by advocating a different patient selection and different observers, but probably they mean that the problem of neurovascular compression cannot be considered as a simple cause-effect mechanism. A central involvement of trigeminal pathways with a delicate balance between abnormal and physiological inputs coming from the damaged root and modified excitability of neurons of the trigeminal nucleus must be considered. The balance between the excitability threshold of wide dynamic range (WDR) and nociceptive specific (NS) neurons of caudalis trigeminal nucleus and pathological input from the damaged trigeminal root is subtle. If the definitive causal role of vascular compression can be disputed, the modulatory role of peripheral pathways on pain perception is universally accepted. In such a modulatory role neurovascular compression must be considered. In the trigeminal root of patients with tic douloureux Kerr found areas of focal demyelination [23], possibly a source of ectopic impulses, "after discharge phenomena" and electric accouplement (ephapses). The physiological imput to the trigeminal nucleus may be altered by electrophysiological changes of fibers in the area of more or less evident cross compression. In patients with a high pain threshold (pharmacologic effect or endogenous factors) even an exaggerated firing of pathological inputs from a grossly compressed root may not be sufficient to evoke pain paroxysms, while in patients with a low pain threshold (i.e. multiple sclerosis, as documented also by high frequency of recurrences after percutaneous treatment and by the high frequency of other paroxysmal manifestations in these patients) even microscopical damage due to pulsatile compression of a small artery or vein on a few root fibers (that others could judge not sufficient to be named neurovascular conflict) can be involved in evoking pain. The concept of a central neuromodulatory role of impulses coming from the area of cross compression also explains the possibility that a long-lasting alteration of discharge modalities of the trigeminal root can primarily lower the pain threshold as sustained by more recent theories and suggested by recent reports on extracranial neurovascular conflicts [33, 34]. Furthermore, there may be other mechanisms cooperating in the developement of this process (aging?) and vascular compression could be only one of those correctable by surgery.

In conclusion, we think that TN has a central origin, in which vascular compression plays a major modulatory role.

Other facial pains and differential diagnosis

Facial pain can be of neurological, vascular and nonvascular, and non-neurological origin.

Facial pain of neurological origin different from typical TN

Vagoglossopharyngeal neuralgia

About one case for every 70 of TNs is vagoglossopharyngeal neuralgia [35]. Pain has the same characteristics observed in TN, but is distributed in the glossopharyngeal and vagus nerves (throat, base of tongue with radiation to ear and neck). The trigger is usually located in the throat and the pain is typically triggered by swallowing. Generally at the beginning of the disease carbamazepine is effective. Syncopal episodes may be observed due to the vagal component. It can be associated to TN. When typical, it has the same physiopathological explanation of TN.

Geniculate neuralgia

It is an exceptional condition, characterized by paroxysmal lancinating pain localized to the distribution area of the nerve of Wrisberg.

Neuropathic trigeminal pain (or atypical facial pain)

The clinical characteristics are constant and unilateral localized facial pain, abnormal or unpleasant dysesthesia described as burning, aching or throbbing pain in an area of clinically detectable sensory deficit, and the presence of allo-dynia. A sympathic component may be observed. If minor demyelination of the trigeminal root entry zone is related to typical tic douloureux, significant distal trigeminal injuries (trauma, tumor, aneurysms) are thought to produce these atypical pain syndromes through a mechanism much like what has been posited for other painful incontinuity nerve injuries [36]. Neurological examination may disclose signs related to compression of other cranial nerves or nervous system.

Postherpetic neuralgia

The ophthalmic division is generally affected. In about 10% of patients painful vesicular cutaneous eruption pain becomes chronic after herpes zoster. Postherpetic neuralgia is usually described as a constant burning and aching; there may be superimposed shocks and jabs. It rarely produces throbbing or cramping pain. The pain is present to some degree at all times with no pain-free intervals. Scars and pigmentary changes from the acute vesicular eruption are generally visible. The involved area may demonstrate hypesthesia, hypalgesia, paresthesias, and dysesthesias.

Facial pain of vascular origin

Cluster headache

The pain is generally severe, unilateral, located around the temple, zygomatic or in the jaw region. The problem is sometimes perceived by the patient as a toothache in a maxillary molar or second premolar. Pain attacks last from 30 min to 3 h, appear at the same time every day in one half the cases, and is ac-companied by flushing (redness) or blanching of the face and conjunctiva, lacrimation, and occlusion of the nostril. These attacks frequently occur at night, during or immediately after an episode of REM sleep. In about 20% of patients, Horner's syndrome occurs coincidentally with the attack. The headaches occur daily for 2 or 3 months and then go into complete remission for months or 1 year before the next episode. Men are typically affected. Attacks can be spontaneous or triggered by alchohol; oxygen inhalation often controls pain.

Chronic paroxysmal hemicrania

Attacks of chronic paroxysmal hemicrania (CPH) resemble those of cluster headache but they last for a shorter time, are more frequent, have no nocturnal preponderance, occur mostly in females, and are absolutely responsive to in-domethacin. The mean duration of attacks is around 15 min. Their frequency may be as high as 40 per 24 h, with a mean of about 12. Sometimes pain can be precipitated by head movements.

Short-lasting unilateral neuralgiforme headache attacks with conjunctival injection, tearing, sweating and rhinorrhea (SUNCT)

May be a new entity which has similarities with cluster headache and CPH. This syndrome has been described by Sjaastad et al. [37]. It is characterized by pain attacks of short duration (usually less than 120 s), localized to the orbital region, with conjunctival injection, tearing and rhinorrhea. Pain can be triggered by head rotation or mechanical stimuli, but without a well-defined trigger zone. Attacks can recur for months and then spontaneously disappear. Only a few cases have been described in the literature up to now; so far all of them are males.

Cluster-tic syndrome

It is characterized by the association of a typical trigeminal pain with facial pain of vascular origin [38]. Usually tic precedes vascular pain. Attaks last about 1 min and recur many times a day.

Temporal or giant cell arteritis

It occurs in patients 55 years of age or older as diffuse, throbbing pain around the ear and temple with malaise, anorexia, weight loss, low grade fever, and night sweats. Palpation of the superficial temporal artery reveals a firm cylinder with no pulse or a flattened, fibrotic mass that is painful to palpation. If the ophtalmic artery is involved, blindness can occur. The ESR is high.

Facial pain of nonvascular and non-neurologic origin

Symptomatic facial pains

Generally they can be easily recognized. Sinusitis, glaucoma, and iridocyclitis sometimes can be confused with a vascular headache, but never with TN. In this group is included all pain of ocular, maxillofacial, odontic, otorhinolaryngological, or rheumatologic origin which can be best treated according to specialist manuals. Among these pains, cancer pain related to facial tissue damage and subsequent ongoing activation of cutaneous or visceral nociceptors (nociceptive pain) or to direct damage of the nervous system (neuropathic pain) can present with subtle and polymorphic clinical aspects which should be promptly referred to a specialist for an early diagnosis and treatment.

Atypical facial pain

All pain with nonvascular and nonneuralgic characters, without a known organic cause, should be considered atypical facial pain. This is generally a wastebasket diagnosis, in which patients affected by trigeminal neuropathic pain and patients with autonomic changes are often erroneously included. The most important discrimination is between unilateral and bilateral atypical facial pain. Bilateral atypical facial or intraoral pain occurs almost exclusively in middle-aged women who are frequently depressed and agitated. The pain is described as constant and burning; it usually is not triggered, and cutaneous stimulation is only uncomfortable, not painful. There is rarely any sensory loss. Although described with great vehemence, the pain does not affect eating or talking. It is not paroxysmal. There are no associated autonomic abnormalities than can be detected clinically. Unilateral atypical facial pain occurs, again, most commonly in women, usually younger than the atypical bilateral facial pain sufferers. They complain of a burning, constant, usually circumscribed pain. Some report a superimposed jabbing component that may be triggered. There is no sensory loss, but touching the skin in the painful area is often very unpleasant. In spite pain-causing behaviors, eating, talking and facial grooming are not often interrupted, as they are in patients with tic douloureux. Significant behavioral and psychosocial dysfunction often predates the onset of the facial pain [39]. Causes are unknown and a psychosomatic origin is supposed.

Diagnosis

Diagnosis is based, above all, on clinical findings. When a cranial nerve neuralgia or neuropathy is suspected, MRI of the head is mandatory to find, in patients with typical facial pain, causes other than neurovascular conflicts (cerebellopontine angle tumors, vascular malformations, multiple sclerosis: for details see etiology) and, in patients with neuropathic pain, any cause of injury throughout the whole course of the nerve. In typical TN a neurovascular conflict can be observed. Specificity and sensitivity of the method in revealing neurovascular conflicts are not clear and surgical exploration often reveals false-negative result. When the facial pain is typical, negative MRI findings for neurovascular compressions is not a contraindication to surgical exploration of the cerebellopontine angle. Surgical surprises such as small tumors not found at MRI examination are not unusual. Cerebral angiography must be performed when a vascular malformation is suspected.

Pharmacological dissection

A useful aid in the diagnostic work-up of patients with facial pain of uncertain origin may be pharmacological dissection. Different tests, during which the patient is asked to describe the pain levels on a visual analog scale can be used to evaluate the effect of intravenous/intrathecal drug/placebo bolus administration. Using drugs acting through different mechanisms, some insights on pain components can be gained: pain of nociceptive origin is responsive to opioids (i.v. bolus of 5-10 mg of morphine or i.t. bolus of morphine at the dose of 0.1-0.5 ml; i.v. bolus of fentanyl at a dose of 1 μg/kg. Both tests, if positive, can be followed by administration of naloxone 0.4 mg: the prompt increase of pain will further confirm the positivity of test), neuropathic pain of peripheral origin can be relieved by i.v. lidocaine (1.5-5 mg/kg administred in 10-15 min); central pain, generally not relieved by opioids, can be responsive to GABA agonists [40] (i.v. bolus of propofol at a dose of 0.2 mg/kg, also predicting outcome of cortical stimulation; or i.t. administration of 2.5 mg midazolam bolus, or i.t baclofen bolus of 50 µg).

Diagnostic and therapeutic blocks

Local infiltrations and anaesthetic blocks are useful for differential diagnoses between somatic and the psychosomatic pain and, especially, of referral pain, neurologic pain, and atypical facial pain. Local blocks may be used to identify the etiologic area in patients with peripheral neurologic or inflammatory disorders, to assist in discriminating between pains that may originate from two different structures and to identify referral of pain. In case of typical TN the denervation of the trigger zones usually provides a short period of pain relief.

References

1   Fromm GH, Graf-Radforg SB, Terrence CF, Sweeth WH (1990) Pre-trigeminal neuralgia Neurology 40:1493-1495
2. Yensen TS, Rasmussen P, Riske-Nielsen E (1982) Association of trigeminal neuralgia with multiple sclerosis: clinical and pathological features. Acta Neurol Scand 65:182-189
3. Brisman R (1987) Bilateral trigeminal neuralgia. J Neurosurg 67:44-48
4. Rushton JG, Olafson RA (1965) Trigeminal neuralgia associated with disseminated sclerosis: report of 35 cases. Arch Neurol 13:383-386
5. Lazar ML, Kirkpatrick JB (1979) Trigeminal neuralgia and multiple sclerosis: demonstration of the plaque in an operative case. Neurosurgery 5:711-715
6. Broggi G, Ferroli P, Franzini A, Servello D, Dones I (1998) Microvascular decompression for trigeminal neuralgia: considerations on a series of 250 cases, including 10 patients with multiple sclerosis. J Neurol Neurosurg Psychiatry (in press)
7. Foix B, Thevenard L, Nicolesco M (1922) Algie faciale d'origine bulbotrigeminale au cours de la syringomyelie: troubles sympathiques. Rev Neurol 38:990-998
8. Conrad B, Mergner T (1979) High cervical neurinoma (C1/C2) diagnosed falsely as multiple sclerosis because of trigeminal neuralgia. Arch Psychiatr Nervenkr 227:33-37
9. Jannetta PJ (1967) Arterial compression of the trigeminal nerve at the pons in patients with trigeminal neuralgia. J Neurosurg 26:159-162
10. Burchiel KJ, Steege TD, Howe JF, Loeser JD (1981) Comparison of percutaneous radiofrequency gangliolysis and microvascular decompression for the surgical management of tic douloureux Neurosurgery 9:111-119
11. Fuad SH, Taha JM (1990) An unusual cause for trigeminal neuralgia: controlateral meningioma of the posterior fossa. Neurosurgery 26:1033-1038
12. Linskey ME, Dong Jho H, Jannetta PJ (1994) Microvascular decompression for trigeminal neuralgia caused by vertebro basilar compression J Neurosurg 81:1-9
13 Nomura T, Ikezaki K, Matsushima T, Fukui M (1994) Trigeminal neuralgia. differentiation between intracranial mass lesions and ordinary vascular compression as causative lesions. Neurosurg Rev 17:51-57

14. Morrıson G, Hegarty WM, Brausch CC, Castele TJ, Whıte RJ (1974) Direct surgıcal obliteration of a persıstent trigemınal artery aneurysm. J Neurosurg 39:249-251
15. Martuzza RL, Ojermann RG, Shillıto J (1981) Facıal paın assocıated wıth a mıddle fossa arachnoıd cyst. Neurosurg 8:712-716
16. Dandy WE (1934) Concernıng the cause of trıgemınal neuralgıa. Am J Surg 24:447-455
17. Clarke CRA, Harrıson MJG (1978) Neurologıcal manıfestatıons of Paget's disease. J Neurol Scı 38:171-178
18. Jannetta PJ (1976) Mıcrosurgıcal approach to the trıgemınal nerve for tıc douloureux. Prog Neurol Surg 7:180-200
19. Sındou M, Amranı F, Mertens P (1990) Décompression vasculaire mıcrochırurgıcale pour névralgie du trijumeau. Comparaıson de deux modalités technıques et déductıon physıopathologıques. Etude sur 120 cas. Neurochırurgie 36:16-26
20. Hamlin PJ, King TT (1992) Neurovascular compression ın trigemınal neuralgıa: a clın-ıcal and anatomical study. J Neurosurg 76:948-954
21. Trousseau A (1853) De la névralgıe épıleptıforme. Arch Gen Med 1:33-44
22. Crue BL, Alvarez-Carregal E, Todd EM (1964) Neuralgıa: consıderatıons of central mechanisms. Bull Los Angeles Neurol Soc 29:107-132
23. Kerr FWL (1967) Evıdence for a pherıpheral etıology of trigeminal neuralgıa. J Neuro-surg 26:168-174
24. Calvın W, Devor M, Howe JF (1982) Can neuralgıa arıse from mınor demyelınation? Spontaneous firing, mechanosensıtıvity and afterdıscharge from conductıng axons. Exp Neurol 75:755-763
25. Howe JF, Loeser JD, Calvın W (1977) Mechanosensıtıvıty of dorsal root ganglıa and cronically ınjured axons: a physiologıcal basıs for the radıcular paın of nerve root com-pressıon. Paın 3:25-41
26. Canavero S, Bonıcalzı V, Pagnı CA (1995) The rıddle of trigemınal neuralgıa [letter] Paın 60:229-230
27. Rappaport ZH, Devor M (1994) Trigemınal neuralgıa: the role of self-sustaınıng dıs-charge in the trigemınal ganglıon. Paın 56:127-138
28. Dubner R, Sharav Y, Gracely RH, Prıce DD (1987) Idıopathıc trigemınal neuralgıa: sen-sory features and pain mechanısms. Pain 31:23-33
29. Fromm GH, Seassle BJ (eds) (1991) Trıgemınal neuralgia: current concepts regardıng pathogenesis and treatment. Butterworth-Heınemann, Boston, pp 1-230
30. Pagnı CA (1993) The origın of tıc douloureux: a unified vıew. J Neurosurg Sci 37:185-194
31. Burchıel KJ, Clarke H, Haglund M, Loeser JD (1988) Long term efficacy of mıcrovascu-lar decompression ın trigemınal neuralgıa. J Neurosurg 69:35-38
32. Adams CBT (1989) Microvascular decompressıon: an alternatıve vıew and hypothesıs. J Neurosurg 57:1-12
33. Franzını A, Scaıolı V, Leocata F, Palazzını E, Broggı G (1995) Paın syndrome and focal myokymia due to anterıor interosseous neurovascular relationshıps: report of a case and neurophysıologıcal consıderatıons. J Neurosurg 82:578-580
34. Scaıolı V, Franzını A, Leocata F, Broggı G (1996) Hand dystonia and neuralgıc paın due to neurovascular contact to cervical spınal root (Letter). Movement Dısord 11:102-104
35 Youmans JR (1982) Neurologıcal surgery, 2nd edn. Saunders, Philadelphıa, pp 3604-3605
36. Burchıel KJ (1993) Trigeminal neuropathic paın. Acta Neurochır (Wıen) 58(Suppl): 145-149
37. Sjaastad O, Kruszewskı P (1992) Trigemınal neuralgıa and "SUNCT" syndrome: sımı-larities and dıfferences ın the clınical pıcture. An overview. Funct Neurol 7:103-107

38. Solomon S, Apfelbaum RI, Guglielmo KM (1985) The cluster-tic syndrome and its surgical therapy. Cephalalgia 5:83-89
39. Weddington WN, Blazer D (1979) Atypical facial pain and trigeminal neuralgia: a comparison study. Psychosomatics 20:348-356
40. Canavero S, Bonicalzi V (1998) The neurochemistry of central pain: evidence from clinical studies, hypothesis and therapeutic implications. Pain 74:109-114

Chapter 15

Trigeminal nerve block and surgery

G. Broggi, A. Franzini, P. Ferroli

The trigeminal nerve is one of the peripheral nerves often involved in painful conditions. It supplies the sensory fibers to the entire face and the anterior two-thirds of the head. It is the target of "tic douloureux", a fascinating disorder, characterized by paroxysmal lancinating pain which is triggered by non-noxious tactile stimulation and which is probably the most tractable chronically painful condition known. Furthermore, along its intra- and extracranial course, the trigeminal nerve is commonly subject to trauma from head injury, tumor, sinus disease, facial trauma, dental procedures and other causes, presenting, like other peripheral nerves, a broad spectrum of associated syndromes of neuropathic pain, often included in the wastebasket diagnosis of "atypical facial pain". Thus, since the early nineteenth century it has been the object of direct surgical attempts to injure this nerve with the aim of pain relief. Some decades later, it was suggested that a peripheral nerve might be destroyed by injecting a toxic substance into it and Bartholow used chloroform for this in 1876 [1]: the dichotomy between open surgery and percutaneous techniques, still debated nowadays, was born. In this chapter techniques, indications and results of trigeminal nerve surgery and block will be described and discussed.

Diagnostic and therapeutic trigeminal nerve blocks

Local infiltrations and anaesthetic blocks are useful for differential diagnoses between somatic and psychosomatic pain, expecially, in case of referral pain, and atypical facial pain. Local blocks may be used to identify the etiology of pain in peripheral neurologic or inflammatory disorders, to assist in discriminating between pain that may originate from two different structures and to identify the referral of pain. In cases of typical trigeminal neuralgia it has long been known that denervation of the triggering zones provides a period of pain relief. However, even in cases of typical trigeminal neuralgia, no neurolytic or ablative procedure should be done without prior diagnostic/prognostic block.

Mandibulary division

Mandibular incisor teeth infiltration

Anaesthetic solution is deposited over the thin cortical bone adjacent to the apices of the four mandibular incisors, producing anaesthesia of the incisor teeth and labial gingiva. A patient with a painful pathologic process at the midline of the mandible or the incisor teeth requires anaesthesia for possible anastomosing nerve fibers from the controlateral side.

Mental nerve block

This procedure is performed at or through the mental foramen, which lies just below the mandibular premolar apices or beneath the second premolar. It is usually located 10-12 mm above the inferior border of the mandible. The mental nerve exits through the mental foramen after traversing the short mental canal from the inferior alveolar canal. The lower lip and the chin can be anaesthetized by deposition of approximately 1.5 ml of anaesthetic solution into or lateral to the mental foramen. To anaesthetize the incisors, the canine, the premolar teeth, the labial gingiva, and the inferior lip effectively, the needle must enter the mental canal for its entire distance of 3-6 mm. The canal projects laterally, posteriorly, and superiorly in the adult; thus, the needle must be directed inward, downward, and forward. The mental nerve block injection techniques, to be completely effective, require that the needle enter the canal, which may require palpating with the needle point.

Long buccal nerve block

A 0.3 to 0.5 ml amount of anaesthetic solution is deposited into the vestibular mucosa just distal to the tooth or the area being investigated. Anaesthesia of the buccal mucosa anterior to the injection site is produced. The long buccal innervation terminates in the area of the mental nerve.

Lingual nerve block

A 0.5 ml amount of anaesthetic solution is deposited in the lateral posterior floor of the mouth, thereby producing discrete anaesthetization of the lingual nerve. The lingual nerve has several normal positions in the posterior floor of the mouth: above and below the mylohyoid muscle and in various positions in the mucosa medial to the third molar. In the posterior floor of the mouth, the lingual nerve may be located just medial to the mandibular third molar. The sensory distribution of the lingual nerve includes the mucous membrane on the floor of the mouth, the lingual gingiva, and the mucous membrane of the anterior two thirds of the tongue.

Inferior alveolar nerve block

This block is performed with the bidigital palpation technique, which takes into account the variability of the size and contours of the rami of mandible in different individuals. Some of the variations are in the total anterior posterior width and in the placement of the inferior alveolar foramen, which may be at, below, or above the general occlusal plane of the mandibular dentition. Cook [2] noted that the mandibular foramen and the sulcus are in a line between the narrowest anterior – posterior dimension of the ramus and two thirds the distance from the anterior to the posterior border. The location of the center of the sulcus, two thirds of the distance from the anterior to the posterior border, was constant within 2 mm limits. With these anatomic facts established, a precise injection technique is possible, whereby the sulcus is located in a line determined by the middle of the thumb and the middle finger. For a right inferior alveolar injection, the center of the palmar surface of the thumb is set at the innermost point of the indentation on the posterior border. With the thumb and the third finger in these positions, the center of the sulcus is in a line between the fingers. A straight line is more easily established with the thumb and the third finger than with any other finger, and this straight line is the essence of this injection. The needle is inserted directly toward the inferior alveolar sulcus. The area anaesthetized by an inferior alveolar nerve block includes, on the same side as the block, the mandibular teeth, the facial gingiva adjacent to the incisors, canine, and premolar teeth, the mucous membrane, the vermilion, and the skin of the lower lip, and the chin. The inferior alveolar nerve has many aberrant pathways and extra trunks [3], which can explain why the usual inferior alveolar nerve block, on rare occasions, is not completely effective.

Intraoral trigeminal third division block

The anaesthetic solutions are deposited near the foramen ovale through an intraoral approach described by Gow-Gates [4] as follows: place the head so that the intertragic notch assumes an upward inclination. Open the mouth as widely as possible. Palpate the anterior border of the ramus with the forefinger. Dry the puncture point on the lateral margin of the pterygomandibular depression and just medial to the medial tendon of the temporalis muscle and paint with antiseptic solution and topical anaesthetic. Align the needle with the plane that extends from the lower borders of the intertragic notches through the corners of the mouth, keeping it parallel to the angulation of the ear to the face. Aim the needle at the posterior border of the tragus and advance it. The depth of penetration will be approximately 25 mm. When the point of the needle reaches bone at the base of the neck of the condyle, withdraw the needle 1 mm. Perform aspiration and deposit the anaesthetic solution rapidly. Keep the mouth open for another 20 s to permit diffusion of the anaesthetic solution.

Extraoral approach to the trigeminal third division block

This form of anaesthesia is initiated by palpating the zygomatic arch and mandibular notch. A point is marked below the arch and a skin wheal of local anaesthetic agent is raised. A 5 cm, 22-gauge needle is inserted perpendicular to the skin and is advanced slowly until either a peripheral nerve response is elicited or bone is encountered. If bone is contacted, it is usually the lateral pterygoid plate and the needle therefore is positioned too far anteriorly. It must be withdrawn and reinserted posteriorly and to a depth no more than 6 mm deeper than that at which the pterygoid plate was contacted; 2-3 ml of anaesthetic solution must be injected. The possible complications are penetration of internal maxillary artery or his branches and penetration of the auditory tube.

Maxillary division

Nasopalatine nerve block

The mucosa overlying the premaxillary area on the palatal side of the dental arch is anaesthetized. The needle is inserted just lateral to the incisive papilla and parallel to the long axis of the maxillary incisor to a distance of approximately 5-19 mm. The injection of 0.25-0.5 ml of solution anaesthetizes the palatal tissue adjacent to the four incisor teeth and perhaps the canine teeth. Some fibers may also partecipate in innervation of the maxillary central and lateral incisor.

Anterior superior alveolar nerve block

The maxillary incisor teeth and the canine teeth are anaesthetized, unless the incisor teeth are innervated by the nasopalatine nerve. Deposition of 0.5-1 ml of anaesthetic solution over the apices of the maxillary incisors produces anaesthesia of the affected teeth and the associated labial soft tissues. In some patients, the clinician may need to give deep injections into the nasopalatine canal and/or intranasal injections to introduce 0.5 ml of anaesthetic solution at the superior end of the nasopalatine canal to produce profound anaesthesia of the incisor dentition.

Maxillary canine tooth infiltration

This technique is performed specifically for the canine tooth because of the possibility of separate and direct innervation from the infraorbital nerve. Deposition of 0.5-1 ml of anaesthetic solution over the apex should produce anaesthesia of the canine and the associated labial gingival tissues.

Middle superior alveolar nerve block

Approximately 1 ml of anaesthetic solution is deposited supraperiosteally through tautly drawn mucosa overlying the second premolar tooth produces anaesthesia of the premolars, the mesiobuccal root of the first molar, and the associated buccal soft tissues.

Posterior superior alveolar nerve block

The anaesthetic solution is delivered with the patient's mouth partially closed to prevent the coronoid process from traversing forward and obscuring the space lateral to the maxillary tuberosity. With the index finger, the clinician palpates the zygomatic process of the maxilla and retracts the cheek. The needle is inserted at a 45° angle to the sagittal plane at a 45° angle to the occlusal plane, to a depth of 12-18 mm. The molar teeth and the associated buccal gingiva, with the exception of the mesiobuccal root of the first molar, are anaesthetized by this injection in most patients.

Infraorbital nerve block

Structures innervated by the middle and anterior superior alveolar nerves are anaesthetized. The infraorbital foramen is located directly below the center of the pupil of the eye as the patient gazes forward and and 3-5 mm below the orbital rim. The infraorbital canal may be entered extraorally from an inferior and medial direction; 0.3 ml of anaesthetic solution is deposited over the area of the infraorbital foramen. The ball of the index finger of the hand that is not manipulating the syringe is placed on the orbital rim just superior to the foramen, the point of the needle is directed approximately 5 mm into the foramen and 0.5 ml of solution is deposited in the canal. By retrograde flow, the other terminal nerves of the maxillary division of the trigeminal nerve may be anaesthetized.

Anterior palatine nerve block

The palatal mucosa is anaesthetized as far anteriorly as the canine teeth. The greater palatine foramen is located approximately 3 or 4 mm anterior to the junction of hard and soft palates. Thus, it lies approximately halfway between the second and the third molars and approximately 10 mm from the bony palatal origin. The direction of the approach is from the opposite side of the mouth. Approximately 0.25-0.5 ml of anaesthetic solution is used.

Intraoral maxillary nerve block

All branches of the maxillary division as well as the pterygopalatine ganglion are anaesthetized. The pterygopalatine fossa is approached intraorally by passing the needle either through the greater palatine foramen and the pterygopalatine canal or posterior to the maxillary tuberosity to the area of the fossa. The maxillary division of the trigeminal nerve is blocked by using the pterygopalatine canal approach via the greater palatine foramen. A drop or two of local anaesthetic is deposited in the mucosa overlying the greater palatine foramen at the junction of the alveolar process and the horizontal roof of the palate, approximately 3 or 4 mm anterior to the junction of the hard and soft palates. The resulting anaesthesia permits probing with the point of the needle to find the orifice of the greater palatine canal. When the canal is located, the needle is advanced in a superior, posterior, and lateral direction. The maximum depth in the canal should not exceed 38 mm. From 1 to 1.8 ml of local anaesthetic solution is deposited in the pterygopalatine fossa and produces a block of the second division of the trigeminal nerve. In some instances, the foramen is too small or too inaccessible or too tortuous and the pterygopalatine approach must be discontinued.

Extraoral maxillary nerve block

A point below the zygomatic arch is marked that is lateral to the sygmoid notch of the mandible. A small wheal of local anaesthesia is raised at the site. A 7.5 cm, 22-gauge, short-beveled needle is inserted through the wheal at 45° angle to the frontal plane and slightly superiorly to the horizontal plane. If the needle contacts the lateral pterygoid plate at depth of approximately 5 cm, it must be withdrawn slightly and redirected more anteriorly. A peripheral nerve response in the distribution of the infraorbital nerve should be elicited, and the needle is withdrawn 1 or 2 mm and 3 ml of solution is deposited. If no response is produced, and if the needle lies at a depth of not greater than 35 mm, then 3-5 ml of local anaesthetic solution is deposited, with the thought that the volume of solution produces the required anaesthesia.

Ophthalmic division

The supraorbital nerve block is performed where the nerve emerges from the orbit and through the supraorbital foramen or notch. The supratroclear nerve emerges just medial to this foramen and usually is anaesthetized by the injection. The supraorbital foramen, infraorbital foramen, and the mental foramen all lie on a straight line when viewed anteriorly. The patient is supine, with the head stabilized. The skin is penetrated just medial to the supraorbital foramen, and 0.2-0.4 ml of solution is deposited as the needle advances to the foramen. The forehead and scalp are anaesthetized posteriorly to the lambdoidal suture area.

Trigeminal nerve surgery: indications and methods

Typical tic douloureux

Trigeminal nerve surgery sould be warranted for typical tic douloureux when a trial of pharmacological therapy has failed or when drugs produce unacceptable side effects or inadequate pain relief. Open surgery, aiming to dissect free trigeminal nerve root from compression of any origin, or percutaneous procedures, causing a more or less controlled damage to the nerve, are available with different indications.

Microvascular decompression (MVD)

The concept of MVD of the trigeminal nerve described by Dandy in 1934 [5], rediscovered by Gardner and Miklos [6] and fully recognized and popularized by Jannetta [7], is a milestone in the management of medically intractable trigeminal neuralgia. In the last 30 years thousands of patients have undergone successful MVD and today it represents one of the most widely used surgical options for trigeminal neuralgia. Several studies and our experience on more than 300 patients agree on the high rate of long-term success.

This is the only method which removes the presumed cause without damaging the trigeminal root. The procedure is performed under general anaesthesia via a small (less than 2 cm in diameter in our experience) lateral retromastoid craniectomy. A classical neuroanaesthesiologic technique is used: induction is performed with thiopental or propofol and anaesthesia is maintained with isoflurane and 50% nitrous oxide in oxygen. Because of the danger of air embolism, the sitting position has been abandoned and the operation is usually performed in park-bench position or in supine position, with the head rotated on the opposite side of neuralgia. Through a 6-7 cm retroauricular skin incision the asterion and the mastoid are exposed. The key-hole craniectomy should expone margins of transverse and sigmoid sinuses. Using the operating microscope, the cerebellum is retracted medially and inferiorly to expose the trigeminal nerve as it courses from Meckel's cave to the pons. The nerve is cautiousely dissected free without unnecessary manipulation. Any compressive arteries are maintained away from the nerve and its entry zone in the pons through little pieces of teflon, dacron or muscle. Compressive veins are electrocoagulated and divided. The usual finding is an ectatic superior cerebellar artery that is trapped under the nerve; this leads to second and third division pain. Most patients with first division pain have a loop of the anterior inferior cerebellar artery impinging upon the caudal parte of the nerve. We found a vascular conflict in all cases, even in patients with multiple sclerosis. In the literature, over 90% of the patients have a clear-cut impingement of the nerve by an artery or vein or sometimes a combination of the two; in the remaining small fraction of patients in whom the offending lesion is not found, a partial rhizotomy is performed by some.

In the early postoperative period pain immediately disappears in more than 90% of patients, sometimes it can fade away slowly. Some of the criticism about MVD is based on presumed high mortality and morbidity. In our experience there was no mortality and no permanent invalidity. Ataxia, disequilibrium and gait disturbances, sometimes observed in the early postoperative period or at hospital discharge (3 days after operation), had disappeared fully within 2 weeks without rehabilitation. According to data from the literature of series of more than 3 000 published cases [8], the mortality rate is 0.3% (12/3 033). Cranial nerve morbidity is reported, but generally diplopia, dysphagia, facial weakness, vertigo and trigeminal hypoesthesia are all transient. Injury to the acoustic branch of the eighth cranial nerve is the only relevant long-term cranial nerve dysfunction reported in many series, ranging from 0.1 to 3% [8]. This is probably the only complication that cannot be prevented in all patients due to the extreme vulnerability of the internal auditory artery and tiny cochlear endings. Other reported complications such as postoperative CSF leak, hemotympanum, sigmoid sinus thrombosis, cerebellar infarct and hematoma can be minimized with a careful surgical technique and perfect hemostasis. In a recent review of our experience [8] we did not find any age-related, statistically significant difference in the incidence of surgical complications and so we perform MVD without an absolute age limit. Furthermore, in elderly patients surgical exposure of the cerebellopontine angle is easier due to atrophy, and the postoperative course is generally uneventful, with early mobilization.

In the literature many series report data on the efficacy of MVD [8]. Direct comparison of results is difficult, however, because of differences in follow-up and differing definitions of operative success. The number of completely pain-free patients at long-term follow-up ranges from 53% to 94%. In our experience, about 80% of patients are pain-free at 5-year follow-up. Barker et al. [9] found 70% of 1 185 patients with an excellent outcome 10 years after surgery.

Female sex, operative findings at MVD, previous destructive surgical treatments, and duration of disease, have been correlated with the outcome. In our experience a clinical history of over 7 years is the only statistically significant prognostic factor.

Percutaneous methods

Among all the percutaneous procedures described for the treatment of trigeminal neuralgia (injection of alchohol, phenol, local anaesthetics, boiling water, cryolysis) [1], only radiofrequency thermorhizotomy, glycerol injection, and balloon microcompression are currently used today. The percutaneous approach to reach the foramen ovale described by Hartel in 1914 [10] is always followed: three anatomic landmarks are chosen on the face:
1. a point 3 cm anterior to the external auditory meatus along the lower border of the zygoma;
2. a point beneath the medial aspect of the pupil;
3. a point 2.5 cm lateral to the labial commissure at which the needle penetrates the skin of the jaw.

The foramen ovale lies on the sagittal plane crossing point 2 and on the coronal plane crossing point 1. All procedures can be performed under local anaesthesia plus sedation with barbiturates (thiopental boli of 2 mg/kg). Under fluoroscopic control, the index finger of a gloved hand is placed into the mouth to avoid unintended penetration of buccal mucosa, while the needle, aiming to the point 1, is directed initially laterally for about 3 cm in the loose cheek and than swung medially towards the sagittal plane, indentified by point 2. Using these landmarks we have been able to penetrate the foramen ovale on the first attempt in most cases and after a simple adjustment in all instances. Entrance of the needle into the foramen is signaled by a wince and a brief contraction of the masseter muscle, indicating contact with the mandibular sensory and motor fibers. Before advancing the needle any further a perfect lateral roentgenogram or fluoroscopy is necessary to control correct positioning of the needle and depth of entry inside the foramen: the needle should be directed toward the point of junction between the petrous apex and the clivus with the apex at the floor of the skull. The risk of skull base vascular and cranial nerve injury is low, but extensively documented with all percutaneous procedures: the needle can unintentionally be inserted into the jugular bulb, into the internal carotid artery as it enters the skull, into the petrous carotid in instances where the bone below was defective, into the carotid in the foramen lacerum, into the internal maxillary artery and its rami; the ninth, tenth and eleventh cranial nerves can be injured in the foramen lacerum, and the third, fourth and sixth cranial nerves in the cavernous sinus or through the inferior orbital fissure and optic nerve through the inferior orbital fissure. Reports of injury to all cranial nerves but the second can be found in the literature. Temporal abscesses and intracranial hemorrhages may also occur. Cases of death are reported [11]. A perfect knowledge of skull base anatomy and its individual variations (canal of Vesalius which lies anteromedially close to the rotundum, innominate canal of Arnold which lies posteriorly, etc.; see [11] for an extensive review) is mandatory for this kind of surgery.

Radiofrequency thermorhizotomy

A controlled radiofrequency (RF) heat lesion was introduced by Sweet and Wespic [12] because heat was shown to cause greater selective injury to A-delta and C fibers [13], sparing the heavily myelinated tactile fibers. However, selective destruction of pain fibers remains something of a myth because, clinically the temperature at the surface of the electrode is higher than at the periphery, thus destroying all fibers adjacent to the electrode before the selective heat reaches the periphery. Nevertheless radiofrequency thermorhizotomy (RFT) is probably the percutaneous technique by which, according to the literature and our experience with more than 1 500 cases, with which the best long-term results can be achieved. The technique requires good cooperation on the part of the patient and must be performed under local anaesthesia and readily reversible sedation. This can be obtained with small boli of thiopental (2 mg/kg), repeated when needed, for analgesia. With the patient in supine position the 20-gauge needle electrode is inserted inside Meckel's cave using the Hartel technique as described above and is stimulated. If the response is detected in the area where the lesion is desired, an incremental lesion is made using heat. Between increments the patient is tested until the desired sensory deficit is inflicted. If the stimulation gives a response in a different area, the electrode with thermocoupling is moved into what is believed to be the desired target and stimulation is repeated. The frequency of electrical stimulation for a sensory response is 100 Hz, with a voltage ranging from 0.05 to 0.2 V. The motor response of the masseter muscle should be evoked with no more than 0.5 V. Facial muscle contraction due to V-VII reflex and eye abduction induced by sixth nerve stimulation should be obtained at 1-1.5 V. After checking the correct placement of the electrode by neurophysiologic means, the tip temperature can be elevated to 65-70 °C to cause the lesion. Sometimes the lesion may appear in a division other than that in which the response was elicited. Occasionally, a lesion in the third division may lap to the first without involving the second and without any prodromal warning to the patient, with unintended corneal anaesthesia and subsequent keratitis (reported incidence in the literature: 0.4%-20%; our experience: 0.4%) [11, 14]. Constant testing of corneal sensation is advisable. Thousands of patients have been treated with this method all over the world and long-term follow-up data are available: 96%-100% of patients have early, complete relief; recurrences requiring operation vary from 7% to 31%; postoperative dysesthesias requiring drugs from 5% to 24% and in 1%-8% are often unbearable and intractable [11]. In our experience [14] with a 9.3-year average follow-up, a recurrence rate of 18.1% was found. A painful dysesthesia developed in 5% of cases. Keratitis requiring tarsorrhaphya was observed in 0.4% of cases, oculomotor palsy in 0.5%. A clear correlation between postoperative sensory deficit and cure rate was found.

Glycerol injection

This technique has been described by Hakanson in 1982 [15]. During the development of a stereotactic technique of trigeminal irradiation he used glycerol as a vehicle to introduce tantalum dust into the trigeminal cistern. Quite unexpectedly he observed that the intracisternal injection of glycerol alone rendered the patient completely pain free without significant sensory loss. The mechanism of action is poorly understood, and evidence is conflicting as to whether there is a selective destruction of nerve fibers and, if selective, which fibers are preferentially destroyed. The procedure is performed under local anaesthesia with the patient sitting on a rotatable chair with radiography available both by fluoroscopy and films. A 22-gauge lumbar puncture needle is inserted into the foramen ovale using the technique of Hartel [10]; CSF must be obtained. If fluoroscopy shows the needle to be in the correct position, less than 1 ml concentrated metrizamide is injected to obtain a trigeminal cisternography and to adjust the amount of glycerol to the volume of the cistern. Contrast is evacuated by gravity drip through the needle and then gravity drainage into the posterior fossa, extending the patient's head for some minutes. On returning to the sitting position, an amount of 0.18-0.3 ml glycerol is introduced. For the first division, the head must be kept forward flexed at 45°, for the second at 25° and for the third in neutral position, slightly bent toward the affected side. The position is maintained for an hour to keep the glycerol mainly in the cistern. Strong paresthesias and pain in one or more divisions may be experienced. RF stimulation can be performed during the procedure to evaluate the needle position. A sensory examination to pinprick after each drop of glycerol injected can be performed to monitor the entity of the sensory deficit. The technique has gained some popularity.

It is currently used in many centers and results have been pubblished by several authors [11]: from 82% to 96% of patients have early, complete relief after one or two glycerol injections; recurrences requiring operation vary from 9% to 30% with a medium follow-up shorter than for thermorhizotomy. Even if the method was introduced with the hope to relief from tic without causing sensory deficits, postoperative dysesthesias, anaesthesia dolorosa, and keratitis are reported at percentages similar to those of other percutaneous methods. We abandoned the method after the first 20 cases because of too many recurrences.

Percutaneous microcompression

Mullan and Lichtor [16] have converted to a percutaneous procedure the open compression of the trigeminal ganglion and root proposed by Shelden et al. in 1955 [17]. Preul et al. [18] showed a uniform, axonal swelling and fragmentation at 7 days after Mullan's technique was performed in 19 adults rabbits and concluded that trigeminal pain is mostly relieved by damage to large myelinated fibers. The corneal reflex is mediated by small fibers from the ophthalmic nerve, which is why keratitis is less likely to occur using this method. We perform this procedure under local anaesthesia with deep sedation while inflating the ballon (thiopental boli of 0.2 mg/kg), but it can also be performed under general anaesthesia because no cooperation from the patient is required. Oxygen is given via nasal prongs and heart rate and blood pressure are monitored throughtout the procedure. To counteract bradycardia and increases in blood pressure often observed during compression, atropine and sodium nitroprusside must be promptly available. A 14-gauge liver biopsy needle is inserted into, but not beyond, the foramen ovale, using the technique of Hartel [10] under fluoroscopic control. A no. 4 Fogarty balloon catheter is then pushed in 1 cm beyond the needle into Meckel's cave and slowly inflated with diluited 50% water-soluble contrast medium (Iopamiro) under fluoroscopy until it assumes a pear shape as it begins to protrude out toward the posterior fossa through the trigeminal porus. Severe braycardia requiring atropine is often observed. Initially the compression was maintained for 3-10 min with a 0.5 to 1 ml volume. Further experience has indicated that, once an appropriated pressure is reached (1 200±240 mmHg), 1 to 3 min of pear-shaped ballon compression is adequate and limits the duration of compression-related cardiovascular instability and the incidence of postoperative dysesthesias [1, 19, 20]. Bradycardia upon distension of the balloon is an indication that a good compression is being achieved [1]. Hyperemia of the conjunctiva indicates a good result, irrespective of the division involved. After deflation of the ballon, the catheter and needle are withdrawn, maintaining pressure on the soft tissues of the cheek for a few minutes to prevent formation of a hematoma should a maxillary vessel be impinged. Rarely, at the beginning of insertion of the needle through the maxillary region a hematoma may commence; after some minutes of soft tissue compression the procedure could be continued. The technique has gained great popularity among the percutaneous methods because it is easy to perform, can be repeated with little disconfort to the patient, and achieves good results with few complications. According to our experience with more than 100 cases and published series [20], this procedure has a recurrence rate that seems to be somewhat higher than that of RFT but with a lower incidence of postoperative dysesthesias, anaesthesia dolorosa and, above all, keratitis. Rare cases of generally transient diplopia have been observed.

Conclusions about surgical treatment of trigeminal tic douloureux

Typical trigeminal tic douloureux can be cured without inflicting any damage only by MVD. According to our extensive experience with both open surgery and percutaneous techniques, MVD should be proposed as first-choice surgery to all patients of all ages. Percutaneous techniques should be reserved for patients with anaesthesiologic contraindications and for patients refusing posterior fossa surgery. The presence of a postoperative sensorial deficit, sometimes well tolerated in comparison with pain, but often annoying and sometimes unbearable, should be stressed. The choice of the percutaneous technique is related to surgical skill and familiarity with different procedures. We currently use thermorhizotomy for patients with pain not involving the first division; in others a ballon compression is performed. The role of MVD in the treatment of patients affected by trigeminal neuralgia and multiple sclerosis is not clear. In our experience of about 10 cases submitted to MVD, we have observed a recurrence rate higher than in patients with the so-called idiopathic form, also when using percutaneous methods. Nevertheless, it may be worthwhile to perform MVD even in these patients to give them the possibility of pain relief without sensory deficits, also considering the possibility of developing contralateral pain during the course of the disease.

Neuropathic trigeminal pain

When a compressing mass injuring the nerve along its course can be detected by radiological means, decompressive trigeminal surgery is mandatory. Some success has been reported following chronic stimulation of the gasserian ganglion [21-23]. The electrode can be introduced either percutaneously or via a temporal craniotomy and connected to a stimulus generator implanted on the chest wall. It is not clear how to select patients for this operation. Trigeminal tractotomy or nucleotomy have also been used with variable results in some patients [24, 25]. All peripheral ablative procedures for chronic neuropathic pain are contraindicated except in cases of cancer pain with brief life expectancy.

Facial pain of vascular origin

Various surgical treatments have been tried: retrogasserian lidocaine block, alcoholization, RF lesions or glycerol injection of the gasserian ganglion, open trigeminal rhizotomy, superficial petrosal neurectomy, division of the nervus intermedius, tractotomy of bulbar descending cephalic pain tract, cryosurgery, or resection of the sphenopalatine ganglion [11]. Indications in this field are not clear and not universally accepted. Probably none of these procedures gives consistent, long-lasting relief and they should therefore not be considered before failure of full trials of medical therapy. At present, in cases of cluster headache, percutaneous alcohol injection or RF lesions to the sphenopalatine ganglion appear to be the most effective and least invasive procedures used in experienced centers. MVD can be useful in cases of TIC-cluster headache.

Cancer pain

The relevance of trigeminal nerve surgery in the treatment of cancer pain is strongly decreased since therapy with spinal intrathecal or intraventricular opioid infusion systems have become available. In cases of intolerance to opioids, ablative procedures, always preceded by a prognostic block, can be used in patients with a brief life expectancy.

References

1. Mullan S, Brown JA (1996) Trigeminal neuralgia. Neurosurgical Q 6:267-288
2. Cook WA (1995) The mandibular field and its control with local anaesthetic Mod Dent 22:11-14
3. Carter RB, Keen EN (1971) The intramandibular course of the inferior alveolar nerve. J Anat 108:433-441
4. Gow-Gates GAE (1973) Mandibular conduction anasthesia: a new technique using extraoral landmarks. Oral Surg Oral Med Oral Pathol 36:328-331
5. Dandy WE (1934) Concerning the cause of trigeminal neuralgia. Am J Surg 24:447-455.
6. Gardner WJ, Miklos MV (1959) Response of trigeminal neuralgia to "decompression" of sensory root. Discussion of cause of trigeminal neuralgia. JAMA 170:1773-1776
7. Jannetta PJ (1967) Arterial compression of the trigeminal nerve at the pons in patients with trigeminal neuralgia. J Neurosurg 26:159-162
8. Broggi G, Ferroli P, Franzini A, Servello D, Dones I (1998) Microvascular decompression for trigeminal neuralgia: considerations on a series of 250 cases, including 10 patients with multiple sclerosis. J Neurol Neurosurg Psychiatry (In press)
9. Barker FG, Jannetta JJ, Bissonette DJ, Larkins MV, Jho HD (1996) The long-term outcome of microvascular decompression for trigeminal neuralgia. N Engl J Med 334:1077-1083
10. Hartel F (1914) Trigeminusneuralgie und ganglion injection. Med Klin 10.582-584
11. Gybels JM, Sweet WH (1989) Neurosurgical treatment of persistent pain Physiological and pathological mechanisms of human pain In: Gildenberg PL (ed) Pain and headache, Vol 11. Karger, Basel, pp 30-40
12. Sweet WH, Wespic JG (1974) Controlled thermocoagulation of trigeminal ganglion and rootlets for differential distruction of pain fibers. J Neurosurg 40:143-156
13. Broggi G, Siegfried J (1977) The effect of graded thermocoagulation on trigeminal evoked potentials in the cat. Acta Neurochir 24(Suppl):175-178

14. Broggi G, Franzini A, Lasio G, Giorgi C, Servello D (1990) Long-term results of percutaneous retrogasserian thermorhizotomy for "essential" trigeminal neuralgia: considerations in 1000 consecutive patients Neurosurgery 26:783-787

15. Hakanson S (1981) Trigeminal neuralgia treated by the injection of glycerol into the trigeminal cistern. Neurosurgery 9:638-646

16. Mullan S, Lichtor T (1983) Percutaneous microcompression of the trigeminal ganglion for trigeminal neuralgia. J Neurosurg 59.1007-1012

17. Shelden CH, Pudewz RH, Freshwater DB (1955) Compression rather than decompression for trigeminal neuralgia. J Neurosurg 12:123-126

18. Preul MC, Long PB, Brown JA, Velasco ME, Weaver MT (1990) Autonomic and histopathological effects of percutaneous trigeminal ganglion compression in the rabbit. J Neurosurg 72:933-940

19. Lobato RD, Rivas JJ, Sarabia R, Lamas E (1990) Percutaneous microcompression of the gasserian ganglion for trigeminal neuralgia J Neurosurg 72:546-553

20. Lichtor T, Mullan JF (1990) A 10-year follow-up review of percutaneous microcompression of the trigeminal ganglion. J Neurosurg 72.49-54

21. Steude U (1984) Radiofrequency electrical stimulation of the gasserian ganglion in patients with atypical trigeminal pain: methods of percutaneous temporary test-stimulation and permanent implantation of stimulation devices. Acta Neurochir 33:S481-S486

22. Meyerson BA, Hakanson S (1986) Suppression of pain in trigeminal neuropathy by electrical stimulation of the Gasserian ganglion. Neurosurgery 18:59-66

23. Meyerson BA, Hakanson S (1980) Alleviation of atypical trigeminal pain by stimulation of the gasserian ganglion via an implanted electrode. Acta Neurochir 30:S303-S309

24. Schvarcz JR (1979) Stereotactic spinal trigeminal nucleotomy for dysesthetic facial pain. Adv Pain Res Ther 3:331-336

25 Nashold BS, Lopes H, Choda Kiewitz J, Bronec P (1986) Trigeminal DREZ for craniofacial pain. In: Samii M (ed) Surgery in and around the brainstem. Springer-Verlag, Berlin Heidelberg New York, pp 53-58

Chapter 16

Cervical plexus block

D. Lugani, A. Casati, G. Fanelli

Regional anaesthesia of the neck was first introduced in order to evaluate the neurological status of the patient during surgical intervention on the carotid artery and during cross-clamping. Cervical plexus block provides safe and effective anaesthesia for all unilateral neck surgical interventions such as CEA (carotid endo-arterectomy), allowing continuous check of cerebral function and perfusion.

Anatomy

The cervical plexus is formed from the ventral rami of C1-C4 spinal nerve roots. Each nerve lies posterior to the vertebral artery, in the groove between anterior and posterior tubercles which can be used as landmarks. C1-C4 roots also provide communicant rami which connect them to the superior cervical sympathetic ganglion (Figs. 1, 2).

There are two sets of cervical plexus branches: the superficial and deep ones. Piercing the cervical fascia anteriorly, superficial branches of plexus emerge along the posterior border of the sternocleidomastoid muscle, providing sensory innervation to the cutaneous district of neck, occipital, shoulder, and upper thoracic regions (Fig. 3). Deep branches supply profound structures of the neck (muscles, bones, joints) and form the phrenic nerve.

Indications and contraindications

Major indications are:
- carotid surgery;
- soft tissue surgery of neck (biopsy, exploration);
- unilateral thyroid and parathyroid surgery;
- diagnosis and therapy of chronic shoulder and neck pain.

Major contraindications are:
- local anestethetics allergy;
- lack of patient consent and/or collaboration;
- severe chronic pulmonary disease;
- infection at the site of injection;

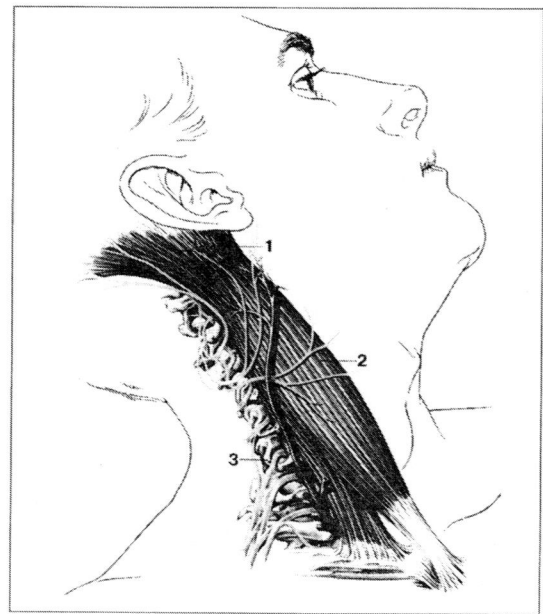

Fig. 1. (1) Mastoıd process; (2) sternocleıdo-mastoıd muscle, (3) Chassaıgnac's tubercle (From [1] wıth permıssıon)

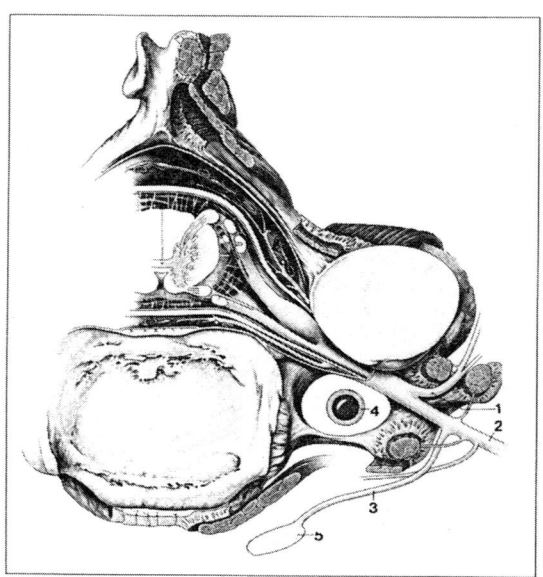

Fig. 2. (1) Prımary posterıor ramus; (2) prımary anterıor ramus; (3) Gray communıcant ramus; (4) vertebral artery, (5) cervıcal superıor ganglıon (From [1] wıth permıssıon)

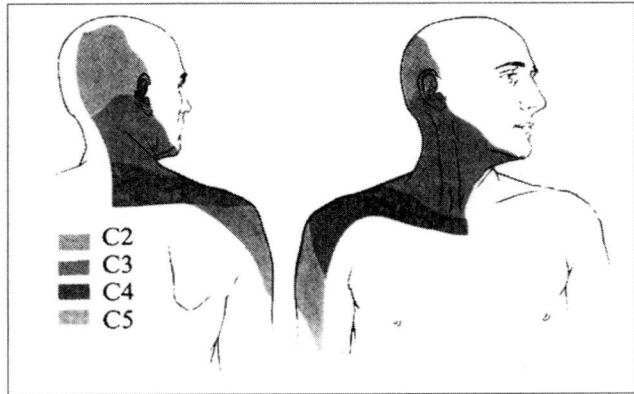

Fig. 3. Distribution of superficial cervical plexus branches. (From [1] with permission)

- coagulopathy;
- preexistent neurologic disease such as multiple sclerosis or polio.

Techniques

The patient is positioned supine with the head turned on the opposite side and the neck slightly extended [2, 3].

Superficial cervical plexus block

A 3.5 to 5 cm long fine needle (25-gauge or a 8.75-cm-long spinal needle) is inserted 1-2 cm deep at the point of crossing between the external jugular vein and posterior border of sternocleidomastoid muscle. After careful aspiration, 10-20 ml of anaesthetic solution (i.e., 1.5% lidocaine) is injected below and along the border of the muscle.

Deep cervical plexus block

A line is drawn between the tip of the mastoid and Chassaignac's tubercle (transverse process of C6 located at the level of the cricoid cartilage). A second line is drawn parallel and 1 cm posterior to this line. The transverse processes to be palpated are located approximately along the second line:
- C2 is 1.0-2.0 cm caudad to the mastoid process (measured on the first line);
- C3 is 1.5 cm caudad to C2;
- C4 is 1.5 cm caudad to C3.
 After raising skin wheals with local anaesthetic a 22-G needle is inserted at each level, with a perpendicular direction to the skin and slight caudad angulation. The needle is advanced until the contact with the transverse process is felt (1.5-3.0 cm deep). After careful aspiration for cerebrospinal fluid or blood,

5-10 ml anaesthetic solution (i.e., 2% mepivacaine) is injected at each level. Occasionally the needle insertion can elicit a paresthesia:
– in the occipital-mastoid region for C2 level;
– in the anterior neck for C3 level;
– in the subclavian region for C4 level.

Complications

1. Intrathechal injection of local anaesthetic with sudden loss of consciousness and respiratory arrest. Hypotension is also frequent. The patient must be immediately treated with artificial ventilation and vasoactive drugs.
2. Epidural injection of local anaesthetic, causing bilateral anaesthesia of upper extremities and thorax. The treatment is aimed to support ventilation (sometimes tracheal intubation and mechanical ventilation are required) and tranquilize the patient with sedative drugs.
3. Intravascular injection of the anaesthetic solution is responsible for CNS toxicity (loss of consciousness, apnea and seizures are possible if the anaesthetic is injected in a vertebral artery) and symptoms of cardiac toxicity (decreased conduction, decreased contractility up to cardiac arrest).
4. Phrenic nerve paralysis with variable respiratory failure more severe in patients affected by chronic obstructive pulmonary diseases (COPDs).
5. Anaesthetic block of other nerves of the neck such as the vagus, glossopharyngeal, recurrent laryngeal can occur. Symptoms can vary from tachycardia to hoarseness or vocal cord dysfunction. Cervical sympathetic nerve block may lead to Horner's syndrome (ptosis, enophtalmus, miosis and anhidrosis).
   A careful aspiration for blood or CSF performed before each anaesthetic injection can avoid intrathecal and intravascular injection.

Use of nerve stimulator

Electric nerve stimulation is often used in regional anaesthesia in order to identify the precise location of the nerve roots and to achieve a better level of anaesthesia with smaller amounts of drug.

Mehta and Juneja [4] describe deep cervical plexus block by Winnie's single injection technique [5] performed with a nerve stimulator (NS). As the cervical plexus is mainly a sensitive nervous structure, the NS cannot elicit muscle twitches as in motor nerves. Slight paresthesias can be obtained by using a more intense current (1.5 mA) in the seeking phase and which must never be decreased below 1 mA (considered to be the minimum level for sensory nerve stimulation). After palpating the groove between anterior and medius scalenus muscles, an 18-G needle is inserted perpendicular to the skin at C4 level in the medial, caudad, and dorsal directions. After connecting the hub of the needle to the NS, paresthesias over the shoulder and upper arm regions, and neck muscle twitches are elicited. After careful aspiration for CSF or blood, 10-15 ml of anaesthetic solution (i.e., 2% mepivacaine) are injected at this level.

The use of NS can offer several advantages compared with simple paresthesia technique; such as a more precise identification of the injection site, the need for smaller volumes of anaesthetic solution and lower anaesthetic drug plasma levels.

Cervical plexus block vs cervical epidural anaesthesia

The placement of an epidural catheter at the C6-C7 or C7-T1 level is a further regional anaesthetic technique for neck surgery [6, 7].

If compared to cervical plexus block, cervical epidural anaesthesia offers some advantages but also important side effects (Table 1).

The most untoward effect of cervical epidural anaesthesia is the risk of total phrenic nerve block: C3-C5 roots involvement can result in pulmonary compromise with reduction of forced expiratory volume in 1s (FEV_1), forced vital capacity reduction (FVC), and maximum inspiratory pressure (MIP) [8]. These respiratory changes can be clinically insignificant in patient without preexisting chronic pulmonary disease [8], while other authors [7] report respiratory failure in COPD-affected patients.

Table 1. Advantages and disadvantages of cervical epidural anaesthesia and cervical plexus block

	Advantages	Disadvantages
Cervical epidural anesthesia	• Better patient comfort during execution of block • Continuous epidural anesthesia for long-lasting surgery and postoperative analgesia	Possible phrenic nerve block Bilateral arm block Bradycardia Asymmetric anesthesia distribution Higher incidence of hypotension Placement and removal of catheter impossible during heparin therapy Adequate training in epidural catheter placement Higher anesthetic drug plasma levels Risk for total spinal block
Cervical plexus block	• Lower incidence of pulmonary side effects • Unilateral block	Higher risk of intravascular or intrathecal injection Discomfort for patient during the execution of the block

Several side effects are possible with cervical epidural anaesthesia: the most frequent are nausea and bradycardia (as a result of bilateral sympathetic block of cardioaccelerator fibers). In the presence of a large extent of anaesthesia spread, hypotension is also possible as a result of splanchnic blood pooling [9]. In contrast, carotid sinus block can enhance the hypertension caused by carotid artery cross-clamping [10].

Plasma levels of local anaesthetics during cervical plexus block

Unless injected intravascularly, plasma levels of local anaesthetic are usually lower than necessary for cardiovascular or neurological toxicity symptoms to develop even after administration of maximal doses of anaesthetic solution [11]. Either lidocaine, mepivacaine, or bupivacaine can be safely used in order to perform the anaesthetic block. Also the mixture of different drugs (e.g., lidocaine and bupivacaine 50% each) has been reported as safe [12] in spite of the cumulative toxic effect [13, 14].

During cervical plexus block, maximum plasma levels are reached rapidly because of the high vascularization of the neck region. The stellate ganglion block is associated to a faster increase in plasma levels probably due to an increased vascularization of the neck [15].

Recently, ropivacaine has been employed for cervical plexus block in carotid surgery [16]. The long duration of this drug allows performance of surgical procedures lasting more than 120 min with the clinical advantage of a lower potential for cardiovascular or CNS toxicity than bupivacaine [17].

References

1. Bruce Scott D (1991) Techniques of regional anaesthesia. Mediglobe, Fribourg
2. Kenneth Davison J, Eckhardt WF, Perese DA (1993) Clinical anaesthesia procedures of the Massachusetts General Hospital. Little Brown, Boston, pp 227-229
3 Hahn MB, McQuillan PM, Sheplock GJ (1996) Loco-regional anaesthesia. Mosby Year Book, New York, pp 69-73
4. Mehta Y, Juneja R (1992) Regional analgesia for carotid artery endarterectomy by Winnie's single injection technique using a nerve detector. J Cardiothorac Vasc Anesth 6:772-773
5. Winnie AP, Ramamurthy S, Durrani Z, Radonjic R (1975) Interscalene cervical plexus block: single injection technique. Anesth Analg 54:370-375
6. Kainuma M, Shimada Y, Matsuura M (1986) Cervical epidural anaesthesia in carotid artery surgery. Anaesthesia 41:1020-1023
7. Bonnet F, Derosier JP, Pluskwa F, Abhay K, Gaillars A (1990) Cervical epidural anaesthesia for carotid artery surgery. Can J Anaesth 37:353-358
8. Stevens RA, Frey K, Sheikh T, Kao TC, Mikat-Stevens M, Morales M (1998) Time course of the effects of cervical epidural anaesthesia on pulmonary function Reg Anesth Pain Med 23:20-24
9. Arndt JO, Hoeck A, Stanton-Hicks M, Stuehmeier KD (1985) Peridural anaesthesia and the distribution of blood in supine humans. Anaesthesiology 63:616-623

10. Bonnet F, Szebely B, AbhayK, Touboul C, Boico O, Saada M (1989) Baroreceptor control after cervical epidural anaesthesia in patients undergoing carotid artery surgery. J Cardiovasc Anesth 3:418-424

11. Tissot S, Frering B, Gagnieu MC, Vallon JJ, Motin J (1997) Plasma concentrations of lidocaine and bupivacaine after cervical plexus block for carotid surgery. Anesth Analg 84:1377-1379

12. De Jong RH, Bonin JD (1981) Mixtures of local anaesthetics are no more toxic than the parent drugs. Anaesthesiology 54:177-181

13. Mets B, Janicki PK, James MF et al (1992) Lidocaine and bupivacaine cardiorespiratory toxicity is addictive: study in rats. Anesth Analg 75:611-614

14. Spiegel DA, Dexter F, Warner DS et al (1992) Central nervous system toxicity of local anaesthetic mixtures in the rat. Anesth Analg 75:992-998

15. Wulf H, Maier C, Schele H, Wabbel W (1991) Plasma concentration of bupivacaine after stellate ganglion block. Anesth Analg 72:546-548

16. Loreggian B, Ruffa D, Greco P, Crespi G, Centemeri MD, Greco S, Servadio G (1998) Cervical plexus block with ropivacaine for carotid endarterectomy. Br J Anaesth 79:A374

17. Markham A, Faulds D (1996) Ropivacaine: a review of its pharmacology and therapeutic use in regional anaesthesia. Drugs 52:429-449

Chapter 17

Neuraxial analgesia: epidural and spinal drugs

N. Rawal

Recent research has demonstrated the increasing importance of the spinal cord in processing and modulating nociceptive input. Since their introduction into clinical practice in 1979 spinal opioids have achieved great international popularity in a variety of clinical settings either as sole analgesic agents or in combination with low-dose local anaesthetic. By bypassing the blood and blood brain barrier, small doses of opioids administered in either the subarachnoid or epidural spaces provide profound and prolonged segmental analgesia. This undoubtedly represents a major breakthrough in pain management. Numerous studies have shown that spinal opioids can provide profound postoperative analgesia with fewer central and systemic adverse effects than opioids administered systemically. A large number of non-opioids have also been administered in the epidural or subarachnoid space to achieve pain relief without the risk of respiratory depression.

Therapeutic application of spinal opioids

Segmental analgesia induced by intraspinal opioids has a role in the management of a wide variety of painful surgical and non-surgical conditions. The technique has been employed successfully to treat intra-operative, postoperative, traumatic, obstetric, chronic and cancer pain (Table 1) [1-3].

The unique feature of spinal opioid analgesia is the lack of sensory, sympathetic, or motor block, which allows patients to walk around without the risk of orthostatic hypotension or motor incoordination usually associated with local anaesthetics administered epidurally or opioids administered parenterally. These advantages of spinal opioids are particularly beneficial in high-risk patients undergoing major surgery, patients with compromised pulmonary or cardiovascular function, grossly obese patients and elderly patients [4-6]. For intrathecal administration, the analgesic doses of morphine are only 2% - 5% of parenteral morphine. Thus, patients can be expected to be less drowsy, more co-operative, and more mobile.

Management of postoperative pain is the commonest indication for spinal opioid analgesia. The technique has been used to provide pain relief following a wide variety of operations such as upper and lower abdominal, thoracic, including cardiac, perineal, and orthopaedic surgery. Spinal opioids have also been used to provide analgesia in different age groups, including children, and are

Table 1. Therapeutic applications of spinal opioid analgesia

Acute pain
- Perioperative pain
- Postoperative pain
- Labour pain
- Trauma pain
- Non-surgical pain (myocardial infarct, angina pectoris, herpes zoster, renal colic, thrombophlebitis etc.)

Cancer pain
- Long-term therapy (subcutaneous ports, implantable pumps)
- Home care

Chronic non-malignant pain
- Intractable pain (ischaemic pain, back pain, intractable angina pectoris etc)

considered particularly beneficial in the elderly high-risk patients. A large number of controlled studies have documented the efficacy of the technique for postoperative pain. In terms of analgesia and restoration of postoperative pulmonary function following abdominal or thoracic surgery, the technique has been found to be superior to alternative methods such as intermittent i.m. injection of opioids, PCA with i.v. opioids, intercostal block or interpleural analgesia [6]. The technique has been applied for treating pain from fractured ribs and in ICU patients with multiple injuries [3].

Combination of opioids and local anaesthetics

The rationale for the combination technique is that these two types of drugs eliminate pain by acting at two distinct sites, the local anaesthetic at the nerve axon and the opioid at the receptor site in the spinal cord. Spinal opioids alone provide good pain relief at rest but may not be adequate during physiotherapy and mobilisation. Although combination therapy is used for postoperative and labour pain, the results are more impressive in labour pain because it is well recognised that labour pain is different from postoperative pain as it is not relieved by epidural opioids alone. Patients receiving epidural injections of local anaesthetics combined with opioids report more rapid onset of analgesia, more profound and long-lasting labour pain relief and less motor blockade than do patients receiving either drug alone. As part of combined spinal epidural (CSE) technique, intrathecal opioids (sufentanil 5-7.5 µg or fentanyl 25 µg) combined with very small doses of local anaesthetic (bupivacaine 1 mg) provide almost instantaneous pain relief to the parturient in labour; the epidural catheter is used if labour is prolonged. These low doses allow parturients to walk around ("walking epidurals"). A 17-nation European survey has shown that the addition of fentanyl or morphine to local anaesthetics for epidural anaesthesia has become routine in many institutions [7].

Patient Controlled Epidural Analgesia (PCEA)

The increasing popularity of the i.v. patient-controlled analgesia (PCA) technique in pain management has generated interest in the use of epidural opioids via a PCA pump. This technique allows the patient to self-titrate epidural opioid or opioid-local anaesthetic combination to desired level of analgesia. Epidural PCA combines the flexibility and convenience of PCA with the superior analgesia of epidural opioids [8].

Spinal administration of non-opioids

Inhibition of afferent nociceptive transmission by mechanisms other than those acting on spinal opioid receptors has been demonstrated in several neurophysiological studies. Non-opioid receptor selective agents such as serotinergic, muscarinic, adenosinergic, γ-aminobutyric acid (GABA), somatostatin agonists and substance P antagonists are believed to inhibit pain modulation at the spinal level. In clinical practice, analgesic effects have been demonstrated following epidural or intrathecal administration of non-opioid drugs such as clonidine, somatostatin, octreotide, ketamine, calcitonin, midazolam, droperidol, neostigmine and adenosine.

Although there is ample evidence that the administration of these drugs in the epidural or subarachnoid space will provide analgesia, many of these drugs are largely experimental at present. The exception is $\alpha2$-agonist clonidine, which is the non-opioid that has been studied most extensively.

Non-opioids such as $\alpha2$-agonists may be more suited as adjuvants rather than sole analgesic agents and their main role lies in reducing the dose requirements of other analgesics. "Balanced spinal analgesia" using a combination of low doses of drugs, with separate but synergistic mechanisms of analgesia, may produce the best results. The optimal drug combinations and dosages remain to be determined.

Safety of spinal opioids

Some of the reported side effects of spinal opioids such as nausea, vomiting, hypotension, somnolence, and early respiratory depression are dose-related and are believed to be due to vascular uptake of opioids. The effects of spinal opioids on gastrointestinal function have also been receiving attention in recent years. The non-systemic and characteristic adverse effects of spinal opioids are pruritus, urinary retention, and late-onset respiratory depression. It is the latter which has major safety and nursing implications.

Respiratory depression

Respiratory depression following spinal opioids has been studied in far greater detail than any other complication related to opioid delivery route. In general, early-onset respiratory depression is a minor problem of epidural opioid analgesia. In contrast, late-onset respiratory depression is potentially more dangerous, since it may occur unexpectedly hours after injection of the opioid.

Delayed respiratory depression is believed to result from the rostral spread of opioids in the CSF. The plasma levels after epidural morphine are relatively low, but CSF concentrations are several hundred times higher. This morphine-laden CSF reaches medullary respiratory centres by diffusion and bulk flow. There is no evidence, either from laboratory or clinical experiments, that has confirmed the hypothesis of sudden respiratory depression because of the arrival of large boluses of intracranial opioid at some distant future time. Today we have a better understanding of the pattern of respiratory depression. It is slow and progressive in onset rather than a sudden apnoeic event.

The true incidence of clinically significant respiratory depression is not known. Data from anecdotal case reports, prospective, controlled studies, and retrospective nation-wide surveys show wide variations in the incidence of respiratory depression because of factors such as differences in patient populations, type of surgery, and pain scores between groups. Because of the rarity of late-onset respiratory depression, small sample sizes and invasive respiratory measurement techniques, the majority of prospective studies of epidural morphine have not detected clinically significant respiratory depression.

Since the introduction of spinal opioids for pain management 19 years ago the technique has been used in hundreds of thousands of patients world-wide. Several anecdotal reports of late-onset respiratory depression and near-misses have been published. Results from large surveys involving thousands of patients suggest that the risk of late onset respiratory depression following epidural morphine is less than 1%; this can be reduced further if certain risk factors are avoided. The risk of respiratory depression following other opioids may or may not be less; current data are inconclusive. What is clear is that respiratory depression following spinal opioids is unpredictable and may be associated with any opioid.

Data obtained over a 2 year period from one institution showed that opioids administered as i.v. PCA or epidurally carry an equally low risk of respiratory depression. Over 15 000 patients were treated either with i.v. morphine (n= 10 019), i.v. fentanyl (n=529) PCA or epidural morphine (n=3 165) and epidural fentanyl (n=1 943). The average duration of treatment was 2.48 days for patients receiving i.v. PCA and 3.76 days for those receiving epidural opioids. Patients were managed on surgical wards under acute pain services (APS) supervision; monitoring consisted of frequent recording of sedation scores and respiratory rates. The incidence of respiratory depression was 0.25% with i.v. PCA and 0.31% with epidural opioids; one i.v. PCA and one epidural patient required intubation and ICU admission [9]. These results support the impression from earlier large studies and surveys that respiratory depression may occur after any opioid irrespective of its route of administration.

It has been demonstrated that simple bedside assessment of level of consciousness and respiratory rate may be superior to sophisticated apnoea monitoring devices. Although the risk should not be underestimated, it is also clear that it is not necessary to nurse most patients in an ICU or postanaesthesia care unit. In 1992 the Swedish Society of Anaesthesiology and Intensive Care issued guidelines for the use of spinal opioids on surgical wards. Irrespective of age, all patients who receive spinal opioids can now be nursed on regular wards. This approval is based on the use of morphine. The observation time is 12 h after every injection. Similar guidelines were proposed by European Society of Regional Anaesthesia (ESRA) in 1996 [10].

Prophylactic antagonist administration

The potential advantage of prophylactic opioid antagonists to patients receiving spinal opioids is that they may prevent respiratory depression that might otherwise go unnoticed if patients are monitored intermittently. This would increase the safety of spinal opioids and allow their use beyond the confines of the ICU and postanaesthesia care unit. Naloxone is effective in reversing respiratory depression associated with administration of spinal opioids, but, its action is of shorter duration than that of most opioids and there is a risk of recurrence of respiratory depression after a single dose. Its short elimination half-life necessitates repeated i.v. injections. This can be overcome by administration of continuous infusion of low-dose naloxone. It has been demonstrated that low-dose naloxone infusion ($0.25 \, \mu g \, kg^{-1} \, h^{-1}$) not only attenuates side effects but may also reduce postoperative opioid requirements [11].

Mixed agonist-antagonist drugs such as nalbuphine or butorphanol have also been used. Both naloxone and nalbuphine require careful dose titration to achieve satisfactory reversal of respiratory depression without reversal of analgesia or precipitating haemodynamic adverse effects. Recently, synthetic analogues of naloxone such as naltrexone and nalmefene have been developed.

Organisation of APS: safety aspects

Analgesia techniques such as patient-controlled analgesia (PCA), spinal opioids alone or in combination with local anaesthetics and other regional analgesia techniques provide superior pain relief as compared to intermittent i.m. injection of opioids but such techniques carry their own risks and therefore require special monitoring. Traditional methods of analgesia are not risk-free either but the risks have rarely been quantified. It is increasingly recognised that the solution to the problems of postoperative pain management lies not so much in the development of new techniques as in development of an organisation to exploit existing expertise. Thus, the safety aspects of newer techniques, whether risk of respiratory depression following spinal or PCA opioids or hypotension, motor block and urinary retention following central blocks are closely related to organisation of APS. The first line of defence against serious complications is an organisation that provides appropriate education and policies that permit nurses and physicians to safely care for patients. Clear instructions should be provided regarding doses of analgesic drugs, treatment of inadequate analgesia, patient monitoring, potential complications (technical or medical) and their management. A well-organised pain service ensures safe pain management [12].

References

1. Cousins MJ, Mather LE (1984) Intrathecal and epidural administration of opioids Anesthesiology 61:276-310
2. Morgan M (1989) The rational use of intrathecal and extradural opioids Br J Anaesth 63:165-188
3. Rawal N (1992) Spinal opioids. In· Raj PP (ed) Practical Management of Pain. Mosby Year Book, New York, pp 829-851
4. Yeager MP, Glass DD, Neff RK et al (1987) Epidural anesthesia and analgesia in high-risk surgical patients. Anesthesiology 66.729-736
5. Rawal N, Sjostrand U, Christoffersson E et al (1984) Comparison of intramuscular and epidural morphine for postoperative analgesia in the grossly obese· influence on postoperative ambulation and pulmonary function Anesth Analg 63:583-592
6. Ballantyne JC, Carr DB, de Ferranti S et al (1988) The comparative effects of postoperative analgesic therapies on pulmonary outcome: cumulative meta-analyses of randomized controlled trials Anesth Analg 86·598-612
7. Rawal N, Allvin R and EuroPain Study Group on Acute Pain (1996) Epidural and intrathecal opioids for postoperative pain management in Europe. A 17-nation questionnaire study of selected hospitals. Acta Anaesth Scand 40:1119-1126
8. Curry PD, Pacsoo C, Heap DG (1994) Patient-controlled epidural analgesia in obstetric anaesthetic practice. Pain 57:125-128
9. Group M, Grass JA, Shrewsbery P, Mekhail N (1998) Incidence of respiratory depression with i.v. PCA and epidural analgesia managed by an acute pain service. Reg Anesth Pain Med 23:A41
10 Aguilar JL, Benhamou D, Bonnet F, Dahl J, Rawal N, Rubin A (1997) ESRA guidelines for the use of epidural opioids Int Monitor Reg Anaesth 9:3-8
11. Gan TJ, Ginsberg B, Glass PSA, Fortney J, Jhaveri R, Perno R (1997) Opioid-sparing effects of a low-dose infusion of naloxone in patient-administered morphine sulphate. Anesth Analg 87:1075-1081
12. Rawal N, Berggren L (1994) Organization of acute pain services – a low cost model. Pain 57: 117-123

Chapter 18

Combined spinal epidural anaesthesia

M. Berti, A. Casati, G. Fanelli

While epidural and spinal blockades are well established regional anaesthetic techniques, combined spinal-epidural anaesthesia (CSE) has become increasingly popular only in last few years. The main reason for this development is the ability of combined spinal-epidural technique to combine the fast onset of spinal block with the possibility to prolong the regional block both intra- and postoperatively.

Spinal anaesthesia is an easy technique, allowing deep blockade of both sensory and motoric nerve roots to be achieved with small doses of local anaesthetic solution. However, when the single-shot technique is used, it is not possible to improve an inadequate block or to prolong the block for postoperative pain relief. On the other hand, compared with epidural blockade, spinal anaesthesia leads to an increased risk for severe and unpredictable hemodynamic side effects and a less predictable spread of the block [1, 2].

The use of a 32-gauge spinal catheter for continuous spinal anaesthesia and post-operative pain management has been reported. However, spinal micro-catheters are often difficult to use and are very expensive [3]. Epidural anaesthesia provides a more predictable control of the central blockade and the insertion of a catheter into the epidural space allows a safe postoperative analgesia with minimal hemodynamic impairment [4]. Disadvantages of the epidural blockade are the risk of an inadequate distribution of the block in 10%-25% of patients (jeopardized epidural anaesthesia).

The rationale for using a combination of the two techniques was to associate the advantages of each technique, minimizing specific disadvantages. The combination of epidural and spinal anaesthesia should provide both short onset and deep blockade of spinal anaesthesia, lower hemodynamic effects by using small doses of spinal anaesthetics with the possibility of improving an inadequate anaesthesia level by means of further top-up epidural doses, and finally a good postoperative pain relief with the epidural catheter.

Various CSE techniques are reported in the literature, and many kits are currently available. Our purpose is to describe the CSE technique and to evaluate the advantages and disadvantages of different technological devices offered to the practical anaesthetist at the present moment.

History

In 1937 Soresi applied an episubdural technique by first injecting local anaesthetic solution in the epidural space and then advancing the needle into the subarachnoid space. This technique did not have great advantages and was not developed further.

In 1979 Curelaru [5], a Swedish anaesthesiologist, introduced an epidural catheter in the epidural space, then, after an epidural test dose had confirmed the correct placement of the epidural catheter, performed a conventional spinal anaesthesia in more caudal interspace. This CSE technique was called double segment or double space technique (DST) and was successfully used during elective Cesarean section by Brownridge [6, 7]. Subsequently, a single space CSE technique (SST) has been reported [8]: after the epidural space was located by a Tuohy needle, a spinal needle 1 cm longer than the Tuohy one was introduced in the subarachnoid space through the Tuohy needle, which was used as an introducer. After the intrathecal injection of local anaesthetic solution, the spinal needle was withdrawn and an epidural catheter was inserted into the epidural space.

Theoretically, this new approach to combined spinal-epidural anaesthesia could produce an increased risk for accidentally placing the epidural catheter into the subarachnoid space through the hole performed in the dura by the spinal needle. Initially, it was suggested the epidural space be located with the hole of the Tuohy needle caudally directed, and then to turn it by 180° before epidural catheter insertion. However, Rawal et al. [9] have demonstrated that this rotation provides no advantages but increases the risk for dural puncture.

Four CSE techniques are available at the present moment:
1. the single needle – single space technique;
2. the double needles – double interspaces technique;
3. the needle through needle technique;
4. the needle beside needle technique.

Double space versus single segment technique

Each CSE technique has its own advantages and disadvantages. The double space technique enables placement of the epidural catheter before the subarachnoid injection is done, providing the feasibility of an epidural test dose before the spinal block is induced. However, if spinal block is induced a few minutes after the epidural test dose, it may be difficult to distinguish between the spinal and epidural blockade, while part of the epidural test dose could compare in the spinal needle hub during dural puncture. Moreover, the epidural catheter can divert the spinal needle during dural puncture or can be perforated by it with the risk of serious damage.

Since it requires only one skin puncture, the single segment technique is less time consuming and better accepted by the patient than the double segment one [10]. This could theoretically also provide a reduction in morbidity from interspinous penetration (including backache and postdural puncture headache) and in the incidence of epidural venous puncture hematoma and infection [4, 11]. The theoretical disadvantages of the single segment approach to CSE may be represented by an increase in the difficulties encountered in identifying the dural sac [12, 13] (i.e., small protrusion of spinal needle beyond the Tuohy needle, or possible deviation from sagittal plane of the Tuohy needle, leading to lateral puncture of dural sac), risk for inadequate distribution of the spinal block if the introduction of the epidural catheter is difficult, impossibility to use the epidural test dose, and the penetration of the epidural catheter into the subarachnoid space through the dural hole produced by the spinal needle. However, it has been reported that the risk for accidentally placing the epidural catheter through the dural hole produced by the spinal needle is very low when fine needles are used [9, 11, 14]. Since the spinal needle is maintained in place only by the dura mater during the intrathecal injection, it can be displaced increasing the rate of failed spinal block [9, 11-13].

While for the double segment technique we can use conventional spinal and epidural needles, special kits are available for single segment techniques:
1. double lumen kit: a Tuohy needle equipped with a parallel tube functioning as a guide for a fine spinal needle. Two parallel tube needles are available: the bent parallel tube (Hanaoka needle) and the straight parallel tube (Eldor needle);
2. tuohy needle with a back hole: technological progress has produced Tuohy needles with an additional hole, through which only a fine spinal needle can be passed;
3. the adjustable system: technological progress has also produced new systems with an adjustable interlocking device, which allows fixation of the spinal needle to the hub of the Tuohy one. These new kits also provide a spinal needle protruding up to 15 mm beyond the tip of the Tuohy needle, allowing an improvement in the success rate of spinal blockade [10, 15].

Indications and contraindications

Combined spinal-epidural anaesthesia has been used alone or with light general anaesthesia in health young patients as well as in high risk, elderly patients in various surgical and nonsurgical procedures, such as abdominal, urological and orthopedic surgical procedures, or during Cesarean section and labor [9, 11].

The contraindications of CSE are the same for either spinal or epidural anaesthesia alone, including low platelet count ($<100\ 000\ mm^3$), impairment of clotting system, severe heart disease such as aortic stenosis or cardiogenic shock, skin infection at the injection site or sepsis, endocranial hypertension, and psychiatric diseases.

The needle through needle technique

With the patient in either the sitting or lateral decubitus position, the epidural space is located with a conventional loss of resistance technique [16] at a lower than L2 interspace. Then, a 27-gauge, pencil point spınal needle is introduced into the Tuohy needle and advanced until either the dural click or free flow of cerebrospinal fluıd (CSF) is observed [17]. Afterward the appropriate dose of local anaesthetic solution is injected. After the spinal needle has been withdrawn, the epidural catheter can be introduced into the epidural space followed by accurate aspiration and injection of 1 ml normal saline to avoid intrathecal or intravascular placement of the epidural catheter, confirming its patency [18]. An epidural test dose should not be administered at this stage, and no epidural anaesthetic should be administered until 15-20 min after spinal injection. If a spinal blockade is produced lower than T_{11}, an epidural top-up (2-5 ml) can be injected to achieve an adequate surgical blockade.

The double segment technique

With the patient in either the sitting or lateral decubitus position, the epidural space is located with a conventional loss of resistance technique [16], then an epidural catheter is introduced into the epidural space through the epidural needle for 4-5 cm. After negative aspıration so as to avoid intrathecal or intravascular placement of the epidural catheter, 3 ml 2% lidocaine can be injected as a test dose. It should be emphasized that, if an epidural test dose is injected, then the anaesthesiologist has to wait an adequate time before inducing spinal block. It has been reported that the onset time for sensory anaesthesia in the S2 segment can be expected within 2 min after intrathecal injection of 3 ml of 1.5% hyperbaric lidocaine [19]; feeling warm feet should not be considered as a reliable indicator of spinal blockade [19]. After a negative epidural test dose, conventional spinal puncture can be performed one or more interspaces below the level of epidural catheter placement, and the appropriate dose of local anaesthetics solution is injected.

The anaesthesiologist must remember that migration of the epidural catheter into the subdural or subarachnoid space is always possible. Thus, each further epidural injection of local anaesthetic solution should be considered as a test dose, avoiding any large volume injection as epidural top-up.

Sequential block

It is well known that both epidural and spinal anaesthesia affect the cardiovascular system due to symphatetic blockade, leading to hypotension and bradycardia [1, 20]. Despite an intravenous preload and the use of vasopressor drugs, it is often difficult maintaining cardiovascular homeostasis when high levels of spinal block are induced, especially in elderly, high risk patients or in pregnant women, in whom prolonged hypotension can lead to an increased fetal risk. To reduce the incidence of hemodynamic complications in high risk patients, a two-stage approach to combined spinal epidural anaesthesia has been suggested [9]. After adequate IV preload (10-15 ml kg^{-1}), a small dose of local anaesthetic solution (i.e., 6-10 mg 0.5% hyperbaric bupivacaine) is injected into the sub-arachnoid space, to achieve a sensory block up to T_8. Then, after 10-15 min, the level of sensory block can be increased by means of small epidural top-up (2-3 ml of local anaesthetic solution) until a T_4 sensory level is reached (Tables 1-6).

Table 1. Level of spinal anaesthesia required for different surgical procedure

Level of block	Surgical procedure
T_4-T_5	Upper abdomen and Cesarean section
T_6-T_8	Urologic and gynecological surgery
T_{10}	TURP, hip surgery and vaginal delivery
L_1	Inferior limb
L_2-L_3	Foot surgery
S_2-S_5	Perineal surgery

Table 2. Site of injection, anaesthetic dose and expected duration for different level of spinal block

Level of block	Site of injection	Dose mg	Expected duration min
S_1-S_5	L_4-L_5	5	40-60
$<L_1$	L_4-L_5	8	60-90
T_{10}	L_3-L_4	10	90-120
T_6	$>L_3$	15	120-180

Table 3. Time and dose of epidural top-up

Drug	Amount per segment ml	Two segment regression min	Epidural top-up min
Lidocaine 2%	1-2	100±40	60
Bupivacaine 0.5%	1-2	200±80	120-180
Ropivacaine 0.5%	1-2	170±20	120-160

Table 4. Dosages in combined spinal epidural anaesthesia for Caesarean section with intrathecal injection of 0.5% hyperbaric bupivacaine

Level of block	Spinal anaesthesia[a] ml	Epidural anaesthesia ml
T_3-T_4	1.3	Bupivacaine 0.5% 10
T_4	1.5-1.6	Bupivacaine 0.25% 8
T_4	1.6-1.8	Bupivacaine 0.5% 10.9
T_4	1 5-2	Bupivacaine 0 5% 0-10
T_4	1.5-2	Bupivacaine 0 5% 6.4 (mean)

[a] 0.5% hyperbaric bupivacaine

Table 5. Epıdural top-up dose

Drugs	Onset min	Two segment regression min	Top-up dose	Time for top-up dose min
2% Lıdocaıne	15	40-60	½ starter	60-90
0.75% Ropıvacaıne	10-20	170±20	½ starter	120-160
0.5% Bupıvacaıne	20-30	120-180	½ starter	120-180

Table 6. Postoperative analgesic solutıons

Drug	Solution %	Loading dose ml	Infusion rate ml/h	Incremental dose ml	Lock out min
Morphıne + Bupıvacaıne *	0.002 0.125	5	4-6	1-2	15-20
Fentanyl + Bupıvacaıne **	0.00025 0.125	5	4-6	1-1.5	15-20
Ropıvacaıne	0.2	5	4-6	1-2	20
Ropıvacaıne + Fentanyl 2.5 g/ml	0.2	5	4-6	1-2	20

* bupıvacaıne 0.5% 25 ml + normal salıne 75 ml + morphyne 2 mg
** bupıvacaıne 0 5% 25 ml + normal salıne 70 + fentanyl 5 ml

CSE for vaginal delivery

The use of CSE has been also reported during management of labor pain [21] by injecting into the subarachnoid space 2 ml 0.25% plain bupivacaine or 1 ml 0.25% plain bupivacaine and either 3 g sufentanil or 12.5 g fentanyl (a lower than 2 ml volume of local anaesthetic solution is recommended [22]). This approach allows for an adequate management of labor pain for 90-120 min without motor blockade. Afterwards, epidural top-up by means of 3-8 ml either 0.1% or 0.125% bupivacaine can be used to prolong pain relief. This technique may be useful in late labor, when the patient asks for analgesia but little time is available before delivery. The extradural catheter may be useful to improve inadequate pain relief or if labor prolongs beyond the duration of spinal analgesia [22].

Postoperative pain management

For postoperative pain relief, continuous epidural infusion should be preferred; otherwise a conventional approach by epidural boluses can be used. Low concentrations of anaesthetic solution (alone or with opioids) can be used.

References

1. Auroy Y, Narchi P, Messiah A et al (1997) Serious complications related to regional anesthesia. Anesthesiology 87:479-486
2. Casati A, Fanelli G, Beccaria P, Aldegheri G, Berti M, Agostoni M, Torri G (1997) Hemodynamic monitoring during alkalinized lidocaine epidural block for lower limb surgery: a comparison with subarachnoid anesthesia. Eur J Anaesth 14:300-306
3. Rundshagen I, Standll T, Kochs E, Muller M, Schulte J (1997) Continuos spinal analgesia. Reg Anesth 22:150-156
4. Rawal N, Van Zundert A, Holmstrom B, Crowhurst JA (1997) Combined spinal epidural technique. Reg Anesth 22:406-423
5. Curelaru I (1979) Long duration subarachnoid anesthesia with continuous epidural block. Prakt Anaesth Wiedebelebung Intensivther 14:71-78
6. Brownridge P (1979) Central neural blockade and Caesarean section. Part I: review and case series. Anaesth Intens Care 7:33
7. Brownridge P (1981) Epidural and subarachnoid anaesthesia for elective Caesarean section. Anaesthesia 36:70
8. Muntaz MH, Daz M, Kuz M (1982) Another single space technique for orthopedic surgery (Letter). Anaesthesia 2:37-90
9. Rawal N, Scholling J, Wesstrom G (1988) Epidural versus combined spinal epidural block for Caesarean section. Acta Anaesthesiol Scand 32:61-66
10. Casati A, D'Ambrosio A, De Negri P, Fanelli G, Tagariello V, Tarantino F (1998) A clinical comparison between needle-through-needle and double-segment techniques for combined spinal/epidural anesthesia. Reg Anesth 23(in press)
11. Felsby S, Juelsgaard P (1995) Combined spinal and epidural anesthesia. Anesth Analg 80:821-826
12. Lyons G, MacDonald R, Mikl B (1992) Combined epidural/spinal anaesthesia for Caesarean section. Through needle or in separate spaces? Anaesthesia 47:199-201
13. Urmey WF, Stanton J, Peterson M, Sharrock NE (1995) Combined spinal-epidural anesthesia for outpatient surgery. Dose response characteristics of intrathecal isobaric lidocaine using a 27-gauge Whitacre spinal needle. Anesthesiology 83:528-534
14. Carrie L (1998) Combined spinal epidural anaesthesia: puzzles problems and fixes. Issues of the annual Meeting of the South African Society of Anesthesia, Durban, pp 560-565
15. Hoffmann VLH, Vercauteren MP, Buczkowski PW, Vanspringel GLJ (1997) A new combined spinal-epidural apparatus: measurement of the distance to the epidural and subarachnoid spaces. Anaesthesia 52:350-355
16. Sabersky L, Kondamury S, Osinubi OY (1997) Identification of epidural space: is loss of resistance to air a safe technique? Reg Anesth 22:3-15
17. Lambert D, Hurley R, Hertwig L, Datta S (1997) Role of needle gauge and tip configuration in the production of lumbar puncture headache. Reg Anesth 22:66-72
18. Mulroy M, Norris M, Liu S (1997) Safety steeps for epidural injection of local anaesthetics: review of the literature and recommandation. Anesth Analg 85:1346-1356
19 Abraham RA, Harris A, Maxwell LG, Kaplow S (1986) The efficacy of 1 5% lidocaine with 7.5% destrose and epinephrine as an epidural test dose for obstetrics. Anesthesiology 64:116-119
20. Carpenter RL, Caplan RA, Brown DL, Stephenson C, Wu R (1992) Incidence and risk factors for side effects of spinal anesthesia. Anesthesiology 76:906-916
21. Gautier P, Debry F, Fanard L, Van Steenberge A, Hody JL (1997) Ambulatory combined spinal epidural blockade analgesia for labor. Reg Anesth 22:143-149
22. Stacey RG, Watt M, Kadim M, Morgan M (1993) Single space combined spinal extradural technique for analgesia in labour. Br J Anaesth 71:499-502

Chapter 19

Imaging for regional block: clinical applications of sympathetic blockade in pain therapy

L. BRANCA

Biomedical imaging began 100 years ago: in 1885 Roentgen discovered X-rays and in the early 1970s computed tomography (CT), in the early 1980s magnetic resonance imaging (MRI), and in the last few years posctron emission tomography (PET) and single photon emission computed tomography (SPECT) have come to be.

The past two decades have seen a revolution in imaging that has had a profound effect on medicine and research; and research is still under way.

In pain therapy, imaging is a fundamental tool in algorithmic clinical diagnostics and therapeutic intervention by invasive techniques [1].

The injection of anaesthetic, neurolytic agents is a medical procedure and thus constitutes a true contract between the anaesthesiologist and patient.

In this context of legal responsibility, the anaesthesiologist undertakes the following:
- to give the most up-to-date care;
- to inform the patient of normally expected consequences of the procedure;
- to record the patient's medical history and to evaluate the indications for the procedure to undertake;
- to provide adequate human and technical resources for the procedure and follow-up.

The practice is inseparable from risk. Risk management requires the recognition that risk exists and that imaging it is a suitable means of diminishing this risk.

Many investigators believe that, for many pain syndromes in which the functional relationship of the sympathetic nervous system causes of chronic pain have been recognized, early treatment by antalgic blocks will decrease the likelihood that chronic intractable pain will ensue.

Moreover, a vast amount of experimental and clinical evidence has accumulated to indicate that interruption of a certain portion of the sympathetic nervous system has beneficial effects on many of these disorders.

Many studies have, however, demonstrated a direct modulation of the sympathetic on afferent fibres, on proprioceptors and on other peripheral receptors, the so-called pain receptors. So the sympathetic system can control pain, allodynia and hyperalgesia.

As far as the action of pain on the sympathetic nervous system is concerned, it has been demonstrated that the action of noxious stimuli at the level of the deep somatic structures may determine the excitation on the sensitive receptors, activating the afferent discharge and inducing a reflex excitation of somatic and vegetative efferent paths. Activation of the somatic efferent fibres determines the phenomenon of muscular contraction and, consequently, further excitation of the sensitive receptors [2].

This is a sudden interruption in the flow of pain information from the periphery to the dorsal horns. In the case of prolonged pain stimulation, it slows the process of genic expression that accompanies the first electrophysiological response. This process, which is one of transcription and can quite justifiably be likened to the long-term potentiation of memory, is responsible for the sensitization of the response, for the broadening of the receptive field, and for the prolongation of the discharge. It starts within a few minutes of repetition of the stimulus (immmediate-early genes) and extends to the entire neuronal chain, including the central section, right up to the somatosensory cerebral cortex [3].

Sympathetic blockade alleviates sympathetically maintained pain, whether the causative lesion is central or peripheral. It probably has an indirect beneficial effect by causing local vasodilatation that improves blood/tissue exchange, with the peroxidation of the products of cellular decomposition and the removal of toxic products (which stimulate pain) [4].

The pathogenesis of this pain is explained by the hypothesis of the "vicious circle" of impulses "periphery – afferent fibres – spinal cord – sympathetic efferent fibres – periphery".

Block of the stellate ganglion and thoracic sympathectomy

Sympathetic blockade at the cervicothoracic level is used for the diagnosis and treatment of painful and other conditions of the head and extremities. One must be as certain as possible that the needle is properly placed; except for C6 anterior tubercle injection, this means the use of radiologic imaging [5].

The stellate (or cervicothoracic) ganglion is the fused inferior cervical and first thoracic sympathetic ganglion. The anterior paratracheal approach to the C6 anterior tubercle is the most popular since it lessens the risk of vascular injection and pleural or vascular injury. This level is chosen for safety reasons and the easy identification of the landmark, not because this is the location of the ganglion.

In vivo imaging with MR shows the ganglion sitting on the anterior surface of the head of the first rib [6]; in transverse planes the distance between the stellate ganglion and the midline varied from 19 and 28 mm (left side) to 21 and 30 mm (right side). In sagittal MRI planes the distance between the stellate ganglion and the dome of the pleura varied from 10 to 40 mm [7].

A relatively large volume of local anaesthetic is required for stellate ganglion blockade in order to fill the fascial compartment around the anterior lateral vertebral column when needle placement is at Chaussaignac's tubercle .

Placement of the needle at the anterior lateral border of C7 provides a higher incidence of successful blockade, causes fewer side effects and requires less local anaesthetic than the conventional method of needle placement at C6 [8].

The needle is inserted two finger-breadths above the sternal notch and 2 lateral from the midline. The needle is inserted slightly mesiad to reach a bony endpoint at the junction of the lateral mass with the vertebral body. There is no anterior process at C7.

Stellate ganglion block at T1 requires a CT scanner; the needle is inserted at an angle determined by the scan to avoid the carotid. There is never any lung at this level.Check with repeated scans as the needle is advanced to the bone; inject anaesthetic mixed with non-ionic contrast, and check a new scan after the first injection to confirm there has been no spread to a vessel or the foramen [6].

In this procedure,the scanner is moved to the level of the stellate ganglion which coincides with the level of the caudal end of the head of the first rib. The distance from the injection site to the medial head of the first rib is measured and the entry angle noted. A laser light is then projected onto the patient to allow localization of the entry site on the skin [9].

Neurolytic thoracic sympathectomy is usually performed at the 2nd and 3rd thoracic level. The thoracic sympathetic chain is related laterally to the pleura and medially to the intravertebral foramina, introducing risks of pneumothorax or either accidental subarachnoid or epidural anaesthesia.

No effective anatomical barrier exists between the sympathetic and somatic nerves in the thoracic region. As a result, extremely precise needle localization and careful limitation of the injected volume are essential to avoid spillage onto somatic roots and consequent risks of segmental numbness, motor weakness, and dysaesthesia [10].

The patient is placed in the prone position with a pillow under the chest, allowing the thoracic curvature of vertebral column to flatten. The landmark is made on the skin using a X-ray image intensifier observing upper ribs and the 1st, 2nd, 3rd and 4th thoracic vertebral bodies. The landmarks include the midline, the transverse line drawn at the midpoints of the 2nd, 3rd, and 4th spinous processes. The points for the insertion of the needles are on the transverse lines, 4-5 cm from the midline.

We must always keep in mind that there is an anatomical relationship between the thoracic sympathetic chain and somatic thoracic roots. They are very close to each other so that the distribution of contrast medium should be confirmed prior to the injection of neurolytic solution [11].

Neurolytic solution should not extend to the 1st thoracic vertebral body. Bonica has developed the paralaminar technique [12]. For the injection of neurolytic solution a 22-gauge short-bevelled needle is used with a 2 ml glass syringe that has been tested to ensure that its wet plunger fits properly so that it can be advanced and withdrawn without any resistence. This is crucial to the second step of determining passage of the bevel of the needle through the superior costotransverse ligament.

To verify the level of the injection it is highly desirable to use an image intensifier and to know the relationship between the spinous process of one vertebra and the lamina to be contacted at the cross-sectional plane.

The needle is inserted only 2 cm lateral to the spinous process and contact is made in the lower portion of the lateral part of the lamina; the second insertion places the bevel of the needle just above the upper surface of the rib below and at some distance below and anterior to the toracic somatic nerve.

Alcoholization of the coeliac ganglia and splanchnic nerves

Neurolytic coeliac plexus block is claimed to be the most satisfactory treatment for pancreatic cancer pain,but its effectiveness and duration remain controversial because of methodological difficulties [13]. The technique chosen for the neurolysis of the coeliac ganglia must be determined according to the local anatomical/pathological condition of the patient, the extent of tumour spread (disclosed by imaging with the patient in a prone or supine position, prior to the execution of the operation), and the clinician's experience and expertise. Recent developments in medical technique allow a safer and more accurate method, minimizing the complication of the block.

Moore et al. [14] studied spread of nerolytic solution in 20 patients and three cadavers and suggested that "CT should be used to improve or confirm our knowledge of needle placement and spread solutions". Nevertheless, other techniques, ranging from no radiographic guidance to CT confirmation, did not alter the quality of block or incidence of complications [15]. Any major complications are rare and can be avoided by a very secure technique.

A consensus could not be reached because of the lack of CT scanners in many hospitals and the latest experience of many anaesthesiologists with the fluoroscopytechnique.

Of course, CT scanning prevents most problems, but even so some surgical interventions as well as some very expanding tumours might disturb the anatomy of the upper abdomen, together with the normal variations in man [16].

In spite of this observation, the less experience one has with the technique of neurolytic coeliac plexus block, the more emphasis should be placed on accurate location of needle position prior to injection of neurolytic solution.

In recent years the fine biopsy needles and the equipment used to control the coeliac plexus position and the needle path (ultrasound, CT) have prompted the "rediscovery" of the old technique [17]. The ultrasonic scanning technique has proved to be a method of reasonable sensitivity for visualizing the intra-abdominal structures; up to now very few communications have been published on this topic, the most comprehensive one being the article by Montero-Matemala et al. [18].

After placing the patient in a supine position and aseptic preparation of skin, the anterior aortic wall and the coeliac axis are localized in transverse scan so as to determine the level of coeliac axis. Then the special ultrasonic transducer with a central canal through which a puncture needle can be introduced is directed longitudinally and angulated until the beam of the oscilloscope screen meets the target. This is the point situated directly below the coeliac axis on the ventral aortic wall. A 22-gauge needle 15 cm long is inserted through the sterile puncture transducer. The needle is advanced up to the characteristic resistance and, (held gently by thumb and long fingers) transmitted pulsation of the aorta is felt [17, 18].

As the ultrasound technique visualizes the injected solution, contrast medium is not necessary. Lastly, sonography shortens the time of the neurolytic procedure.

Using this technique there has been no evidence of posterior spread of neurolytic solution toward the lumbar plexus, lumbar sympathetic chain or epidural space, so the complications described in the posterior techniques do not occur.

There are also techniques used by anaesthesiologists and radiologists guided by ultrasound or an other imaging method, that pass "very thin" needles through the anterior abdominal wall, stomach, intestines, and pancreas to allow the needle tip to be positioned in its desired anterocrural location [19].

A technique for CT guidance of coeliac ganglia blocks was originally introduced by Haaga et al. [20]; for that procedure a 22-gauge needle 15 cm long is inserted from the point of entry in the upper abdominal wall perpendicular to the spinous process of L1 and is located over the coeliac plexus in the preaortic area. The correct position of the needle is verified by the spread of the contrast [17].

The method mostly used world-wide is a fluoroscopy-guided block in a patient in the prone or the lateral decubitus position. Biplanar fluoroscopy is used to confirm the correct position of the needle by injecting 2-4 ml of radio-opaque dye. Contrast medium spread and the image seen in the postero-anterior and lateral radiologic views will depend on the technique utilized: retrocrural, transcrural or transaortic.

If an anterocrural technique is utilized, radiographic guidance is imperative, since there are no algorithms that allow consistent percutaneous placement.

Contrast-enhanced CT scans demonstrate the difficulties involved in confining the neurolytic agent to the anterior, peri-aortic and precrural regions.

With Ischia's transaortic technique [21] (a needle which passes through the aorta and reaches a point above the coeliac trunk), the antero-posterior image shows a patch of contrast medium extending from T12 to L2 in a midline location anterior to the bodies of the vertebrae, which often gives rise to irregular lateral images along the costovertebral groove due to spread of the iodate solution along the ventral surface of the medial and intermediate crura of the diaphram. In the lateral projection, the needle penetrates at the level of the midpoint of the body of L1; the contrast medium forms a mainly pre-aortic patch extending to the upper edge of L3. These images appear as a dorsal extension of the pre and peri-aortic patches.

CT scan demonstrated that the iodate solution spreads around the aorta, predominantly in the pre-aortic region.

Singler [22] has described the transcrural technique (two needles located in the para-aortic position, very close to the origin of the coeliac trunk); the approach offers a similar precrural, peri-aortic spread, but it is technically more laborious and depends heavily upon the systematic use of CT.

A retrocrural block, the longest used with a classical description, involves a deep splanchnic nerve block. This results in the spread of solution cephalad and posterior to the diaphragmatic crura.

Some investigators recommend a diagnostic block before a neurolytic block; the advantages of a diagnostic block include evaluation of the effectiveness and physiological consequences of the block and observation of the patient's response. There are differences in local diffusion.

Individual patients with pancreatic cancer were more likely to have a right retrocrural space which was predicted to be unreachable during a classical retrocrural block than were patients without cancer. This predicted unreachability seems to be due to a higher percentage of patients with pancreatic cancer having a retrocrural cross-sectional area of less than 1.0 cm^2. Such individual differences in anatomy may contribute to the incomplete analgesia following retrocrural block of the coeliac plexus [23].

In general, in patients with extreme tumour masses in the upper abdomen, the spread of neurolytic/contrast medium – solution is not ideal – not the "H" as shown in the classical procedures, depending an anatomical possibilities to spread [16].

Boas has indicated a preference for thoracic splanchnic nerve block rather than coeliac plexus block because it has the advantage of a true compartmental block, thus being safer for the patient [24]. This block may be particularly useful when the retroperitoneum is widely infiltrated by tumour or after failed coeliac block. This technique requires a smaller volume of neurolytic agent and entails a lower risk of complications.

Splanchnic nerve block technique differs little from the classical retrocrural approach to the coeliac plexus, except that the needles are aimed more cephalad at a site that correspond to the anterolateral margin of the T12 vertebral body [10]. The needle is introduced through the skin wheal and directed anteriorly and medially so that its shaft makes an angle of 45° with the midsagittal plane. The needle is advanced until the posterolateral surface of the upper part of the body of the T12 vertebra is contacted. The needle is reinserted in a slightly more lateral direction,which places the bevel of the needle just lateral to the anterolateral surface of the body of the vertebra. Biplanar fluoroscopy-guided block is used to confirm the correct position of the needle by injecting 2-4 ml of radioopaque dye. The posteroanterior radiological view shows a linear spread of contrast medium medially to the lateral surface of the vertebral body. In anterolateral view, correct placement of the needle is confirmed by a linear spread of the contrast along the anterolateral aspect of the vertebral body.

Superior hypogastric plexus block

This is a retroperitoneal structure located bilaterally at the level of the lower third of the fifth lumbar vertebral body and upper third of the first sacral vertebral body at the sacral promontory and in proximity to the bifurcation of the common iliac vessels.

Analgesia to the organs in the pelvis is possible because the afferent fibres innervating these structures travel in the sympathetic nerves, trunk, ganglia and rami.

A recent study has suggested that, even in advanced stages, visceral pain is an important component of the cancer pain syndrome experienced by patients with cancer of the pelvis [25].

Neurolytic superior hypogastric plexus block is an effective technique for the relief of pelvic cancer pain in a high proportion of patients. Plancarte et al. [26] described the technique of blocking the superior hypogastric plexus. In this block the two 22-G needles are inserted on each side 5-7 cm from the midline at the level of L4-L5 interspace. The needle is inserted perpendicular in all planes to the skin, oriented about 30° caudad and 45° mesiad so that its tip is directed towards the anterolateral aspect of the L5 vertebral body.

Blockade through the transdiscal and transvascular approach is a useful alternative [27].

Biplanar fluoroscopy and 2-3 ml of water-soluble contrast medium is used to verify accurate placement of the needles and to rule out intravascular injection.

Postero-anterior radiographs show bilateral correct needle placement and contrast medium occupyng all of the L5-S1 retroperitoneal space. Accurate placement of the needles is determined by the collection of contrast medium just anterior to the L5-S1 intervertebral space.

Lumbar paravertebral sympathetic ganglion block

Before the recent introduction of superior hypogastric plexus block, lumbar sympathetic block had been used with some frequency to treat lower abdominal, pelvic, and some perineal pain problems [10]. The sympathetic chain in the lumbar area lies along the anterolateral surface of the vertebral bodies. The location of the ganglia on the lumbar vertebral column at the level of the second and third lumbar vertebral bodies was studied in cadavers. This location was identified in four portions such as rostral, mid, caudal one third and intervertebral portion in human cadavers [28].

Because it is necessary to destroy the ganglia themselves with neurolytic solutions in order to obtain an excellent and long-lasting sympathetic denervating effect, neurolytic solutions must cover these portions, including even the intervertebral space where the sympathetic ganglia are located. Therefore, it is necessary to predict the distribution of neurolytic solution by contrast medium prior to the injection [11].

If the aspiration is negative, 0.5 ml contrast solution is injected under image intensifier monitoring using the lateral view. If each needle is in the correct position, the contrast medium spreads in a thin linear fashion that conforms to the anterior edge of the vertebra. The appearance of a "blob" or fuzzy patch of the contrast medium indicates that the injection was made into the psoas muscle or fascia. Some authors first identify the psoas muscle by injecting 0.5 ml of dye (the "psoas stripe" is visualized) and then advance the needle until it is anterior to the psoas muscle [29].

Side effects of chemical lumbar sympathectomy with alcohol or phenol can be sensory deficits or deafferentation pain of varying incidence in the area of paravertebral nerves, e.g., genitofemoral neuralgia, which occurs in 5%-7% of patients. These complications should be considered as contraindications in young patients with nonmalignant disease such as reflex sympathetic dystrophy. In these cases a continuous block with local anaesthetics via a catheter may be an alternative [30].

An 18-G Tuohy needle was placed in L2, 5 cm lateral to the midline of the vertebra. The needle was advanced anteromedially (X-ray control, image intensifier) until contact with the lateral side of the lumbar vertebra. When the needle passed through the psoas fascia, a lack of resistence could be felt. The correct needle position was controlled by radiographic contrast medium. Then a 22-G polyethylene catheter was placed through the needle tip (X-ray control whith radiographic contrast medium in lateral and posteroanterior view).

Ganglion impar block (ganglion of Walther)

The ganglion impar is a solitary retroperitoneal structure located at the level of the sacrococcygeal junction. This ganglion marks the end of the two sympathetic chains.

To perform the technique, the needle is inserted through the skin wheal with its concavity oriented posteriorly, and, under fluoroscopic guidance, it is directed anteriorly to the coccyx, closely approximating the anterior surface of the bone, until its tip is observed to have reached the sacrococcygeal junction [10].

De Leon-Casaola [31] uses the litothomy position: with the patient in this position, local anaesthestic is injected at the level of the anococcygeal ligament. A spinal needle is then utilized to reach the sacrococcygeal junction while efforts are made to remain in midline and outside the posterior rectal wall. Water-soluble contrast medium is then injected to verify adequate needle placement in the retroperitoneal area.

References

1.   Branca L (1996) Imaging di blocco nervoso nella terapia del dolore. Edizioni & Tecnologie, Napoli, pp 17-163
2.   Zucchi PL, Gedda L, Ischia S, Vecchiet L (1995) Pain anamnesis. clinical semeiological aspects. In. Zucchi PL (ed) Compendium of pain semantics. Institute for the Study and Therapy of Pain, Florence, p 269
3.   Ferro Milone F (1993) Chronic pain. a separate entity with its main origin in the central nervous system? Early treatment by antalgic block (Comment). Pain Ther 1·23-28
4.   Procacci P, Maresca M, Cersosimo RM (1989) Sympathetically-dependent pain· pathophysiological and clinical aspects. Algologia 1:2-6

5. Jain S, Shah N, Bedford R (1991) Needle position for paravertebral and sympathetic nerve block: radiologic confirmation is needed. Anaesth Analg 72:S125

6. Hogan Q (1995) Lumbar and cervical sympathetic blocks. Twentieth Annual Meeting of the American Society of Regional Anaesthesia. Asra, Orlando, pp 40-43

7. Cornelisse HM, Slappendel R et al (1995) MR guided localization of the stellate ganglion. Reg Anaesth 20(Suppl 2):142

8. Ackerman WE, Racz GB (1995) A comparison of two techniques for stellate ganglion blockade. Reg Anaesth 20(Suppl 2):147

9. Benzon HT (1994) Sympathetic and somatic nerve blocks: O'Hare (ed) In Comprehensive Review of Pain Management. Asra, pp 405-419

10. Montero A (1994) Is there any future for the use of neurolytic blocks? In: Van Zundert A (ed) Highlights in regional anaesthesia and pain therapy. Permanyer, Barcelona, pp 289-298

11. Ogaw S (1991) Neurolytic sympathectomy. Int J Pain Ther 2:95-100

12. Bonica JJ (1990) Regional analgesia with local anaesthetics. In: The management of pain. Lea and Febiger, Philadelphia, pp 1941-1944

13. Mercadante S (1993) Celiac plexus block versus analgesics in pancreatic cancer pain. Pain 52:187-192

14. Moore DC, Bush WH, Burnett LL (1980) Celiac plexus block: a roentgenographic, anatomic study of technique and spread of solution in patients and corpses. Anaesth Analg 60:369-379

15. Brown DL, Bulley K, Quiel EL (1987) Neurolytic celiac plexus block for pancreatic cancer pain. Anaesth Analg 66:869-873

16. Vielvoye-Kerkmeer PE (1995) Percutaneous celiac plexus block for chronic pain in malignant and non malignant disease. Int J Pain Ther 3(4):131-142

17. Hilgier M (1991) Coeliac plexus neurolysis by anterior approach. Int J Pain Ther 2:101-115

18. Montero-Matemala A, Vidal F, Sanchez A, Bach D (1989) Percutaneous anterior approach to coeliac plexus using ultrasound. Br J Anaesth 62:637-640

19. Brown D (1995) Celiac plexus block Twentieth Annual Meeting of the American Society of Regional Anaesthesia Asra, Orlando, pp 145-154

20. Haaga JR, Reich NE, Havrilla TR, Alfidi RJ (1977) Interventional CT scanning. Radiol Clin North Am 15:456-469

21. Ischia S, Luzzani A, Ischia A, Faggion S (1983) A new approach to the neurolytic block of the coeliac plexus: the transaortic technique. Pain 16:333-341

22. Singler RL (1982) An improved technique for alcohol neurolysis of the celiac plexus. Anestesiology 56:137-141

23 Weber JG, Brown DL, Stephens DH, Wong GY (1995) Celiac plexus block: does pancreatic cancer alter retrocrural computerized tomographic anatomy? Reg Anaesth 20(Suppl 2).146

24. Boas RA (1983) The sympathetic nervous system and pain relief. In Swerdlow M (ed) Relief of intractable pain Elsevier, Amsterdam, pp 215-237

25. De Leon-Casaola OA, Kent E, Lema MJ (1993) Neurolytic superior hypogastric plexus block for chronic pelvic pain associated with cancer. Pain 54.145-151

26. Plancarte R, Amescua C, Patt RB et al (1990) Superior hypogastric plexus block for pelvic cancer pain Anesteriology 73.236-239

27 Plancarte R, De Leon-Casaola OA, Allende S, Lema MJ (1995) The clinical effectiveness of two alternative approaches for neurolytic superior hypogastric plexus blocks in patients with pelvic pain associated with extensive retroperitoneal cancer. Reg Anaesth 20(Suppl 2):90

28. Umeda S, Arai T, Hatano Y, Mori K, Hoshino K (1987) Cadaver anatomic analysis of the best site for chemical lumbar sympathectomy. Anaesth Analg 66:643-646
29. Sprague RS, Ramamurthy S (1990) Identification of the anterior psoas sheath as a landmark for lumbar sympathetic block. Reg Anaesth 15:253-255
30. Strumpf M, Zenz M, Donner B, Tryba M (1994) Continuous block of the lumbar sympathetic trunk via catheter. Pain Digest 1:21-28
31. De Leon-Casaola OA (1996) Invasive strategies for chronic pain associated with cancer In: Van Zundert A (ed) Highlights in pain therapy and regional anaestesia. Permanyer, Barcelona, pp 95-101

Chapter 20

Postoperative advantages of regional anaesthesia

F. Nicosia, M. Nolli

Since facilitating surgery is the traditional aim of anaesthesia, the role of regional anaesthesia (RA) in terms of intraoperative and postoperative advantages has
hardly been considered.

Though anaesthesia is recognised to consist of different components, every single components of anaesthesia can hardly be defined since analgesia, hypnosis,
muscle relaxation and vital function support are not separable during the surgical
procedure. In addition the role of the anaesthesiologist is far from being recognised
by the patients; thus, in a hypothetical project for patient education about the
anaesthesiologist's role as a perioperative physician [1], we undoubtedly seek sensitive instruments that can measure the quality of care the patients feel has been provided with the anaesthesiologist's contribution. During the preoperative visit, we
can focus the patient's attention on postoperative facilities for pain control and
early rehabilitation that RA can offer. In fact, in addition to facilitating surgery at
least three anaesthetic benefits can be "purchased" by the patients: postoperative
functional pain relief, accelerated discharge time, and minimised side effects and
risks. In all these RA can play an important role by improving the clinical outcome
and minimising immediate and long the term costs.

In very recent years there has not been a single issue in the medical journals
that didn't deal with economics, while before 1992 only 1.5% of the scientific
journal publicised reports from the annual meeting of the ASA about the cost-
effectiveness of anaesthesia and presented data in terms of dollars [2]. Analysing
the costs and their determinants in anaesthesia, as well as any cost containment,
has therefore been increasingly important as long as the quality of treatment is
kept constant and, hopefully, improved. Moreover, the administrative involvement in hospitals is nowadays considered necessary and it is one of the new re-
sponsibilities the modern anaesthesiologist is asked to face [3].

Some attempts have been made to compare the low cost of different anaesthesia techniques. When the costs of anaesthesia are compared, the variable costs
for drugs and devices necessary for general anaesthesia (GA) are slightly different than those for RA, being the fixed costs (personnel costs, monitoring, operating room material and sterilisation, administrative services and medical
equipment maintenance) much more relevant, but unchangeable, and the same
for the two techniques. However, Narbone et al. [4] calculated the costs for total
knee replacement with three different anaesthetic techniques and found that
epidural anaesthesia is less expensive than GA (9.8 vs 12.7 $/h) and the combi-

nation of GA plus epidural was as expensive as 15.6 $/h. However, the intraoperative quality of treatment is far from being itemised during anaesthesia, making the detection of economic differences even more complicated. Making the operating time as short as possible turns out to be the most important determinant factor for cost reduction in the operating theatre [2]; consequently, any intraoperative difference between anaesthesia cost components is likely to be less consistent than we think, whilst the organisational attitude and the surgical speed probably are far more crucial for saving time.

Immediate postoperative advantages

Reduced potential complications after RA have been proven in several studies, which demonstrated:
- less need for intensive postanaesthesia care unit time when RA is performed as compared with GA [5];
- early arousal and less pronounced episodic oxygen desaturation [6]; when RA is used as postoperative technique compared with i.v. opioids;
- minimised postoperative protein break-down without compromising whole protein body synthesis, by maintaining extradural block for 24 h after surgery [7];
- patients undergoing arterial reconstructive surgery receive beneficial effects on coagulation status when epidural anaesthesia and analgesia are associated, compared with intermittent opioid analgesia administered on demand [8];
- extensive use of RA and postoperative analgesia are discussed among the positive factors that may have contributed to changes in mortality rate after total hip arthroplasty [9];
- however, since single studies are rarely conclusive, two major periodical reviews of the effects of RA on postsurgical morbidity [10] and postoperative organ dysfunction [11];
- have been published, although the criteria for such meta-analyses have not been fulfilled in all parameters for morbidity and recovery. The former concluded that RA appears to reduce early postoperative mortality after acute hip surgery for fracture, while long-term survival is dependent on factors other than the choice of anaesthesia. The large amount of data suggest that RA should be used whenever possible. The latter, a more recent review, confirms what the previous study underlined: reduced mortality appears to have been demonstrated under an epidural regimen for postoperative analgesia in high risk patients undergoing thoracic, abdominal and vascular procedures.

The reduction of costs consequent to the reduction of morbidity, even though broadly accepted, have not yet been calculated, however.

Early enrolment in postoperative rehabilitation

The beneficial impact of RA on the postoperative period appears more attractive when the concept of early recovery and function restoration is taken into account. Pain, lying in bed and hypoxemia are considered the major cause for potential complications and for prolonged hospital stay after the most common interventions. An effective way to drastically reduce in those factors, otherwise limiting early mobilisation, is RA and aggressive postoperative pain treatment [12]. Recent reports on early discharge after oncologic surgery in high risk elderly patients treated with aggressive RA [13] opened a kind of debate on the utility of the huge investment for endoscopic devices to get similar result in terms of spared time to discharge. Doubts on such investments were raised recently after the publication of a well-designed, controlled study comparing laparoscopic versus small-incision cholecystectomy [14] in which no difference was found in terms of recovery time, hospital stay and return to work. The conclusion was that laparoscopic cholecystectomy does not provide better outcome than mini-laparotomy and it is more expensive.

Our investments in new laparoscopic instrument, imaging systems and surgical strategies should be rethought since cost-effective anaesthetic techniques can actually shorten the recovery time after some kinds of surgery as well as laparoscopic techniques do. For reducing costs the proposal to modify the surgical attitude and standards both in minor surgery (1-day surgical procedures) and in major surgery by organising accelerated surgical programs [15] is more interesting. GA combined with RA is apparently more expensive considering the intraoperative cost, but the total expenditures are lower due to shorter patient recovery time and hospital stay according to some recent studies [16, 17]. Since after abdominal surgery one of the most common side effects is intestinal paralysis, the administration of peridural local anaesthetic has been advocated to counteract stress-induced hyper sympathetic activity which is transferred to the bowel over a few to several days. Early intestinal function postoperatively is the result, thus contributing to an early patient recovery.

Long-term outcome

It is generally known that functional residual capacity (FRC) is the most important intraoperative respiratory parameter. It is also accepted that after upper abdominal surgery FRC stays impaired for days. RA shows clear benefits in the postoperative period, helping the patient recover previous pulmonary function, provided that he/she is encouraged to take advantage of postoperative pain relief [15]. In a recent meta-analysis carried out by Ballantyne and her group [18] postoperative pulmonary complications were researched, comparing 121 studies in which patients were treated after surgery with systemic drugs vs epidural opioids, epidural local anaesthetics, intercostal local anaesthetic and other blockades. The statistical analysis of several studies which used the same method showed a clear trend to significant advantages in terms of fewer pulmonary complications by administering epidural opioids or local anaesthetics when compared with systemic opioids. The weak point of the meta-analysis seems to be the oxygenation support, which appears not to be controlled in many studies. In conclusion, the authors confirm with their results that postoperative epidural pain control can significantly decrease the incidence of pulmonary morbidity.

As a comment to the above-mentioned study, it is important to remember that the surgical and anaesthesiological traditions do not take advantage of the entire potential for patient pain control, which allows early mobilisation and early nutrition. We can conclude by saying that RA helps patients be enrolled in accelerated postsurgical programs and match early discharge criteria [19]. Hospital administrators and managers should be aware of the tremendous potential RA may have in helping patients recover faster. The calculated nationwide lack of postsurgical recovery rooms is probably the background determinant for physicians sceptical attitude towards postoperative pain treatment.

References

1. Editorial (1996) More or better-Educating the patient about the Anaesthesiologist's role as Perioperative Physician. Anaesth Analg 83:671-672
2. Johnstone RE, Martinec CL (1993) Costs of Anaesthesia. Anaesth Analg 76:840-848
3. Editorial views (1996) Evolution of Anaesthesiology. Anaesthesiology 85:1-3
4. Narbone RF, Hopkins EM, McCarthy RJ, Ivankovich AD (1993) Cost-effectivenes analysis of anaesthetic usage pattern for total knee replacement. Anaesthesiology 79:A1065
5. Dexter F, Tinker JH (1995) Analysis of strategies to decrease postanaesthesia care unit costs. Anaesthesiology 82:94-101
6. Catley DM, Thornton C, Jordan C, Lehane JR, Royston D, Jones JG (1985) Pronounced episodic oxygen desaturation in the postoperative period: its association with ventilatory pattern and analgesic regimen. Anaesthesiology 63:20-28
7. Carli F, Webster J, Pearson M, Pearson J, Bartlett S, Bannister P, Halliday D (1991) Protein metabolism after abdominal surgery: effect of 24 h extradural block local anaesthetic. Br J Anaesth 67:729-734
8   Tuman KJ, McCarthy RJ, March RJ, DeLaria GA, Patel RV, Ivankovich AD (1991) Effect of epidural anaesthesia and analgesia on coagulation and outcome after major vascular surgery. Anaesth Analg 73.696-704
9. Sharrock NE, Cazan MG, Hargett MJ, Russo PW, Wilson PD (1995) Changes in mortality after total hip and knee arthroplasty over a ten-year period. Anaesth Analg 80:242-248
10. Scott NB, Kehlet H (1988) Regional anaesthesia and surgical morbidity. Br J Surg 75:299-304
11. Liu S, Carpenter R, Neal JM (1995) Epidural anaesthesia and analgesia Their role in postoperative outcome. Anaesthesiology 82:1474-1506
12. Grass JA (1993) Surgical outcome. Regional anaesthesia and analgesia versus general anaesthesia. Anaesth Rev 20:117-125
13. De Leon Casasola O, Parker BM, Lema M, Groth RI, Orsini-Fuentes J (1994) Epidural analgesia versus intravenous patient controlled analgesia: differences in the postoperative course of cancer patients. Reg Anaesth 19:307-315
14 Majeed AW, Troy G, Nichol JP, Smythe A, Reed MWR, Stoddard CJ, Peacock J, Johnson AG (1996) Randomised, prospective, single-blinded comparison of laparoscopic versus small-incision cholecystectomy. Lancet 347:989-994

15. Khelet H (1994) Postoperative pain relief. A look from the other side. Reg Anaesth 19: 369-377
16. De Leon Casasola O, Lema MG, Karabella D, Harrison P (1995) Postoperative myocardial ischemia – epidural versus intravenous patient-controlled analgesia – a pilot study. Reg Anaesth 20:105-112
17. Liu S, Carpenter R et al (1995) Effect of perioperative analgesic technique on rate of recovery after colon surgery. Anaesthesiology 83:757-765
18. Ballantyne J et al (1998) The comparative effects of postoperative analgesic therapies on pulmonary outcome: cumulative meta-analyses of randomised, controlled trials. Anaesth Analg 86:598-612
19. Khelet H (1997) Multimodal approach to control postoperative pathophysiology and rehabilitation. Br J Anaesth 78:606-617

ORGANIZATION OF PAIN SERVICE

Chapter 21

Organization of acute pain services

N. Rawal

Recent years have seen the development of new analgesic drugs and sophisticated drug delivery systems. Pain management modalities such as patient controlled analgesia (PCA), epidural analgesia with opioids and/or local anaesthetic drugs and regional blocks are being increasingly used. However, in general the obstacles to bringing research to the bedside have not been overcome. The most common technique for providing postoperative analgesia has been and still is the use of i.m. opioids prescribed by surgeons and administered by ward nurses on an as-needed basis. The inadequacies of this method of pain management are well recognised.

Newer analgesia techniques such as PCA, spinal opioids and regional analgesia techniques provide superior pain relief as compared to intermittent i.m. opioids but such techniques have their own risks and therefore require special monitoring. Traditional methods of analgesia are not risk-free either but the risks have rarely been quantified. It is becoming increasingly clear that the solution to the problems of postoperative pain management lies not so much in the development of new techniques as in development of an organisation to exploit existing expertise. This is one of the main conclusions of interdisciplinary expert committee reports by National Health and Medical Research Council of Australia, Royal College of Surgeons of England and the College of Anaesthetists US Department of Health and Human Services and International Association for the study of Pain (IASP). These reports also published guidelines which recommend actions such as using pain assessment tools, frequent pain assessment and evaluation of treatment efficacy, bedside pain documentation system. One of the most important recommendations of these reports is that there is a need for an effective organisation for postoperative pain service which is based on a team approach.

In the USA 24 h acute pain services provide good quality analgesia by using PCA and epidural techniques in increasing number of surgical patients [1]. Almost all major institutions in the USA have APS. Such comprehensive pain management teams usually consist of staff anaesthesiologists, resident anaesthesiologists, specially trained nurses and pharmacists. Sometimes physiotherapists are also included. Patients under the care of APS are visited and assessed regularly by one or more members of the team. A pain fellow or anaesthesiology resident is on-call for emergencies and "non-regular" working hours.

Problems with anaesthesiologist-based APS (USA style)

Anaesthesiologist-based APS organisation models usually provide "high-tech" pain management services. This is not surprising because anaesthesiologists have special expertise in the field of advanced analgesic techniques such as epidural and PCA. Therefore most APS in the USA are essentially PCA and/or epidural services only.

Although the implementation of anaesthesiologist-based APS has had a considerable impact on pain management on surgical wards, only a small percentage of patients receive the benefits of such APS. A good APS organisation is one which ensures optimal pain management for every patient who undergoes surgery, including children and those undergoing surgery on an outpatient basis. Furthermore, the record of USA-style APS in implementing hospital-wide quality assurance measures such as frequent recording of pain intensity ("make pain visible") and recording of treatment efficacy (visual analogic scale, VAS, before and after treatment) has been generally unimpressive so far. Additionally, the costs of USA-style APS are very high ($100-$300 per patient). It is not surprising that such costs are being increasingly questioned by payers. A downsizing of many APS is taking place in USA, and further reductions are predicted by many. A more important issue with anaesthesiologist-based APS is one of professional satisfaction.

Once the APS has been organised and is running satisfactorily, the daily routine of the staff (senior) anaesthesiologist is quite monotonous and rather understimulating. There is also a lack of continuity because the anaesthesiologist performing preoperative evaluation (which includes patient information about proposed postoperative analgesic technique) and epidural block is not the same physician who provides pain management postoperatively. Essentially the surgeon decides which patients the APS anaesthesiologist can treat. To quote Bridenbaugh "it is not the function of the anaesthesiologist to run around the hospital filling up epidural catheters with various analgesic mixtures or setting infusion pumps. Far better that this time be used in teaching or performing regional nerve blocks appropriate for acute pain relief" [2].

The role of an anaesthesiologist in any APS model will be pivotal. In the opinion of this author such a role is professionally more satisfying as a teacher, pain expert and performer of regional blocks in a nurse-based, anaesthesiologist-supervised model.

Development of a low-cost model

It is becoming increasingly clear that simpler and less expensive models have to be developed if the aim is to improve the quality of postoperative analgesia for every patient who undergoes surgery. The organisation should also include patients who undergo day-care surgery. Furthermore, in countries with state-financed health services and current budgetary restraints the USA-style anaesthesiology-based, comprehensive, multidisciplinary postoperative pain control teams appear unrealistic for most institutions. It is generally recognised that effective analgesia alone will not improve postoperative outcome. Improved pain relief allows more postoperative activity and has to be exploited in an aggressive postoperative rehabilitation programme which includes physiotherapy, active mobilisation routines and early enteral feeding. If an institution does not have an organisation to implement such rehabilitation programmes, it is doubtful that "high-tech" epidural combination techniques should be used at all since less invasive and simpler techniques can provide comparable analgesia.

At Orebro Medical Centre Hospital a nurse-based, anaesthesiologist-supervised acute pain service was introduced in February 1991. Our APS is based on the concept that postoperative pain relief can be greatly improved by provision of in-service training for medical and nursing staff, regular recording of pain intensity and treatment efficacy, optimal use of systemic opioids (including use of PCA) and peripherally acting analgesics and use of epidural technique and regional blocks in appropriate patients.

It is emphasised that the majority of patients undergoing surgery do not require PCA or epidural analgesia. The role of simple analgesic techniques should not be overlooked or underestimated. With attentive nursing, greater flexibility of administration, better understanding of pharmacokinetics of prescribed analgesics and regular pain scoring, i.m. or i.v. opioids and/or non-opioids can provide excellent analgesia. Furthermore, quality assurance measures such as frequent recording of pain intensity can no longer be ignored.

At the time of preoperative evaluation, patients are informed about pain assessment by VAS and about pain management techniques that are available and the rationale underlying their use. Every patient who has undergone surgery (under general or regional anaesthesia) is asked to grade his or her pain severity on VAS. This is done every 3 h and recorded on a specially reserved place on the vital sign chart. The idea is to emphasise that routine pain scoring is as important as recording of temperature, heart rate and blood pressure. To evaluate effect of prescribed treatment pain intensity is also scored before and about 45 min after treatment. Pain intensity is recorded more frequently (every hour) in the following categories of patients: a) patients on ICU, b) patients on PACU, c) patients undergoing day-care surgery, and d) patients receiving PCA or epidural opioids.

Appropriate protocols, pain management guidelines, standard orders and monitoring routines have been developed in co-operation with surgeons for each surgical section. A specially trained acute pain nurse (APN) makes daily rounds of all surgery departments. Her duties are described in Tables 1 and 2. In this organisation the treatment of individual patients is based on standard orders and protocols developed jointly by the section anaesthesiologist, surgeon and ward nurse. This gives nurses the flexibility to administer the analgesics when necessary. In Sweden, nurses are allowed to inject drugs i.v. and in epidural catheters. The duties of the section anaesthesiologist consist of providing anaesthesia services as well as acute pain services (Table 1). He selects patients for special pain therapies such as PCA and epidural, and peripheral nerve blocks. During regular working hours this anaesthesiologist is available for consultation or any emergency; later, the anaesthesiologist on-call fulfils the same function.

To facilitate implementation of pain management guidelines and monitoring routines on the wards two ward nurses from each surgical department (day nurse and night nurse) are also included (Table 1). There is a clear understanding between surgeons and anaesthesiologists regarding responsibility so as to avoid the problems of conflicting orders. To reduce the risk of errors and to standardise clinical care, hospital-wide printed protocols and standard orders have been developed jointly to permit the use of opioids by i.m., i.v., s.c. (through in-dwelling butterfly cannula), i.v. PCA and epidural route on surgical wards. At our hospital major abdominal and thoracic surgery has been routinely performed under a combination of epidural block and general anaesthesia for almost 20 years. Major knee and hip surgery is routinely performed under combined spinal epidural (CSE) block. In all such patients postoperative analgesia is provided by epidural local anaesthetics and/or opioids. All epidural catheters are placed preoperatively in the operating room holding area. PCA is initiated in the PACU and continued on the wards.

Table 1. Patients are treated on the basis of standard orders and protocols developed jointly by chiefs of anaesthesiology, surgery and nursing sections. Pain representatives (named) meet every 3 months to discuss and implement improvements in pain management routines. This organisation benefits about 20 000 patients a year (VAS <3); it has been functioning satisfactorily since 1991 (Organization of acute pain services at Orebro Medical Centre Hospital, Orebro, Sweden)

Health care member "pain representatives" (named)	Responsibility
Section anaesthesiologist	Responsible for pre-, peri- and postoperative care (including postop pain) for his/her surgical section
"Pain representative" ward surgeon	Responsible for pain management on his/her ward and for implementing active postop rehab program
"Pain representative" day nurse and "Pain representative" night nurse	Responsible for implementation of pain management guidelines and monitoring routines on the ward
Acute pain nurse (nurse anaesthetist)	Daily rounds of all surgical wards Check VAS recording on charts (every patient VAS <3) "Trouble-shoot" technical problems (PCA, epidural) Refer problem patients to section anaesthesiologist (liaison between surgical ward and anaesthesiologist)
Acute pain anaesthesiologist	Responsible for co-ordinating hospital-wide acute pain services and in-service teaching

Table 2. Why a nurse-based acute pain service?

- Traditionally, the nurse's role is crucial in pain management
- Routine pain management does not require anaesthesiologist involvement (standard orders, protocols are important)
- Nurses identify better with nurses (less threatening)
- Enhanced continuity of patient care[a]: same anaesthesiologist pre-, peri- and postoperative (regional blocks)
- APN provides (daily ward rounds)
  - effective liaison between surgeon, anaesthesiologist and ward nurse
  - in-service training, "trouble shooting" (epidural, PCA)
  - checks pain assessment (VAS) documentation
- Once running, APS requires little extra personnel (1-1.5 APN for 20 000 patients)
- Less expensive (APN cost $2-3 per patient)
- Positive experience with nurse-based APS so far (since 1991)[b]
- Facilitates implementation of aggressive postoperative rehabilitation programmes (depends on APS model)
- Neither APN nor anaesthesiologist guarantees good pain management on wards - ward nurse quality crucial

The main role of the anaesthesiologist is to teach and train ward nurses, to supervise APN and to maintain a co-operative spirit among disciplines ("pain representative" meetings)

[a] Versus physician who has APS function only. APN, acute pain nurse; PCA, patient-controlled analgesia; VAS, visual analogue scale
[b] Similar nurse-based APS available currently in many Swedish hospitals and several European hospitals

The acute pain anaesthesiologist and APN co-ordinate pain management routines between the surgical sections and chair quarterly "pain representative" meetings of section anaesthesiologists, surgeons and day and night ward nurses (Table 1). The usual discussion topics at these meetings are practical pain problems, protocol modifications, suggestions for improvement of services and introduction of newer techniques.

In the organisation described above the only additional cost is that of the APNs. At our hospital about 20 000 surgical procedures are performed annually; all of these patients can be expected to benefit from this organisation. The cost of 1.5 APNs is about 45 000 US dollars or less than $3 per patient (excluding drug and equipment costs). The APS were introduced gradually on a department-by-department basis. The implementation of the services for the whole hospital took about 18 months. The routine recording of VAS on surgical wards as described above has demonstrated for surgeons and ward nurses that even repeated injections of i.m. opioids may be unable to maintain VAS scores that are considered acceptable (VAS <3) for the department, this is particularly valid in patients with severe pain, such as those undergoing upper abdominal, thoracic or knee surgery. This has resulted in increased requests for and better acceptance of techniques such as PCA and epidural techniques on the surgical wards. The development of a structured program with readily available assistance is appreciated by nurses and surgeons on the ward. Since surgeons are active members in this organisation, it is easier to implement aggressive postoperative rehabilitation programmes to exploit the full potential of improved analgesia. Although all anaesthesiologists are involved with postoperative pain management of their patients the section anaesthesiologists (Table 1) are responsible for developing protocols and standard orders for their section. This system is professionally more stimulating because the anaesthesiologist provides continuity of patient care since he or she is routinely involved in preoperative assessment, intraoperative management and postoperative follow-up.

An independent audit of patient opinion and personnel routines regarding pain management showed that about 95% of patients are satisfied with postoperative pain treatment (unpublished data). At present many Swedish hospitals have nurse-based, anaesthesiologist-supervised APS, similar to be one described above [3]. In small hospitals APN's work part-time with APS. Similar models are being increasingly established in many European hospitals. Nurse-based models have also been described by others [4-6].

APS in Europe

Few European hospitals have organised APS. The USA model is not transferrable to most European hospitals because of state-run health services and cost issues. Except for the work of a few enthusiasts the situation in Europe is generally unsatisfactory. Models for APS have been proposed from Germany [6], UK [4, 5, 7], Switzerland, Norway [8], and Sweden [3]. However, these models are from individual institutions and their impact on pain management on a country-wide basis is unclear. After the publication of the report by a joint working party of Royal College of Surgeons and College of Anaesthetists in 1990 there has been considerable interest in improving postoperative pain relief in the UK. This has centred around development of high dependency units (HDU), acute pain teams and expansion in the use of techniques such as PCA. It has been estimated that less than 30% of British hospitals have a HDU; therefore, if complex analgesia techniques such as epidural, PCA, regional blocks are restricted to HDUs there would be little improvement in the quality of pain relief for the majority of patients undergoing surgery [4]. A few nurse-based APS have been successfully implemented in the UK. The lack of organised APS at most institutions is mainly due to administrative difficulties and financial restrictions. Even when resources are available it may be difficult to introduce new analgesia techniques on surgical wards due to practical constraints, communication problems and, perhaps most importantly, nursing policies [7].

There seems to be an awakening of interest in establishing APS in European hospitals. This was one of the conclusions of a 17-nation European survey that included Austria, Belgium, Denmark, Finland, France, Germany, Greece, Iceland, Ireland, Italy, Netherlands, Norway, Portugal, Spain, Sweden, Switzerland and the UK [9]. Of the 105 hospitals surveyed only 37% (range 10-80%) had some kind of APS. Less than 10% of participating hospitals had a formal organisation that would meet the requirements of a good APS. The availability of special units ("intermediate ward", "step-down" unit) for patients requiring prolonged pain relief by techniques such as epidural and PCA varied considerably. Overall, a majority of European anaesthesiologists were dissatisfied with pain management on surgical wards; the situation was considered satisfactory on PACUs. Many anaesthesiologists (20%-67%) reported economic reasons for their inability to provide analgesic treatment of choice. These results are similar to those of a UK survey by Semple et al. [10] and a Canadian survey by Zimmermann and Stewart [11]. The 17-nation European survey also showed that anaesthesiologists had responsibility for acute pain services in 50% of hospitals, an advisory role in 42% of hospitals and no role at all in 8% of hospitals. None of the participating hospitals had anaesthesiology-based, comprehensive USA-style APS.

In summary, there are several problems with USA-style anaesthesiologist-based comprehensive, multidisciplinary APS these include: a) lack of anaesthesiologist continuity, b) APS benefits selected patients only, c) high expense and d) professionally understimulating. A nurse-based (anaesthesiologist-supervised) model is presented that eliminates the problems described above. Furthermore, every surgical patient's pain is recorded frequently with the aim of maintaining a VAS of <3 in accordance with hospital-wide pain policy. In this model the anaesthesiologists' main function is performing regional blocks in appropriate patients, teaching and training ward nurses and supervising the APN.

References

1. Ready LB, Oden Rollin Chadwick HS, Benedetti C, Rooke GA, Caplan R, Wild LM (1988) Development of an anaesthesiology-based postoperative pain management service. Anaesthesiology 68:100-106

2. Bridenbaugh DL (1990) Acute pain therapy: whose responsibility? Reg Anaesth 15:219-222

3. Rawal N (1994) Organization of Acute Pain Services· a low-cost model. Pain 57 117-123

4 Wheatley RG, Madej TH, Jackson IJB, Hunter D (1991) The first years experience of an acute pain service. Br J Anaesth 67:353-359

5. Gould TH, Crosby DL, Harmer M, Lloyd SM, Lunn JN, Rees GAD, Roberts DE, Webster JA (1992) Policy for controlling pain after surgery: effect of sequential changes in management Br Med J 305:1187-1193

6 Maier C, Kibbel K, Mercher S, Wulf H (1994) Postoperative Schmerztherapie auf Allgemeinen Krankenflegestationen: Analyse der achtjahrigen Tatigkeit eines Anasthesiologischen, Akut-Schmerzdienstes (Postoperative pain therapy on normal wards. Eight years experience with an Acute Pain Service). Anaesthesist 43:385-397

7 Cartwright PD, Helfinger RG, Howell JJ, Siepmann KK (1991) Introducing an acute pain service. Anaesthesia 46:188-191

8 Breivik H, Hogstrom H, Niemi G, Stalder B, Hofer S, Fjellstad B, Haugtomt H, Thomson D (1995) Safe and effective post-operative pain relief: introduction and continuous quality improvement of comprehensive post-operative pain management programmes. Ballieres Clin Anaesth 9·423-460

9. Rawal N (1995) Acute pain services in Europe: a 17-nation survey. Reg Anaesth 20·S85
10. Semple P, Jackson IJB (1991) Postoperative pain control. A survey of current practice. Anaesthesia 46:1074-1076
11. Zimmermann DL, Stewart J (1993) Postoperative pain management and acute pain services activity in Canada. Can J Anaesth 40:568-575

REGIONAL ANAESTHESIA IN SPECIALTIES

Chapter 22

Regional analgesia and anaesthesia in obstetrics

C. Benedetti, M. Mercieri

Bonica, in the mid-forties, realized the importance of providing safe analgesia and anaesthesia for parturients. In 1947, he developed the first obstetrical anaesthesia service in the world to provide continuous analgesia and anaesthesia care to these patients [1]. The need of proper pain control during parturition, which John Bonica perceived through his clinical observation and acumen, was confirmed several decades later by the research of Melzack. In 1994, Melzack published a study which demonstrated that, in the majority of women, the pain associated with parturition is more intense than neoplastic pain and pain secondary to a bone fracture [2]. This paper also brought to the forefront a concept seldom understood by most physicians. The assessment of the intensity of pain is often overlooked by clinicians and until they realize the enormous difference existing between tolerable and intolerable pain as rated by each individual patient, pain will continue to be inappropriately treated. For instance, when we speak of labor analgesia the aim is not to produce a completely pain-free parturition, but to reduce the pain to an acceptable level. A proper level of analgesia will allow the mother to actively participate in the labor while being spared the atrocity of uncontrolled, intolerable pain.

The so-called biological "function" of labor pain has not found significant scientific support. Proponents of the natural childbirth affirm that labor pain improves the relationship between mother and child, the maternal wellbeing, as well as showing a favorable impact on the psychological and physiological development of the child [3]. This is however a very controversial argument especially in the light of the data which have been published during the last 30 years: it is well known that if severe pain is not alleviated, it can provoke deleterious effects on the mother, the fetus and the neonate [4].

Numerous studies have shown that the pain associated with uterine contractions can increase ventilation by 5 to 20 times the basal frequency, with the possibility of a severe respiratory alkalosis. This, in turn, will lead to a left shift of the haemoglobin dissociation curve and a consequent reduced release of O_2 to the fetus. Furthermore, intense acute pain causes a significant increase in the sympathetic activity with release of adrenergic hormones. These hormones cause a 50% to 150% increase in cardiac output, a 20% to 40% increase in arterial blood pressure, and a 35% to 70% decrease in uterine blood flow. All these alterations cause an increase in metabolism and oxygen consumption. The increase in oxygen consumption together with the loss of bicarbonates, which are excreted by kidneys to compensate for the respiratory alkalosis, cause a progressive metabolic acidosis that is for the mother transferred to the fetus. A further consequence of intense pain for the mother is the reduction of gastrointestinal motility with an increased risk of aspiration of the gastric content.

In conclusion, since about 20% of parturients report tolerable pain during labor and delivery, we can not state that every parturient must receive analgesia. However, obstetrical analgesia and anaesthesia represent an undeniable progress in the quality of the care given to obstetrical patients by providing comfort to the mother. They, sometimes are a therapeutic necessity that can improve the outcome of both the mother and the neonate. This is especially true if the mother suffers from severe cardiac or vascular diseases or when utero-placental insufficiency is present.

Basic concepts of labor pain

Parturition is divided in three stages: the first, or dilatation stage, the second, or expulsion stage, and the third, or placental stage. The first stage consists of two phases: a longer, latent one and a shorter, active one; it starts at the beginning of labor and ends at full cervical dilatation (10 cm). During this phase pain is mainly visceral and, when contractions are mild, is transmitted by T10 and T11 spinal nerves. However, as contractions become more intense, and pain more severe, also the two adjacent segments become involved. The visceral pain caused by uterine contractions is referred anteriorly to the skin and the abdominal wall between the umbilicus and the pubic symphysis, laterally to the skin and the subcutaneous tissues above the iliac crests, and posteriorly to the skin and the subcutaneous tissues above the last four lumbar vertebrae and the upper half of the sacrum.

The second stage, or expulsion stage, starts after the complete dilatation of the cervix and the formation of the birth canal. At this point uterine contractions are accompanied by a reduction of uterine volume due to the descent of the fetus in the birth canal. In this period pain is principally somatic due to the dilatation and stretching of the soft perineal tissues and is mostly carried by the pudendal nerves at the level of S2, S3, and S4.

The third stage, or placental stage, stars after the neonate is delivered and ends with the delivery of the placenta and the membranes. This stage is not associated with significant spontaneous pain; however, soon after the end of this stage, the mother may experience pain for the suturing of the episiotomy or the repair of the perineal and vaginal lacerations which may have occurred during delivery.

In summary, labor pain usually starts at low intensity and increases slowly during the latent phase of the first stage. During the active phase and the second stage, pain increases with a fast crescendo and reaches levels of severe to excruciating intensity. The use of oxytocin, to increase uterine contractions and deliberate the rupture of the membranes, also causes significantly more intense labor pain. It is this wide range of pain intensity degrees, that quickly go from mild to excruciating, which is responsible for the need of different types of medications. Intraspinal opioids are effective in relieving mild to moderate pain, but for severe to excruciating pain local anaesthetics are needed.

Analgesia and anaesthesia in obstetrics

Analgesia for parturition

Epidural block

Lumbar epidural blocks are the most widely utilized technique for providing effective analgesia during parturition. This technique allows the continuous infusion of analgesics and an easy control of the duration and the intensity of analgesia. It is nevertheless associated with several possible limitations, side effects, and complications, including: a partially effective block, maternal hypotension, and accidental puncture of the dura with possible postpartum headache.

Limitations. To obtain a good analgesic coverage for both labor and delivery, analgesia should extend from T10 to S5. Unfortunately, due to the positioning of the epidural catheter in the upper segments of the lumbar or the lower segments of the thoracic spine, the anaesthetic agents tend to diffuse cranially if the parturient is in a supine position; as a consequence the sacral roots are sometimes not easily blocked (10%-20% of the cases). This results in an incomplete analgesia during delivery. To overcome this problem the patients should be in a reclining position when injecting a bolus of analgesic medication or during continuous infusion. According to our experience 10% of parturients report unsatisfactory perineal analgesia in delivery. In this situation the injection of 5ml of 2% lidocaine via the epidural catheter or a pudendal nerve block performed by the obstetrician can provide good perineal pain relief. In case of very rapid second stage, the i.v. injection of 15-25 mg of ketamine can provide the needed relief.

To provide effective segmental blocks the use of two epidural catheters – a lumbar one and a caudal one – has been described. With this technique the lumbar catheter is used for the first stage while the caudal catheter is used for the second stage. In this way the patient can obtain impeccable analgesia with relatively low dosage of local anaesthetic.

One of the disadvantages of the epidural technique described in the literature is the slow "onset" of analgesia. This problem can be particularly important for women in severe pain or needing an emergency Caesarean section. However we should remember the in the great majority of parturients the intensity of pain increases gradually over a period of several hours. Therefore, if we follow the patient carefully, we should be able to provide the proper analgesia in a timely fashion. There are, however, a few cases in which it is difficult to either predict the duration of the first stage of labor or the parturient's request of analgesia at the end of the first stage. In these situations, the relatively slow onset of analgesia may prevent the establishment of an effective block before delivery.

Side effects. Some obstetricians believe that if epidural analgesia is administered when cervical dilatation is <5 cm this may cause an increase in the incidence of Caesarean sections because of the higher frequency of distocia [5]. However, even thought the incidence of Caesarean sections is around 20% in the major industrialized countries, the causes and effects having not yet been proven. Chestnut et al. [6] have conducted a study on two groups of patients. The patients of the first group received epidural analgesia when cervical dilatation was 3 to 4 cm. In the second group epidural analgesia was administered when the dilatation of the cervix was >5 cm. This study, shoud not increase in the incidence of forceps deliveries, Caesarean sections, or prolongation of the second stage in the two groups of parturients. This study further emphasizes the discrepancy of the data at our disposal. Indeed, after the onset of an epidural block [7] a transitory reduction of uterine activity occurs which lasts 10-15 min. This decreased activity mostly refers to the intensity of the contractions rather than to their frequency, and uterine activity returns normal within 30 min. The majority of the studies demonstrate a reduction in the duration of the first stage of labor after the beginning of epidural analgesia [8, 9], and a prolongation of the second stage [9, 10]. It is interesting to note that there is a tendency toward better fetal condition when the second stage is prolonged in the presence of epidural analgesia [11].

Intrathecal block.

A single-dose subarachnoid or intrathecal block is not indicated for labor analgesia mostly because of its short duration that makes it inadequate for most labors; a more intense sympathetic block with possible hypotension; and possible postspinal headache.

In the late '80s, the development of a 32-G intrathecal catheter that could pass through a 25-26 G spinal needle reintroduced continuous intrathecal block for obstetrical analgesia and anaesthesia. This technique combined the effectiveness of intrathecal block with the flexibility of continuous block and the major advantage of this microcatheter is that it greatly reduces the incidence of postspinal headache [12, 13]. The development of cauda equina syndrome in several elderly patients after the use of 5% hyperbaric lidocaine injected via these devises caused the recall of these catheters, and nowadays they are not available for clinical use. The insertion of epidural catheter in the intrathecal space is not done routinely because of the high incidence of severe postspinal headache.

Combined subarachnoid epidural blocks

In the early '80s, some anaesthesiologists proposed the combined use of intrathecal and epidural block. By this technique, one drug is injected intrathecally and, simultaneously, an epidural catheter is placed to assure the possibility to supplement anaesthesia. After the unavailability of intrathecal microcatheters, anaesthesiologists began to use more frequently this technique called combined spinal epidural (CSE) block. It has been used ever more frequently during the last several years not only for obstetrical analgesia and anaesthesia but also for other surgical procedures. A recent international study made in seventeen European countries, with data obtained from 105 hospitals, has shown that CSE is used in every nation, even though the frequency varies greatly: from 0.2% in Ireland to 60% in Holland (the data from Italy has not been published). CSE is most frequently used for the following surgical procedures: femoral prosthesis (28.2%), hysterectomy (19%), knee surgery (14.4%), Caesarean section (14%), urgent Caesarean section (13%), femur fracture in the elderly (7.2%), prostatectomy (5.6%) [14, 15].

CSE blocks have the advantages of both techniques while decreasing the disadvantages. They offer the rapid onset, efficacy, and minimal toxicity of the spinal block as well as the possibility of improving an inadequate block or prolonging the duration of analgesia with epidural supplement both during and after surgery. When used for labor analgesia, CSE allows the administration of low doses of both local anaesthetics and opioids, thus creating a highly selective sensory block with minimal motor block. This may allow the patient to walk during the first stage of the labor. In a study of 300 parturients, CSE has provided a good analgesia while allowing some parturients to walk during their labor [16]. Even though it is not yet demonstrated that deambulation during labor reduces its duration, a meta-analysis of several studies suggests that, if the patient walks, the request for analgesic medication is reduced, and that women appreciate the possibility of walking even for brief periods of time during labor [15]. A study designed for testing the hypothesis that CSE blocks, which allow deambulation, could reduce the incidence of dystocia when compared to epidural block, has failed to demonstrate that CSE is associated with a decreased incidence in forceps delivery or Caesarean section [17]. Therefore, CSE does not offer any advantage in this with respect to epidural block.

The technique of combined subarachnoid epidural block

Combined Spinal/Epidural block can be performed in different ways: double interspace, by which each block is performed at two different interspaces, or single-space technique with either needle through needle – a specially designed Tuohy needle with a hole on the bottom (back eye) – or double-barrel needle. Most commonly, the technique is preferably performed with the patient in a sitting position or in a lateral decubitus. An epidural needle is inserted at a desired intravertebral level (below L2) until the epidural space is identified. A 25-27G long spinal needle, which protrudes 13-15 mm from the tip of the Tuohy needle, is inserted through the epidural needle and advanced until the dura is perforated. Aspiration of cerebral spinal fluid (CSF) before injecting the analgesic/anaesthetic solution will confirm the intrathecal placement of the needle. Once the spinal needle is removed, the epidural catheter is inserted 4 to 5 cm in the epidural space through the epidural needle. Some anaesthesiologists have voiced the concern that spinal analgesia/anaesthesia could mask paresthesia, which may occur during the insertion of the epidural catheter. This is an important concern since the unrecognized neural trauma caused by the catheter or the injection of local anaesthetic into a nerve is associated with severe neurological sequelae [18]. However, Levine and Datta [19] have demonstrated that during labor analgesia with CSE, which induces a limited sensory block, the incidence of paresthesia is not altered by the intrathecal block (30.7% in the epidural block group and 32.2% in the CSE group). When the intrathecal block is of such intensity to provide surgical anaesthesia, this problem can be theoretically avoided if the catheter is inserted before the spinal block is performed at a different interspace (technique described by Brownridge) [20]. However, even this technique has its own problems. Since the final direction of the epidural catheter is not predictable, as demonstrated by epiduroscopic studies [21], the epidural catheter may interfere with the performance of the spinal block, or the spinal needle may perforate it. To obviate this problem, a double-barrel Tuohy needle, which allows the placement of the epidural catheter before the spinal block, has been developed. The single technique also causes less discomfort and trauma to the patient, and decreases complications such as postspinal headaches, puncture of an epidural vein, hematoma, infection and technical difficulty [22]. This technique, however, requires a cooperating patient and more time to perform than a single intrathecal block. In fact, an expert regional anaesthesiologist takes 4-6 minutes to complete the placement of CSE blocks [15]. If a patient has intense pain, the best option is to first perform a spinal block to obtain a rapid analgesia and then introduce an epidural catheter when the patient is more calm and cooperative.

Technical concerns

Length of the needle. The distance between the ligamentum flavum and the dura mater varies from patient to patient and the range is between 3 and 10.5 mm. Moreover, the anterior/posterior diameter of the dural sac varies during extension and flexion of the vertebral column. At the L3-4 interspace the diameter increases from an average of 14.5 mm in extension to an average of 18 mm in flexion. In some kits for CSE block the spinal needle extends from the tip of the Tuohy needle by a fixed length (10 mm for Vygon, 13 mm for Braun). A recent study reported a 15% failure rate when a spinal needle protruding by 10 mm from the tip of the epidural needle was used and the authors concluded that the protrusion should be of at least 13 mm [22]. In the B-D Durasaf the 27-G spinal needle protrudes by 15 mm.

Migration of the epidural catheter. If the epidural catheter migrates at the subdural level, its migration is not recognized [23] and the injection of a normal epidural dose of local anaesthetic can cause a total spinal anaesthesia. A study, in which dura mater from cadavers was used, has shown that it is impossible to push an 18-G Portex epidural catheter through a hole produced by a 26-27 G spinal needle, and it is difficult to push it through the holes produced by 22 or 25 G needles. An epiduroscopic study [21] has shown that a 22-G needle may produce holes sufficiently large to allow passage of the catheter. However, even when five different holes were produced in the same area with a 25-G spinal needle, penetration of the catheter occurred only once in 20 attempts. On the contrary, after an intentional dura puncture with a Tuohy needle, the penetration of the catheter occurred in 45% of the cases. Penetration of the catheter in the intrathecal space or in the vessel may occur as the catheter erodes the epidural vessel or the dura. In general, however, the migration of a catheter is easily identifiable through a simple aspiration.

Rotations of the epidural needle. It has been suggested that, if the needle-through-needle technique is used, the 180-degree rotation of the Tuohy needle after the subarachnoid injection will allow the epidural catheter to be inserted farther from the dural puncture, thus avoiding intrathecal insertion of the epidural catheter. However, it has been reported that this maneuver may actually puncture the dura, increasing the incidence of complications from 3% to 17% after rotation of the needle [24].

Percentage of failures. In a study which compared the needle-through-needle technique with that of double interspace, a higher rate of spinal block failure was reported for the needle-through-needle technique (13%) [25]. But this is the only study that reports such a high percentage of failure. It has been estimated that when useing single spinal or epidural technique for Caesarian section, an alternative technique is required in about 4% of cases [15]. On the contrary, Lyons et al. have reported that of 900 Caesarian sections performed with CSE blocks, general anaesthesia was necessary in only one case[26].

Risk of post spinal headache. The risk of post-dural puncture headache is one of the major causes of postanaesthesia morbidity in parturients. Even the use of fine 25-G diamond-tipped spinal needles can cause postspinal headache (PSH) in 14.5% of parturients [27]. This high incidence of PSH can be drastically reduced by using a pencil-point needle such as the Sprotte. Studies conducted with this type of needle have reported a low incidence of PSH, ranging from 1.5% to 0% [27-29]. No controlled, randomized studies exist that compare the incidence of PSH after the CSE technique and after intrathecal blocks. Paradoxically enough, several authors have reported very low or no incidence of post-dural puncture headache after CSE. In a retrospective study of 6 000 parturients who underwent a CSE technique with 27-G Whittaker needle, Cox et al. reported an incidence of 0.13% [30]. Brownridge studied over 1 000 patients and reported not a single case of post-dural puncture headache [31]. Dennison has described only two cases after 400 CSE blocks performed for Caesarean section (0.5%) [32]. Possible explanations for this are:
– Tuohy needle acts as an introducer and avoids multiple attempts;

- the technique allows the use of very fine needles;
- less CSF is lost because of the increased epidural pressure;
- with a single-needle technique the spinal needle exits from the Tuohy slightly curved. In this case there is a decreased possibility that the holes in the dura mater and the arachnoid are aligned, thus reducing the risk of CSF loss;
- some anaesthesiologists assert that epidural opioids may prevent PSH while others deny that they have prophylactic effect [33]; however, epidural morphine has been successfully utilized for the treatment of PSH [34].

Norris et al. [35] compared CSE patients and epidural patients and reported that the risk of post-dural puncture headache does not increase in case of CSE. Indeed, in their study the patients who received epidural analgesia had a higher incidence of post-dural puncture headache after an unintentional puncture of the dura mater with the epidural needle. This result is not explainable since, to perform a CSE block, the epidural space has to be identified as in an epidural block.

Medications used for combined spinal epidural blocks

Intrathecal sufentanil at the dose of 10 µg is widely used. It produces an analgesia that lasts 90-120 min, but is associated to a higher incidence of nausea and vomiting [36]. The results obtained with an intrathecal dose of 5 µg are variable [37]. Gautier et al. [38] suggest a technique using intrathecal injection of 5 µg sufentanil, 1 mg bupivacaine and 25 µg epinephrine in 1.5 ml normal saline. This technique produces optimal analgesia that lasts 142±54 min with minimal or no motor block. The addition of a vasoconstrictor is used to prolong the analgesia through a reduced absorption of the injected medication. It is hypothesized that the drug will be at higher concentrations near the nerve to be blocked. However, this hypothesis has not been confirmed. On the contrary, some studies have demonstrated that the plasma concentration of the injected drug does not decrease after the addition of epinephrine [39]. Therefore, a direct effect on the spinal nociceptive system may be assumed [39]. Ossipov et al. [40] have demonstrated that epinephrine increases the analgesic affect of spinal opioids through a mechanism that may be caused by the simultaneous activation of opioid and adrenergic receptors. However, in Gautier's study, the incidence of hypotension was not different from that usually reported (20%-44%) [41, 42]. Kartawiadi et al. [43] have utilized the same anaesthetic mixture for a study which compares CSE blocks with epidural analgesia. Also in this study the onset of analgesia after CSE blocks was faster and lasted longer (137±11 min) but the hemodynamic response was similar in the two groups.

In order to reduce the risk of severe hypotension Rawal et al. have developed a sequential CSE technique that differs from the one previously described for the following reasons [44, 45]:
- the patient is in a sitting position, not in lateral decubitus;
- the dose of hyperbaric spinal 0.5% bupivacaine is 1.5 ml because the aim is to obtain a block from T8-9 to S5;
- the patient is then placed supine with a left lateral uterine displacement.

After the spinal block is set (approximately 15 min) it is extended to T4 by injecting small doses of local anaesthetic via the epidural catheter (1.5-2 ml for each non-block segment). While this technique requires more time, the use of minimal concentrations of local anaesthetic and, more important, the gradual slow development of sympathetic blockade reduce the frequency and severity of maternal hypotension when compared with intrathecal or epidural techniques in which the block develops rapidly [46, 47]. In fact, the low incidence of maternal hypotension has to be attributed to a slower action of the low supplemental epidural dose, which allows the necessary time for the compensatory mechanism to be efficacious. This technique, therefore, is particularly useful in high-risk parturients. In order to identify the optimal intrathecal dose of bupivacaine; Fan et al. [48] compared four different doses of hyperbaric bupivacaine (2.5, 5, 7.5, 10 mg) in patients who had to undergo Caesarean section using sequential CSE blocks. The authors have shown that 5 mg of hyperbaric bupivacaine combined with appropriate dosages of epidural lidocaine produced adequate analgesia. Higher doses of bupivacaine were associated with side effects such as hypotension, nausea, vomiting and dyspnea.

The transdural transport of drugs

We have shown that CSE blocks allow the anaesthesiologist to inject smaller amounts of intrathecal drugs so that the incidence and severity of maternal hypotension is reduced. Doses of intrathecal bupivacaine ranging from 7.5 to 10 mg produce a good anaesthesia in patients who undergo Caesarean section. However, some patients may require a supplemental dose of epidural anaesthetic to expand the intrathecal block. A few authors [45, 49] have noted a rapid expansion of the intrathecal block after relatively low dosages of epidural local anaesthetic. The reason for this event is still unknown. The rapid spreading of the block negates the hypothesis of a slow seepage of the drug through the dura mater, even though this could be possible. The following hypothesis have been proposed:
- passage of the local anaesthetic from the epidural to the intrathecal space through the dural hole caused by the insertion of the intrathecal needle [50];
- continued diffusion of the initial intrathecal block;
- presence of "subclinical" analgesia in the higher thoracic dermatomes which becomes more intense after the diffusion of the epidural local anaesthetic [51];
- changes in epidural pressure. The pressure becomes atmospheric, which can cause a better diffusion of the local anaesthetic for an effect on the volume and circulation of the CSF [49];
- compression of the subarachnoid space caused by the epidural catheter and the volume of the local anaesthetic, which determines an increased flow of CSF and a more extensive diffusion of the intrathecal local anaesthetic [45, 52].

Experimental studies have shown that epidurally injected medications may pass intrathecally through a dural hole and the amount of medication passing through the hole is directly proportional to it's size. Suzuki et al. [53] have shown that after a dural puncture with a 26-G spinal needle, the injection of 18 ml of 2% mepivacaine through an epidural catheter causes a 2-dermatome increase of the sacral blockade after 15 min. However, the cranial diffusion appears to be more important but more variable since the spread of the block may increase up to 9 dermatomes.

Another reason that is worth considering is the increase of the volume in the epidural space. Blumgart et al. [54] have noted an increase in the cranial diffusion of the intrathecal block, by injecting in the lumbar epidural space either 10 ml of normal saline or 10 ml of local anaesthetic. Such cranial expansion of the block did not occur in the control group that did not receive an epidural injection. However, Steinstra et al. [55] noted that the cranial expansion of the block is greater in patients who receive local anaesthetic when compared to those receiving normal saline. However, it must be mentioned, that the increase in the extension of the intrathecal block obtained by increasing the volume of the epidural space is possible only until the block is not fixed (15 to 20 min). Afterward the influence of the epidural injection saline on the intrathecal block is not demonstrable. In parturients the increase of epidural venous pressure increases the epidural space with a consequent decrease in the volume of CSF. This is believed to be the major reason for the decreased amount of local anaesthetic necessary in parturients. Furthermore, the injection of a 10 ml bolus of local anaesthetic in the epidural space causes a transient increase in CSF pressure by up to 12 mmHg [56].

In conclusion, one must be cautious when large volumes of drugs are rapidly injected in the epidural space, because the negative pressure usually present in the epidural space may become positive. Both during a CSE technique and after an inadvertent dural puncture with a Tuohy needle, it is safer to use solutions containing low concentrations of drugs and to inject them slowly.

Test dose

For labor analgesia, the use of a traditional test dose, after the placement of the epidural catheter in the CSE technique is a controversial topic. Some authors assert that since low dosages of local anaesthetic and/or opioids are used in the CSE blocks, the epidural test dose is not necessary [57]. They are also concerned that the test dose to determine a decrease in the motor functions are necessary for deambulation. Since with the CSE technique for labor analgesia, the dosages of epidural local anaesthetic mixed with low dose of opioids are small, an intravascular or even an intrathecal injection would not cause serious sequelae. The i.v. injections can produce minimal analgesia and minimal side effects to the mother and fetus. If the dose is injected intrathecally it will produce a more noticeable motor block with minimal loss of sympathetic tone [13]. A study of 8 000 deliveries has demonstrated that with the CSE technique, the test dose is not necessary[57]. However, it must be emphasized that if a labor CSE analgesia technique must be converted into epidural anaesthesia for Caesarean section, small amounts (5 ml) of local anaesthetic should be injected every 5 min until the desired level and intensity of block is reached.

Hypotension, nausea and vomiting

The possibility of hypotension after epidural or intrathecal local anaesthetic and opioids is widely reported. Some studies have shown that a systolic pressure <90 mmHg was present in 17% to 28% of parturients after epidural analgesia [58]. Furthermore, systolic hypotension <90 mmHg was also reported in 14% of the parturients who received intrathecal fentanyl-morphine [59] and after intrathecal sufentanil [60] for labor analgesia. The mechanisms of hypotension after administration of intrathecal opioids is not well understood. Some authors hypothesize that intrathecal sufentanil may cause decrease in arterial pressure through its actions on receptors localized on the pregangliar sympathetic fibers [61], or by producing a mild local anaesthetic effect [60]. However, in humans the sympathetic activity is unchanged 30 min after the intrathecal injection of 0.4 mg morphine [62]. Furthermore, intrathecal opioids may impair the release or the action of substance P and reduce the maternal blood pressure variation caused by the reflex pressor responses [63]. In a study reported by Norris et al. [35], on 924 patients who underwent either CSE or epidural analgesia (536 vs 388), both techniques had a similar effect on arterial pressure. However, pruritus, nausea and vomiting were more frequent in the CSE group. The incidence of pruritus after intrathecal morphine may be as high as 100% in parturients [64], while after sufentanil the incidence varies between 33% to 95% [60, 65, 66]. The incidence of pruritus in Norris et al. study [35], who used intrathecal sufentanil, was 43.7%. Some parturients complained of facial or generalized pruritus, while others stated that the pruritus was localized in the perineal area and on legs. Most of times this symptom is temporary and not severe and therefore does not require any specific treatment [35]. Thomas et al. [67] hypothesize that the facial pruritus is mediated by specific opioid receptors present in the dorsal horn. The pruritus seemed less common after administration of intrathecal meperidine [67] and is antagonized by local anaesthetic injected in the intrathecal space [68].

In animals, sufentanil is found in samples of CSF obtained from the cisterna magna within 1 min after its epidural injection [69]. The drug therefore enters the CSF rapidly and produces central effects. Frequently, it is possible to observe sedation, euphoria, dysphasia, respiratory depression, and slurred speech after the intrathecal injection of 10 µg of sufentanil [35]. For this reason some authors [70] have tried to limit the cranial diffusion of intrathecal sufentanil. To reach this objective they have compared the effects of administering hyperbaric sufentanil with the patient in a reclining position (10-30 degrees from the horizontal plane) or with the tip of the needle oriented either cranially or caudally. While the direction of the tip of the needle had no influence on the analgesia, the hyperbaric sufentanil produced no or minimal analgesia for labor. The authors concluded that a site of analgesic action of sufentanil is supraspinal.

Anaesthesia for Caesarean section

When a Caesarean section is indicated, regional anaesthesia is the technique of choice except for very few particular situations. However, lumbar epidural anaesthesia is not the technique of choice for elective or emergency Caesarean section because a large dose of local anaesthetic is sometimes necessary to produce the profound and extensive block required by the surgical procedure. This large dose of local anaesthetic can produce severe toxic effect. Furthermore, for emergency sections the onset of anaesthesia is too slow. However, if a labor epidural is providing effective analgesia and a non-urgent Caesarean section is indicated, the epidural block can be converted into effective anaesthesia in the great majority of cases. In our institution the failure rate of converting an epidural analgesia into anaesthesia is 3%, however, several studies have reported that epidural anaesthesia for Caesarean section is inadequate in 25% of the cases [71-73]. This high failure rate is difficult to explain.

Intrathecal technique

Intrathecal block is the technique of choice for Caesarean sections even if precautions must be taken, especially with regard of preventing or rapidly correcting severe hypotension. For a Caesarean section, a sensory block extending from T4 to S5 is required. Such an extensive block is associated with a relatively high incidence of severe hypotension. There are several factors contributing to its development. The high sympathetic blockade is a major factor as well as the rapid onset of the block. Prophylactic measures such as preblock hydration, left lateral uterine displacement are not always effective in maintaining normal arterial pressure. It is important to remember that, when a parturient is in a supine position, the pregnant uterus compresses the inferior vena cava and, in so doing, causes a significant decrease of cardiac pre-load which may lead to hypotension even in the absence of a significant sympathetic block. All women who have received an intrathecal or epidural block should lie laterally or, if supine, should have left uterine displacement to prevent the compression of the inferior vena cava. It is also extremely important to routinely and frequently monitor maternal blood pressure to be able to rapidly correct the severe hypotension which may occur, since it can have serious consequences not only for the mother but also for the fetus. Maternal hypotension may cause maternal cerebral hypoperfusion, which may lead to respiratory arrest, and a relative high parasympathetic tone may induce nausea, vomiting and bradicardia. Furthermore, if it is not corrected, hypotension may cause fetal hypoxia and acidosis secondary to uteroplacental hypoperfusion. The use of vasopressors, such as ephedrine 5-10 mg i.v., and placing the patient in the Trendelenburg's position, if the intrathecal block is fixed, are the treatments of choice for this condition. If the hypotension is associated with bradicardia, 0.4-0.6 mg atropine i.v. is indicated.

Combined spinal epidural blocks

Besides the high incidence of hypotension intrathecal anaesthesia through a single-shot technique, has the particular limitation of not being able to improve an inadequate block or to provide postoperative analgesia. The CSE technique overcomes these problems. The intrathecal injection of a relatively low dose of local anaesthetic (5-7.5 mg of 0.75% hyperbaric bupivacaine -0.65-1.0 ml) causes, in most parturients, a rapid anaesthesia that may be sufficient for the Caesarean section. If the intrathecal block is inadequate, it can be supplemented by injecting via the epidural catheter 3-5 ml 2% lidocaine repeated as needed to produce adequate anaesthesia. For postoperative pain control a slow continuous infusion of epidural opioid (i.e. 250-300 μg/h of preservative-free morphine) for 24-48 h will provide excellent postoperative pain control in most parturients.

Contraindications of regional anaesthesia/analgesia in obstetrics

There are few contraindications to the use of regional anaesthesia in obstetrics, and they are:
- patient's refusal;
- hypovolemia or hemorrage;
- coagulation abnormalities, including low platelet;
- infection over the site of the block or septicemia;
- extremely urgent Caesarean section.

In these situations, whenever an instrumental or surgical delivery is indicated, general anaesthesia should be employed. General anaesthesia in obstetrics is quite challenging. All parturients have to be considered "full stomach", regardless how long they have not eaten, and "rapid induction" safeguards must be employed. The pregnant uterus and the other abdominal organs displace the diaphragm higher in the thoracic cavity, significantly decreasing the functional residual capacity (FRC). A short period of apnea, even after proper preoxygenation, leads to low oxygen saturation as it is now frequently observed, since the mandatory use of pulse oxymeter, during induction of general anaesthesia. Finally, tracheal intubation is often more difficult in parturients, especially the morbidly obese, due to changes which occur in the larynx. This may include a larger epiglottis and a smaller opening between the vocal cords. The use of 6.0 endotracheal tube often allows an easier and more rapid intubation than with a 7.0-8.0 tube.

The care of obstetrical patients in our institution

The Ohio State Medical Center is an academic institution and a regional center designated for high-risk obstetrical patients. Over 4 000 deliveries occur every year and 78% of our labor patients receive labor analgesia in the form of lumbar epidural. Elective or urgent Caesarean sections are done under intrathecal anaesthesia. Our analgesic protocols for parturients is as follows.

- When the patient is committed to active labor, either spontaneous or induced, a lumbar epidural catheter is placed, and the catheter is tested with 3 ml of 1.5 i.v. lidocaine + 1:200 000 epinephrine for intrathecal or intravascular placement. Care is taken to inject the test dose at the end of a contraction as the tachicardia induced by the pain of the contraction starts to abate. This is necessary to prevent a false positive test for intravascular injection caused by the painful contraction. If the test dose is negative, 3.3 ml aliquots of an analgesic solution are injected epidurally every 3 min up to 10 ml. The analgesic solution contains 0.125% bupivacaine, 0.5 μg sufentanil, and 1:200 000 epinephrine. A continuos epidural infusion of a solution containing 0.0625% bupivacaine, 0.5 μg sufentanil, and 1:200 000 epinephrine is administered at a variable rate of 8-14 ml/h (average 10 ml/h). The patient is continuously monitored by the obstetrical nurse for progression of labor, status of the fetus, maternal heart rate and blood pressure, level and intensity of analgesic block and physical and psychological comfort. If the block becomes too profound or too high, the epidural infusion is decreased or stopped for a period of time; in other words, the analgesia is carefully titrated to effect. As mentioned above, if a labor epidural is providing effective analgesia and a non-urgent Caesarean section is indicated, the epidural block is converted to effective anaesthesia by injecting 5 ml of 2% lidocaine every 3-5 min up to a total of 20 ml. This is highly effective in the great majority of cases since the failure rate of converting an epidural analgesia to anaesthesia is of 3%. For postoperative pain control, a single epidural bolus of 3 mg of preservative-free morphine has proven effective to provide a very comfortable postoperative period.
- For elective or urgent Caesarean section an intrathecal block is performed below the L2 interspace using a 24-G Sprotte needle, 10 mg of 0.75% hyperbaric bupivacaine and 0.3 mg of preservative-free morphine. Slight changes in the extension of the block can be accomplished by carefully changing the patient position in relation to the horizontal plane. This technique has been very effective for us. The addition of morphine to the solution provides postoperative analgesia for 24-36 h [74] at which time the patient is given oral analgesics for postoperative pain control.
- Patients with severe cardiovascular diseases are monitored invasively and the analgesic/anaesthetic care adjusted accordingly.

Conclusions

In this chapter we have described the three regional anaesthetic techniques most frequently used in obstetrics. The epidural and intrathecal blocks have been used for decades parturition with great success. Continuous intrathecal block provides the best analgesic/anaesthetic care for parturients but the unavailability of proper equipment makes the routine use of this technique presently not feasible. CSE blocks have gained popularity worldwide because of the above-mentioned advantages. However, proper anaesthesia/analgesia obstetrical care is provided by relatively few centers in the world, even in highly industrialized countries. Therefore, in our opinion, improvement in obstetrical care will not occur through the application of any specific technique – available or to be developed in the future – but through a change in philosophy; a philosophy according to which the proper treatment of the pain associated with parturition is mandatory. Considering the amount of pain associated with parturition and the need for anaesthesia in instrumental deliveries and Caesarean sections, an Obstetrical Anaesthesia and Analgesia Service is required in each hospital which wishes to provide Obstetrical Care. An Obstetrical Anaesthesia Service has the responsibility of caring for two human beings simultaneously (the mother and fetus) with a combined life expectancy of about 140 years. Any untoward anaesthetic complication may have dire and long-lasting consequences for both patients. This service has to provide impeccable anaesthesia care including properly titrated and safe analgesia during parturition and safe anaesthesia for Caesarean section and, therefore, it has to be 24 h staffed every day of the year. The anaesthesiologists and supportive staff must be highly skilled in obstetrical and regional anaesthesia, and have at their disposal the most up to date anaesthetic and monitoring equipment.

Probably the most foretelling comment came from a foreign anaesthesiologist visiting our obstetrical unit. He commented on how quiet our unit was, compared to the one in his hospital where the screams from the parturients were a constant reminder of the physical suffering and humiliation that these patients were condemned to endure. The unavailability of pain control during parturition raises ethical issues. While all civilized countries affirm that torture is not acceptable even for the worst criminal, on many occasions, and, in some countries more than others, we subject women to intolerable pain, which is equivalent to torture. Since proper obstetrical analgesia has been proven, when properly applied, to be very safe and effective, not providing it when needed is unethical.

We should all remember a remark of Primo Levi: "If pain and suffering can be alleviated and we do nothing about it we, ourselves, are torturers"!

References

1   Benedetti C, Chapman CR, Bonica JJ (1990) A life dedicated to the alleviation of human suffering. In: Benedetti C, Chapman CR, Giron G (eds) Opioid analgesia recent advances in systemic administration. Advances in Pain Research and Therapy. Raven Press, New York, pp 16-17
2   Melzack R (1984) The myth of painless childbirth. Pain 19:321-337
3. Wagner A, Grenom A, Pierre F, Soutoul JH, Fabre-Nys C, Krebhiel D (1989) Maternal

behaviour toward her newborn infant Potential modification by peridural analgesia or childbirth preparation. Rev Fr Gynecol Obstetr 84:29-35

4   Bonica JJ (1980) Obstetric analgesia and anaesthesia. World Federation of Societies of Anaesthesiologists, Amsterdam

5.   Thorp JA, Hu DH, Albin RM, McNitt J, Meyer BA, Cohen GR, Yeast JD (1993) The effect of intrapartum epidural analgesia on nulliparous labor. a randomized, controlled prospective trial. Am J Obstet Gynecol 169:851-858

6.   Chestnut DH, McGrath JM, Vincent RD et al (1994) Does early administration of epidural analgesia affect obstetric outcome in nulliparous women who are in spontaneous labor. Anaesthesiology 80:1201-1208

7.   Raabe N, Belfrage P (1976) Lumbar epidural analgesia in labour. A clinical analysis Acta Obstet Gynecol Scand 55:125-129

8   Hall WL (1977) Epidural analgesia and its effect on the normal progress of labor. Am J Obstet Gynecol 129:316

9.   Crawford JS (1972) The second thousand epidural blocks in an obstetric hospital practice. Br J Anaesth 44:1277

10.   Crawford JS (1972) Lumbar epidural block in labor· a clinical analysis. Br J Anaesth 44:66

11.   Maresh M et al (1983) Delayed pushing with lumbar epidural analgesia in labour Br J Obstet Gynecol 90:623

12   Benedetti C, Tiengo M (1990) Continuous subarachnoid analgesia in labour Lancet 335·225

13.   Morton CP, Armstrong PJ, McClure JH (1993) Continuous subarachnoid infusion of local anaesthetic. Anaesthesia 48:333-336

14.   Rawal N (1995) European trends in the use of combined spinal epidural technique - a 17 nation survey. Reg Anaesth 20:162

15.   Rawal N, Van Zundert A, Holmstrom B, Crowhurst JA (1997) Combined spinal-epidural technique. Reg Anaesth 22:406-423

16.   Collis RE, Baxandall ML, Srikantharajah ID, Edge G, Kadim MY, Morgan BM (1993) Combined spinal epidural analgesia with ability to walk throughout labour. Lancet 341:767-768

17.   Nageotte MP, Larson D, Rumney PJ, Sidhu M, Hollenbach K (1997) Epidural analgesia compared with combined spinal-epidural analgesia during labor in nulliparous women. N Engl J Med 337:1715-1719

18.   Katz N, Hurley R (1993) Epidural anaesthesia complicated by fluid collection within the spinal cord. Anaesth Analg 77:1064-1065

19.   Levin A, Segal S, Datta S (1998) Does combined spinal-epidural analgesia alter the incidence of paresthesia during epidural catheter placement? Anaesth Analg 86:445-446

20.   Brownridge P (1981) Epidural and subarachnoid analgesia for elective Caesarean section. Anaesthesia 36·70

21.   Holmstrom B, Rawal N, Axelsson K, Nydahl PA (1995) Risk of catheter migration during combined spinal epidural block-percutaneous epiduroscopy study. Anaesth Analg 80:747-753

22.   Joshi G, McCaroll S (1994) Evaluation of combined spinal-epidural anaesthesia using two different techniques. Reg Anaesth 19:169-174

23.   Reynoids F, Speedy H (1990) The subdural space: the third place to go astray. Anaesthesia 45.120-123

24   Carter LC, Popat MT, Wallace DH (1992) Epidural needle rotation and inadvertent dural puncture with catheter. Anaesthesia 47:447-448

25.   Lyons G, MacDonald R, Mikl B (1992) Combined epidural spinal anaesthesia for Caesarean section. Through the needle or in separate spaces? Anaesthesia 47:199-201

26. Lyons G (1995) Epidural is an outmoded form of regional anaesthesia for elective. Caesarean section. Int J Obst Anaesth 4:34-39

27. Cesarini M, Torrielli R, Lahaye F, Mene JM, Cabiro C (1990) Sprotte needle for intrathecal anaesthesia for Caesarean section: incidence of post-dural puncture headache. Anaesthesia 45:656-658

28. Ross BK, Chadwick HS, Mancuso JJ, Benedetti C (1992) Sprotte needle for obstetric anaesthesia: decreased incidence of post dural puncture headache. Reg Anaesth 17:29-33

29. Sears DH, Leeman MI, O'Donnell RH et al (1990) Incidence of postdural puncture headache in Caesarean section patients using the 24 G Sprotte needle. Anesthesiology 73:A1003

30. Cox M, Lawton G, Gowrie-Mohan S, Priest T, Arnold A, Morgan BM (1995) Ambulatory extradural analgesia. Br J Anaesth 74:114

31. Brownridge P (1991) Spinal anaesthesia in obstetrics. Br J Anaesth 67:663

32. Dennison B (1987) Combined subarachnoid and epidural block for Caesarean section. Can Anaesth Soc J 34:105-106

33. Abboud T, Zhu J, Reyes A, Miller H, Steffens Z, Afrasiabi K, Afrasiabi A, Sherman G, Emershad B (1992) Effect of subarachnoid morphine on the incidence of spinal headache. Reg Anaesth 17:34-36

34. Eldor J, Guedj P, Cotev S (1990) Epidural morphine injections for the treatment of postspinal headache. Can J Anaesth 37:710-711

35. Norris MC, Grieco WM, Borkowski M, Leighton BL, Arkoosh VA, Huffnagle HJ, Huffnagle S (1994) Complications of labor analgesia: epidural versus combined spinal epidural techniques. Anaesth Analg 79:529-537

36. Camann WR, Minzter BH, Denney RA, Datta S (1993) Intrathecal sufentanil for labor analgesia. Effects of added epinephrine. Anaesthesiology 78:870-874

37. Van Decar T, Callicot R, Jones R, Herman MD (1994) Determination of a dose response curve for intrathecal sufentanil in labor. Anesthesiology 81:A1148

38. Gautier PE, Debry F, Fanard L, Van Steenberge A, Hody JL (1997) Ambulatory combined spinal epidural analgesia for labor. Influence of epinephrine on bupivacaine-sufentanil combination. Reg Anaesth 22:143-149

39. Yaksh T, Reddy SVR (1981) Studies in the primate on the analgesic effects associated with intrathecal action of opiates, alpha-adrenergic agonists and baclofen. Anaesthesiology 54:451-467

40. Ossipov MH, Suarez IJ, Spaulding TC (1989) Antinociceptive interactions between alpha-2 adrenergic and opiate agonists at the spinal level in rodents. Anesth Analg 68:194-200

41 Segal S, Eappen S, Datta S (1997) Superiority of multi-orifice over single-orifice epidural catheters for labor analgesia and Caesarean delivery J Clin Anaesth 9:109-112

42. Robin SH, Hew E, Ogilvie G (1987) A comparison of two types of epidural catheters. Can J Anaesth 34:459-461

43. Kartawladi SL, Vercauteren MP, Van Steenberge AL, Adriaensen HA (1996) Spinal analgesia during labor with low-dose bupivacaine, sufentanil, and epinephrine. A comparison with epidural analgesia. Reg Anaesth 21·191-196

44. Rawal N (1986) Single segment combined spinal epidural block for Caesarean section. Can Anaesth Soc J 33.254-255

45. Rawal N, Schollin J, Wesstrom G (1988) Epidural versus combined spinal epidural block for Caesarean section. Acta Anaesthesiol Scand 32 61-66

46 Thoren T, Holmstrom B, Rawal N, Schollin J, Lindeberg S, Skeppner G (1994) Sequential combined spinal epidural block versus spinal block for Caesarean section· effects on maternal hypotension and neurobehavioral function of the newborn. Anaesth Analg 78:1087-1092

47. Swami A, McHale S, Abbott P, Morgan B (1993) Low dose spinal anaesthesia for Caesarean section using combined spinal-epidural (CSE) technique. (Abstract) Anaesth Analg 76:S423

48. Fan S-Z, Susetio L, Wang Y-P, Liu CC (1994) Low dose of intrathecal hyperbaric bupivacaine combined with epidural lidocaine for Caesarean section – a balance block technique. Anaesth Analg 78:474-477

49. Kumar C (1987) Combined subarachnoid and epidural block for Caesarean section. Can J Anaesth 34:329-330

50. Bernards CM, Kopacz DJ, Michel MZ (1994) Effect of needle puncture on morphine and lidocaine flux through the spinal meninges of the monkey in vitro. Implications for combined spinal-epidural anaesthesia. Anaesthesiology 80:853-858

51. Zaric D, Axelsson K, Haligren S, Nydahl P-A, Philipson L, Samuelsson L (1996) Evaluation of epidural sensory motor blockade by thermostimulation, laser stimulation and recording of somatosensory evoked potentials Reg Anaesth 21:124-130

52. Bromage P (1975) Mechanism of action of extradural anaesthesia. Br J Anaesth 47:199-212

53. Suzuki N, Koganemaru M, Onizuka S, Takasaki M (1996) Dural puncture with a 26 gauge spinal needle affects spread of epidural anaesthesia. Anaesth Analg 82:1040-1042

54. Blumgart CH, Ryall D, Dennison B, Thompson-Hill LM (1992) Mechanism of extension of spinal anaesthesia by extradural injection of local anaesthetic. Br J Anaesth 69:457-460

55. Steinstra R, Dahan A, Alhadi ZRB, van Kleef JW, Burm AGL (1996) Mechanism of action of an epidural top-up in combined spinal epidural anaesthesia. Anaesth Analg 83:382-386

56. Ramsay M (1991) Epidural injection does cause an increase in CSF pressure. Anaesth Analg 73:668

57. Morgan BM (1995) Is an epidural test dose necessary? Eur J Obstet Gynecol 59:559-560

58. Ong B, Cohen MM, Cumming M, Palahniuk RJ (1987) Obstetrical anaesthesia at Winnipeg Women's Hospital 1975-83: anaesthetic technique and complications. Can J Anaesth 34:294-299

59. Ducey JP, Knape KG, Talbot J et al (1992) Intrathecal narcotics for labor cause hypotension Anaesthesiology 77:A997

60. Cohen SE, Cherry CM, Holbrook RH Jr et al (1993) Intrathecal sufentanil for labor analgesia – sensory changes, side effects, and fetal heart rate changes Anaesth Analg 77:1155-1160

61. Anderson M, D'Angelo R, Philip J et al (1993) Intrathecal sufentanil compared to epidural bupivacaine for labor analgesia. Anaesthesiology 79:A970

62. Kirno K, Lundin S, Elam M (1993) Effects of intrathecal morphine and spinal anaesthesia on sympathetic nerve activity in humans. Acta Anaesth Scand 37:54-59

63. Hill JM, Kaufman MP (1990) Attenuation of reflex pressor and ventilatory responses to static muscular contraction by intrathecal opioids. J Appl Physiol 68:2466-2472

64. Abboud TK, Shnider SM, Dailey PA et al (1984) Intrathecal administration of hyperbaric morphine for the relief of pain labor. Br J Anaesth 56:1351-1359

65. Camann WR, Denney RA, Holby ED, Datta S (1989) A comparison of intrathecal, epidural, and intravenous sufentanil for labor analgesia. Anaesthesiology 77:884-887

66. Camann WR, Minzter BH, Denney RA, Datta S (1993) Intrathecal sufentanil for labor analgesia Effects of added epinephrine. Anaesthesiology 78:870-874

67. Thomas DA, Williams GM, Iwata K et al (1993) The medullary dorsal horn A site of action of morphine in producing facial scratching in monkeys. Anaesthesiology 79:548-554

68. Scott PV, Fischer HB (1982) Intraspinal opiates and itching: a new reflex? Br Med J 284:1015-1016
69. Stevens RA, Petty RH, Hill HF et al (1993) Redistribution of sufentanil to cerebrospinal fluid and systemic circulation after epidural administration in dogs. Anaesth Analg 767:323-327
70. Ferouz F, Norris MC, Arkoosh VA, Leighton BL, Boxer LM, Corba RJ (1997) Baricity, needle direction, and intrathecal sufentanil labor analgesia. Anesthesiology 86:592-598
71. Kileff ME, James FM, Dewan DM, Floyd RB (1984) Neonatal neurobehaviour responses after epidural anaesthesia for caesarean section using lidocaine and bupivacaine. Anaesth Analg 63:413-417
72. Larsen JV (1982) Obstetric analgesia anaesthesia. Clin Obstet Gynecol 9:685-709
73. Morgan BM, Aulakh JM, Barker JP, Goroszeniuk T, Trojanowski A (1983) Anaesthesia for Caesarean section – a medical audit of junior anaesthetic staff practice. Br J Anaesth 55:885-889
74. Abboud T, Dror A, Mossad P (1988) Mini-dose intrathecal morphine for relief of post-caesarean section pain. Anaesth Analg 67:370-374

Chapter 23

Regional anaesthetic techniques in orthopaedics

F. Bonnet, M. Osman, A. Babinet-Berthier

Orthopaedic surgery aims to recover functional capacity in patients but it carries a specific morbidity and mortality. Orthopaedic surgery conveys several challenges for the anaesthesiologist, including prevention of thromboembolic complications, reduction of peri- and postoperative bleeding and management of autologus blood transfusion and postoperative pain. Orthopaedic surgery is the place where the most dramatic developments in regional anaesthetic techniques have occurred. These techniques have been evaluated in terms of advantages and drawbacks compared to general anaesthesia. In addition, the techniques themselves have changed over the past years, the main trends being the development of peripheral blocks for the anaesthesia itself and the postoperative analgesia as well. Thus, anaesthesia in orthopaedics is a very large topic, but this review will only focus on specific problems related to the use of regional anaesthetic techniques.

Considerations about the techniques of regional blocks

In Europe, there has been extensive development in peripheral blocks related to the use of nerve stimulators. Even if a nerve stimulator does not improve the reliability of a skilful expert in nerve blockade, it improves teaching of the techniques and offers new opportunity to experiment with new techniques. Nerve stimulation is especially useful for deep blocks such as lumbar plexus block via the posterior approach or sciatic nerve block. Nerve stimulation also allows identification of distal nerves whatever their location. The description of brachial plexus block at the humeral canal is thus related to the introduction of nerve stimulation. Nerve stimulation has introduced a new concept in the practice of peripheral block. Without stimulation, the principle of nerve blockade is to identify a nerve structure with the help of superficial anatomical landmarks and then the induction of paraesthesia. Since paraesthesia is worrisome for the patient, once it occurs, a given amount of the anaesthetic solution is injected without precise identification of all the nerve structures. The principle is to administer a large amount of solution which diffuses inside the virtual space limited by nerve sheath. In contrast, nerve stimulation allows precise identification of each nerve structure in a plexus. For example, at the axillary level, anterior (median and ulnar nerves) and posterior (radial nerve) responses can be identified by muscle contractions from stimulation of structures inside the common axillary vascular sheath, but motor response can also be elicited from nerves outside the sheath (musculocutaneous nerve) [1]. With precise location of each nerve structure only a limited amount of the anaesthetic solution must be given to achieve a specific blockade and to be confident in the result, provided the nerve stimulator is used properly. The approach of the upper limb nerve at the midhumeral level is one of the techniques recently described as a result of nerve stimulation [2]. Briefly, the needle is inserted at the junction between the upper and the middle third of the arm, just against the brachial artery, almost tangential to the skin to locate the median nerve. Once the appropriate motor activity is evoked, the needle is reoriented to become perpendicular to the horizontal plan, just medial to the humeral artery, and is advanced to stimulate the ulnar nerve. The needle is then reoriented, the tip being placed inside the biceps muscle to achieve stimulation of the musculocutaneous nerve. Thereafter, the needle is introduced so that the tip slips under the humerus where the radial nerve lies in a groove. Complementary subcutaneous infiltration is performed to block the cutaneous medial nerves of the arm and the forearm. Selective stimulation of the four main nerves of the arms allows a more complete blockade to be achieved than the one obtained with axillary block [2]. Other interesting techniques of lower limb plexus, and nerve blocks are also extensively practised through nerve stimulation. For example, the posterior approach of the lumbar plexus which was introduced to achieve a more extensive blockade than the classical "3-in-1" technique, used a Tuohy needle and the "loss of resistance" technique [3-5]. This method of localization, although commonly effective, is not as reliable as nerve stimulation, which significantly increases the success rate of the procedure [6]. Whatever the landmarks used, the posterior approach of the lumbar plexus does not allow complete block of the sacral plexus. Since combined blockade of the lumbar and of the sacral plexus is necessary for surgery of the knee or above the knee, large amounts of local anaesthetic solution are administered to the patient in these conditions. Precise localization of the lumbar plexus and sciatic nerve with the nerve stimulator lead to decreases in the amount of local anaesthetic given to the patient without compromising the reliability of the block. Moreover, a more distal approach to the sciatic nerve is possible with reliability. For example, with a lateral popliteal approach, surgery of the foot and ankle can be performed [7-10]. The block is completed by a subcutaneous infiltration of the saphenous nerve under the head of the tibial bone to allow the placement of a tourniquet when necessary. Finally, nerve stimulation also improves the success rate of nerve blocks, facilitating a distal approach for selective nerves incompletely blocked by the proximal approach (i.e., ulnar nerve after interscalene block or radial nerve after axillary block).

Interscalene block and shoulder surgery

Elective shoulder surgery is an indication for interscalene block. The benefits of regional anaesthesia include a better patient acceptance [11] and a more rapid turnover in the recovery room. The brachial plexus is identified in the interscalene space, and a C6 motor response (flexion of the arm) is elicited. Bupivacaine 40 ml in 0.5% solution are injected. Skin infiltration is required for posterior portals or for surgical incisions extending toward the axilla (T2 innervation). Interscalene block leads to ipsilateral diaphragm paresis, which is well tolerated in most patients [12, 13]; however, it is commonly recommended to give supplemental oxygen to the patient and to monitor SaO_2. Anterior diffusion of the anaesthetic solution is responsible for cervical sympathectomy with unilateral Horner's syndrome, stuffy nose, change in voice and sometimes hearing loss [14]. Complications of the block such as epidural or subarachnoid spread of the solution are fortunately extremely rare. Acute bradycardia and hypotension have been described in about 20% of patients in the sitting position [15]. This so-called Bezold-Jarisch reflex is attributed to the increased circulating adrenaline levels in patients receiving adrenaline-containing solutions.

There is commonly a controversy between surgeons and anaesthetists concerning the risk of neurological complications. When such a risk could be related to the operative procedure, surgeons commonly prefer to check motor and sensory functions at the end of the surgical procedure. In this case it is preferable to use interscalene block for postoperative analgesia. This can be done either by bolus injection of clonidine-containing solution (in order to prolong the duration of analgesia) or by a continuous infusion of local anaesthetic through a short catheter [16]. An alternative solution for postoperative analgesia is to perform a suprascapular block with a limited (10 ml) amount of local anaesthetic [17]. The suprascapular nerve indeed supplies 70% of the sensory nerve supply of the shoulder joint, including the superior and the postero-superior regions of the joint, capsule and overlying skin. This nerve block result in a 50% reduction in opioid demand after shoulder arthroscopy [17].

Spinal anaesthesia for orthopaedic surgery

Spinal anaesthesia is commonly used in orthopaedic surgery and there is no specific consideration concerning the technique itself in this case, except that pencil point needles convey the possibility to reduce the incidence of postdural puncture headache and make the technique acceptable for younger patients. Orthopaedic surgery has specific requirements which guides the choice of the anaesthetic solution and adjuvants. First of all the placement of a tourniquet is responsible for tourniquet pain, a phenomenon which appears after a delay of 45-60 min, increasing with the maintenance of tourniquet and sometimes requiring the shift to general anaesthesia if the tourniquet cannot be deflated. Tourniquet pain is thought to be related to increasing discharges of C fibres overwhelming the anaesthetic blocks. The incidence of tourniquet pain is decreased by increasing the dose of local anaesthetic, by choosing bupivacaine [18], isobaric solution instead of hyperbaric ones [19-21]. The incidence of tourniquet pain is also dramatically decreased by the addition of opioids or clonidine [20] to the local anaesthetic solution. Since opioids and clonidine strengthen the local anaesthetic block, they are commonly used as adjuvants in orthopaedic patients. Over the past years the doses given have been reduced to avoid side effects. Recommended doses are in the range of 0.1-0.3 mg for morphine, 10-20 µg for fentanyl, 5-10 µg for sufentanil and 30-75 µg for clonidine. The limitation of opioid doses has reduced the risk of respiratory depression, but side effects such as nausea, pruritus and urinary retention persist. Clonidine avoids the risk of urinary retention related to the use of opioid but it worsens the incidence of hypotension and bradycardia. Clonidine also reduces the incidence of shivering associated with central blocks. Clonidine could be preferred to opioids when a very effective block is required, for example, because of tourniquet placement; conversely, when one would like to benefit from a prolonged analgesic effect, morphine is the favoured drug.

Peripheral blocks for postoperative analgesia

Orthopaedic patients are submitted to some painful procedures and, consequently, require effective postoperative analgesia. It is especially important for patients who require active physiotherapy and mobilization, which are impossible without the help of analgesic treatments [22]. Peripheral blocks achieve a better pain relief in this setting than parenteral opioid administration or intravenous patient-controlled analgesia (PCA) [23, 24] and are equally as effective as epidural analgesia but simpler [25]. Continuous local anaesthetic infusion (bupivacaine 0.125%, most of the time) is performed after insertion of short catheters. Catheters can be placed in the interscalene place, in the axillary groove, under the fascia iliaca close to the femoral nerve, in the lumbar region in the psoas compartment, or even in the popliteal space. Although the technique is reliable, it requires careful monitoring and training of nurses in the ward. Catheter displacement is the main cause of failure or incomplete analgesia. Interscalene continuous block is used for shoulder surgery [26], axillary block for hand surgery [27], femoral block for surgery of the hip or the knee [23, 24, 28] and sciatic block at the knee for foot surgery [9, 29]. Some problems with femoral block for postoperative analgesia after knee surgery result from the fact that the nerves which supply the posterior aspect of the knee derive from the sciatic plexus. Supplemental parenteral analgesia is therefore required in that case. More recently it has been suggested that the principle of PCA could be applied with the technique of peripheral blocks. Patients self-administer a bolus of local anaesthetic (for example, 5 ml bupivacaine 0.125% with a 30-min lock-out interval) according to their need, and especially before mobilization of the operated joint.

Bolus injection is a simpler technique although analgesia is shorter in duration than continuous infusion. To avoid this limitation a combination of local anaesthetics with adjuvants has been suggested. There is, today, no definite evidence supporting the efficacy of opioids in combination with local anaesthetics in peripheral blocks. This was documented by a recent meta-analysis [30]. Conversely, there are several studies which document that clonidine actually prolongs the duration of analgesia for several hours when combined with local anaesthetics for peripheral blocks [31-33]. Since a limited dose of clonidine (<150 µg) is usually given to the patient via this route of administration, and probably due to a limited plasma resorption, side effects of clonidine (hypotension, bradycardia, sedation) are rare. Nevertheless, incomplete motor blockade may sometimes persists for hours. The bolus technique is less effective than the continuous infusion but, when supplemented with parenteral analgesia, it permits satisfactory analgesia, especially after hip or shoulder surgery. The administration of clonidine-containing bupivacaine (0.25%) solution provides analgesia which usually includes the first 24 postoperative hours, whatever the site of administration. A second injection may eventually prolong the duration of analgesia over the second postoperative day.

The practice of peripheral nerve blocks for postoperative analgesia is maturing. These techniques provide the same quality of analgesia as epidural technique but probably with fewer side effects. Patient self-administration of boluses via this route offers a great flexibility and adaptation to postoperative physiotherapy.

Intra-articular analgesia

Local anaesthetics were initially administered intra-articularly to perform surgery but anaesthesia was never completely satisfactory and did not compare favourably with other regional techniques such as spinal anaesthesia or peripheral blocks. Intra-articular administration was then dedicated to postoperative analgesia instead of anaesthesia. A 20-to-40 ml injection of 0.25% bupivacaine rapidly achieves analgesia, which lasts no more than 4-6 h [34-37].

Moreover, the evidence of a local analgesic action of morphine has provided a new opportunity to promote a safe and efficient analgesic technique. Stein et al. demonstrated, indeed, that the administration of morphine into the knee joint allowed postoperative pain to be reduced more than i.m. morphine did [38]. Several clinical and laboratory studies from the same group have supported the hypothesis that peripheral opioids were the target of intra-articular morphine. A recent meta-analysis of all the published studies since the pioneer report of Stein et al. concluded that intra-articular morphine actually induces analgesia [39]. Bupivacaine has the advantage over morphine of allowing the development of analgesia within a short delay [40, 41] while morphine induces analgesia of longer duration. The combination of the two is therefore supposed to benefit from the effects of each agent taken separately [35, 37, 42, 43]. Finally, other agents such as non steroid anti-inflammatory drugs [44] and clonidine [45], have been documented to induce efficient postoperative analgesia after intra-articular injection.

Intra-articular analgesia is usually suggested as an analgesic technique for knee surgery but it can also be used following shoulder arthroscopy. To be effective, the technique must be used properly, and it is especially advised to keep the tourniquet inflated for several minutes after injection of the analgesic solution [46]. Extensive destruction of the joint by the surgical process is a contra-indication of the technique because of leakage of the solution out of the knee. In addition, intra-articular administration of an analgesic agent is less effective than other regional anaesthetic techniques and especially than regional blocks [47]. For more painful procedures, this technique could only be considered as an adjuvant.

Haemostasis disorders and central blocks

The practice of central blocks in patients with haemostatic disorders [48] is still controversial. Nevertheless, there are different clinical situations corresponding to this problem. In some instances the technique of central block must be changed; in others the antiaggregant or anticoagulant treatment must be adapted; in yet others, central block must be cancelled to the benefit of general anaesthesia; and, finally, in many cases neither the regional anaesthetic technique nor the anticoagulant treatment have to be changed.

The main risk is the occurrence of an epidural or subdural haematoma, leading to permanent neurological deficit. The incidence of such complications is between 1/10 000 and 1/50 000. Epidural haematoma may also occur spontaneously in patients receiving anticoagulant but not epidural anaesthesia and in patients with central blocks but no haemostasis disorder. Considering the low incidence of this complication, the additional risk resulting from the combination of antiaggregant, anticoagulant and central blocks is difficult to estimate. Nevertheless case-report studies point out that patients who suffered from epidural haematoma frequently had difficult punctures, more frequently epidural than spinal anaesthesia, and associated haemostasis disorders (i.e., anticoagulant in patients with liver cirrhosis or renal failure and decreased platelet aggregation). Special attention must be paid in these circumstances to avoid regional anaesthesia.

The increased risk associated with difficult puncture and the fact that epidural is more risky than spinal anaesthesia stress the point of the responsibility of the mechanical trauma. In patients receiving antiaggregants or anticoagulants it is wise to choose the less traumatic technique, i.e. to prefer spinal to epidural anaesthesia and to prefer single-shot technique to the placement of a catheter. In agreement, the FDA has recently warned against the use of epidural catheters in patients receiving low-molecular-weight heparin for thromboprophylaxis. Central block can be performed in these patients but a significant delay, accounting for the pharmacokinetics of each heparin, must occur between the heparin injection and the needle puncture. This is especially the case when a preoperative injection of low-molecular-weight heparin is performed.

Case reports of epidural haematoma associated with antiaggregants are extremely rare, apart from those case where antiaggregants were combined with anticoagulants. Interruption of ticlopidine is justified because harmful perioperative bleeding has been described. Interruption of aspirin does not seem to be justified before the performance of a central block [49, 50]. This is also the case for non-steroidal anti-inflammatory drugs, which are reversible inhibitors of cyclo-oxygenase. In addition, the bleeding time is a non-specific and non-sensitive examination, meaning that a normal preoperative bleeding time in a patient taking aspirin does not guarantee that there is no risk of increased bleeding, and the correction of a prolonged bleeding time by desmopressin is not a reliable technique. Finally, there are obvious contraindications to regional anaesthesia, i.e. the use of fibrinolytic agents, effective anticoagulation at the time of needle puncture or catheter handling (insertion or withdrawal) and associated haemostasis disorders. There is always an alternative solution to the use of regional anaesthesia and persisting unwillingness to use other techniques when encountering difficulties cannot be supported. At the other extreme, focusing on the risk of bleeding when there are other more worrying problems (i.e., difficult intubation or allergy to anaesthetic agents) is not of benefit to the patient. A cost-benefit analysis is therefore always recommended in any clinical setting.

Morbidity, mortality and regional anaesthesia

For many years it has been suggested or even asserted that regional anaesthesia may improve morbidity and mortality in orthopaedic surgery (and in other circumstances as well). Thus, epidural and spinal anaesthesia have been reported to decrease perioperative bleeding, to prevent thromboembolic complications, to improve recovery of mental function in elderly people, and to shorten hospital stay.

Epidural anaesthesia and operative bleeding

Most of the studies concerning operative bleeding focus on hip surgery. Operative bleeding has been studied in patients suffering from femoral neck fracture (FNF) and in those scheduled for total hip replacement (THR). All the studies concerning FNF fail to report a reduction in bleeding related to the use of spinal anaesthesia compared to general anaesthesia. The main reason is that this type of surgery exposes the patient to the loss of a small amount of blood (300-500 ml) and thus the number of patients included is the different studies is not large enough to point out a significant difference. Anyway, even if a difference exists, it is not clinically relevant. In the case of THR, in contrast, the amount of blood loss is more important (1 000-1 500 ml). Thus, most of the studies found out that epidural anaesthesia reduces either the amount of bleeding or the need for transfusion [51]. A significant benefit of central block would be more appreciated in case of redux surgery of the hip because in this case major blood loss occurs. Nevertheless, there are other means to reduce blood loss in that case such as the use of aprotinin, but a comparison with epidural anaesthesia has never been made.

Prophylaxis of thromboembolic complications

It has long been demonstrated that epidural/spinal anaesthesia reduces the risk of venous thrombosis, especially after hip surgery [52-56]. This effect could be related to an inhibition of platelet aggregation by the local anaesthetic agents, to an improvement in rhoeologic conditions related to haemodilution and to an increase in calf blood flow related to the sympatholytic effect of central blocks. A 50% reduction of venous thrombosis is thus documented after hip or knee surgery. Nevertheless, there is growing evidence that lower limb vein thrombosis may occur not only during the surgical procedure but also in the days and even the weeks following the procedure. It is therefore unlikely that a technique limited to the surgical period will ensure a prolonged prevention. In agreement, it is noteworthy noticing that the per cent thrombotic risk reduction achieved with epidural anaesthesia is less than the one obtained with the use of anticoagulants (80% risk reduction with low-molecular-weight heparin). A recent study comparing epidural anaesthesia to general anaesthesia and low-molecular-weight heparin documents that the risk is far less in the second group of patients. Today, there is no worthy reason to avoid central blocks in patients receiving anticoagulants for thromboprophylaxis not is the prevention of thromboembolic complications a good reason to select epidural anaesthesia for a patient scheduled for hip or knee replacement.

Mental function

Mental disturbances (disorientation, confusion) are occasionally observed in elderly people following general anaesthesia and some of these patients may complain of loss of memory, difficulty in keeping attention or other related disorders of superior mental functions. Despite preservation of consciousness, epidural or spinal anaesthesia does not result in less mental disturbances than general anaesthesia. Most of the studies, in fact, document that, despite some minor disturbance in the first postoperative hours or days, most of the patients recover rapidly and fully their mental function [57, 58]. Moreover, most of the time, mental function tests had improved over preoperative performances. Consequently, the anaesthetic technique cannot be implicated in disturbances in mental function, except for the early postoperative period.

Postoperative recovery

More rapid recovery depends on mobilization and postoperative re-education; the regional anaesthetic technique used in the postoperative period may facilitate postoperative recovery through effective analgesia [22, 58]. Intravenous PCA has never been demonstrated to improve recovery. Conversely, some studies document that epidural analgesia is associated with more rapid achievement of convalescence and shorter hospital stay [59, 60]. No data are available concerning peripheral block because these techniques were not introduced on a large scale until recently but one may expect favourable results in the near future. In contrast, prospective studies failed to demonstrate that central blocks improve mortality following hip surgery [61-65]. Mortality depends more on specific factors such as the delay between fracture and surgery in the case of FNF than on the anaesthetic technique [66].

Conclusions

Regional anaesthesia, including central and peripheral blocks, can been used extensively in patients scheduled for orthopaedic surgery. Nerve stimulation gives the opportunity to improve the techniques in terms of reliability and to describe new approaches of nerve blockade. The main advantage of these techniques is simplicity while in the postoperative course they provide very efficient analgesia, which may benefit patient comfort and recovery.

References

1. Lavoie J, Tétrault MR, Côté DJ, Colas MJ (1992) Axillary plexus block using a peripheral nerve stimulator: single or multiple injections. Anaesth Analg 39:583-586
2. Bouaziz H, Narchi P, Mercier FJ et al (1997) Comparison between conventional axillary block and a new approach at the midhumeral level. Anaesth Analg 84:1058-1062
3. Winnie AP, Ramamurthy S, Durrani Z (1974) Plexus block for lower extremity surgery. Anaesthesiol Rev 1:11-16
4. Chayen D, Nathan H, Chayen M (1976) The psoas compartment block. Anaesthesiology 45:95-99
5. Parkinson SK, Mueller JB, Little WL et al (1989) Extent of blockade with various approaches of the lumbar plexus. Anaesth Analg 68:243-248
6. Dalens B, Tanguy A, Vanneuville G (1988) Lumbar plexus block in children. a comparison of two procedures in 50 patients. Anaesth Analg 67.750-758
7. McLeod D, Wong D, Claridge RJ, Merrick PM (1994) Lateral popliteal sciatic nerve block compared with subcutaneous infiltration for analgesia following foot surgery Can J Anaesth 41:673-675
8. McLeod D, Wong D, Vaghadia H et al (1995) Lateral popliteal sciatic nerve block compared with ankle block for analgesia following foot surgery. Can J Anaesth 42:765-769
9. Singelyn FJ, Aye F, Gouverneur JM (1997) Continuous popliteal nerve block: an original technique to provide postoperative analgesia after foot surgery. Anaesth Analg 84:383-386
10 Singelyn FJ, Gouverneur JA, Gribomont BF (1991) Popliteal sciatic nerve block aided by a nerve stimulator. a reliable technique for foot and ankle surgery Reg Anaesth 16 278-281
11 Tetzlaff JE, Yoon HJ, Brems J (1993) Patient acceptance of interscalene block for shoulder surgery Reg Anaesth 18·30-33

12. Urmey WF, Talts KH, Sharrock NE (1991) One hundred percent incidence of hemidiaphragmatic paresis associated with interscalene brachial plexus anaesthesia diagnose by ultrasonography. Anaesth Analg 72:498-503

13. Fujimura N, Namba H, Tsunoda K et al (1995) Effect of hemidiaphragmatic paresis caused by interscalene brachial plexus block on breathing pattern, chest wall mechanics and arterial blood gases. Anaesth Analg 81:962-966

14. Rosenberg PH, Lamberg TS, Tarkkila P et al (1995) Auditory disturbance associated with interscalene brachial plexus block. Br J Anaesth 74:89-91

15. D'Alessio JG, Weller RS (1995) Activation of the Bezold-Jarisch reflex in the sitting position for shoulder arthroscopy using interscalene block. Anaesth Analg 80:27-32

16. Tuominen M, Haasio J, Hekali R, Rosenberg PH (1989) Continuous interscalene brachial plexus block: clinical efficacy, technical problems and bupivacaine plasma concentrations. Acta Anaesthesiol Scand 33:84-88

17. Ritchie ED, Tong D, Chung F et al (1997) Suprascapular nerve block for postoperative pain relief in arthroscopic shoulder surgery: a new modality? Anaesth Analg 84:1306-1312

18. Conception MA, Lambert DH, Welch KA, Covino BG (1986) Tourniquet pain during spinal anaesthesia: a comparison of plain solutions of tetracaine and bupivacaine. Anaesth Analg 67:828-832

19. Bridenbaugh PO, Hagenouw RR, Gielen MJ, Edstrom HH (1986) Addition of glucose to bupivacaine in spinal anaesthesia increases incidence of tourniquet pain. Anaesth Analg 65:1181-1185

20. Bonnet F, Diallo A, Belon M et al (1989) Prevention of tourniquet pain by spinal isobaric bupivacaine plus clonidine. Br J Anaesth 63:93-96

21. Bonnet F, Zozime JP, Marcandoro J et al (1988) Tourniquet pain during spinal anaesthesia: isobaric versus hyperbaric intrathecal tetracaine. Reg Anaesth 13·29-33

22. Shoji H, Solomonow M, Yoshino S et al (1990) Factors affecting postoperative flexion in total knee arthroplasty. Orthopedics 13:643-649

23 Edwards ND, Wright EM (1992) Continuous low-dose 3-in-1 nerve blockade for postoperative pain relief after total knee replacement. Anaesth Analg 75:265-267

24. Serpell MG, Milar FA, Thompson MF (1991) Comparison of lumbar plexus block versus conventional opioid analgesia after total knee replacement. Anaesthesia 46:275-277

25. Schultz P, Christensen EF, Anker-Moller E et al (1991) Postoperative pain treatment after open knee surgery: continuous lumbar plexus block with bupivacaine versus epidural morphine. Reg Anaesth 16:34-37

26. Tuominen M, Pitkanen M, Rosenberg P (1987) Postoperative pain relief and bupivacaine plasma levels during continuous interscalene brachial plexus block. Acta Anaesthesiol Scand 31:276-278

27. Gaumann DM, Lennon RL, Wedel DJ (1988) Continuous axillary block for postoperative pain management. Reg Anaesth 13:77-82

28. Dahl JB, Christiansen CL, Daugaard JJ et al (1988) Continuous blockade of the lumbar plexus after knee surgery postoperative analgesia and bupivacaine plasma concentrations. Anaesthesia 43:1015-1018

29. Picard PR, Tramer MR, McQuay HJ, Moore R (1997) Analgesic efficacy of peripheral opioids (all except intra-articular): a qualitative systematic review of randomised controlled trials. Pain 72:309-318

30. Singelyn FJ, Dangoisse M, Bartholomée S, Gouverneur JM (1992) Adding clonidine to mepivacaine prolongs the duration of anaesthesia and analgesia after axillary brachial plexus block. Reg Anaesth 17:148-150

31. Singelyn FJ, Gouverneur JM, Robert A (1996) A minimum dose of clonidine added to

mepivacaine prolongs the duration of anaesthesia and analgesia after axillary brachial plexus block. Anaesth Analg 83:1046-1050

32. Gaumann D, Forster A, Griessen M et al (1992) Comparison between clonidine and epinephrine admixture to lidocaine in brachial plexus block. Anaesth Analg 75:69-74

33. Joshi GP, McCarroll SM, Cooney CM et al (1992) Intra-articular morphine for pain relief after knee arthroscopy. J Bone Joint Surg 74:749-751

34. Joshi GP, McCarroll SM, O'Brien TM, Lenane P (1993) Intraarticular analgesia following knee arthroscopy. Anaesth Analg 76:333-336

35. Gyrn JP, Olsen S, Appelqvist E, Chraemmer-Jorgensen B, Duus B, Hansen LB (1992) Intra-articular bupivacaine plus adrenaline for arthroscopic surgery of the knee. Acta Anaesthesiol Scand 36:643-646

36. Haynes TK, Appadurai IR, Power I et al (1994) Intraarticular morphine and bupivacaine analgesia after arthroscopic knee surgery. Anaesthesia 49:54-56

37. Stein C, Comisel K, Yassouridis A, Lehrberger K, Herz A, Peter K (1991) Analgesic effect of intraarticular morphine after arthroscopic knee surgery. N Engl J Med 325:1123-1126

38. Kalso E, Tramer MR, Caroll D et al (1997) Pain relief from intra-articular morphine after knee surgery: a qualitative systemic review. Pain 71:127-134

39. Heard SO, Edwards WT, Ferrari D et al (1992) Analgesic effect of intraarticular bupivacaine or morphine after arthroscopic knee surgery: a randomized prospective, double-blind study. Anaesth Analg 74:822-826

40. Raja SN, Dickstein RE, Johnson CA (1992) Comparison of postoperative analgesic effects of intraarticular bupivacaine and morphine following arthroscopic knee surgery. Anaesthesiology 77:1143-1147

41. Khoury GF, Andrew C, Garland DE, Stein C (1992) Intraarticular morphine, bupivacaine, and morphine/bupivacaine for pain control after knee videoarthroscopy. Anaesthesiology 77:263-266

42. Allen GC, Amand MA, Lui ACP et al (1993) Postarthroscopy analgesia with intraarticular bupivacaine/morphine. A randomized clinical trial. Anaesthesiology 79:475-480

43. Smith I, Shively R, White PF (1992) Effects of ketorolac and bupivacaine on recovery after outpatient arthroscopy. Anaesth Analg 75:208-212

44. Gentili M, Juhel A, Bonnet F (1996) Peripheral analgesic effect of intraarticular clonidine. Pain 64:593-596

45. Witford A, Healy M, Joshi GP et al (1997) The effect of tourniquet release on the analgesic efficacy of intraarticular morphine after arthroscopic knee surgery. Anaesth Analg 84:791-793

46. De Andres J, Bellever J, Barrera L et al (1993) A comparative study of analgesia after knee surgery with intraarticular bupivacaine, intraarticular morphine, and lumbar plexus block. Anaesth Analg 77:727-730

47. McDonald R (1991) Aspirin and extradural blocks. Br J Anaesth 66:1-3

48. Vandermeulen EP, Van Aken H, Vermylen J (1994) Anticoagulants and spinal-epidural anaesthesia. Anaesth Analg 79:1165-1177

49. Horlocker TT, Wedel DJ, Schroeder DR et al (1995) Preoperative antiplatelet therapy does not increase the risk of spinal hematoma associated with regional anaesthesia. Anaesth Analg 80:303-309

50   Chin SP, Abou-Madi MN, Eurin B et al (1982) Blood loss in total hip replacement: role of epidural and general anaesthesia. Br J Anaesth 54:491-494

51. Modig J, Borg T, Karlstrom G, Maripuu E, Sahlstedt B (1983) Thromboembolism after total hip replacement: role of epidural and general anaesthesia. Anaesth Analg 62:174-180

52   Modig J, Maripuu E, Sahlstedt B (1986) Thromboembolism following total hip replacement. a prospective investigation of 94 patients with emphasis on the efficacy of lumbar epidural anaesthesia in prophylaxis. Reg Anaesth 11:72-79

53   Davis FM, Quince M, Laurensson M (1980) Deep vein thrombosis and anaesthesia technique in emergency hip fracture. Br Med J 281:1528-1529

54.   McKenzie PJ, Wishart HY, Gray I et al (1985) Effect of anaesthetic technique on deep venous thrombosis: a comparison of subarachnoid and general anaesthesia. Br J Anaesth 57:853-857

55.   Prins MH, Hirsh J (1990) A comparison of general anaesthesia and regional anaesthesia as a risk factor for deep vein thrombosis following hip surgery· a critical review. Thromb Haemost 64.497-500

56   Bigler D, Adeehloj B, Petring OU et al (1985) Mental function and morbidity after acute hip replacement during spinal and general anaesthesia. Anaesthesia 40:672-676

57.   Jones MJT, Piggot SE, Vaughan RS et al (1990) Cognitive and functional competence after anaesthesia in patients aged over 60· controlled trial of general and regional anaesthesia for elective hip or knee arthroplasty. Br Med J 300:1683-1687

58   Moiniche S, Hjortso NC, Hansen BL et al (1994) The effect of balanced analgesia on early convalescence after major orthopaedic surgery. Acta Anaesthesiol Scand 38:328-335

59   Mahoney OM, Noble PC, Davidson J, Tullos HS (1990) The effect of continuous epidural analgesia on postoperative pain, rehabilitation and duration of hospitalization in total knee arthroplasty Clin Orthop 260:30-37

60.   Williams-Russo P, Sharrock N, Haas S et al (1996) Randomized trial of epidural versus general anaesthesia· outcomes after primary total knee replacement. Clin Orthop 331:199-208

61   McKenzie PJ, Woshart HY, Dewar I et al (1980) Comparison of the effect of spinal anaesthesia and general anaesthesia on postoperative oxygenation and perioperative mortality. Br J Anaesth 52:49-54

62.   Hole A, Terjesen T, Breivik H (1980) Epidural versus general anaesthesia for total hip arthroplasty in elderly patients. Acta Anaesthesiol Scand 24·279-287

63.   Davis FM, Woolner DF, Frampton C et al (1987) Prospective, multi-centre trial of mortality following general or spinal surgery in the elderly. Br J Anaesth 59:1080-1088

64.   Sorenson RM, Pace NL (1992) Anaesthesic technique during surgical repair of femoral neck fractures. a meat-analysis. Anaesthesiology 77:1095-1104

65.   Sutcliffe A, Parker M (1994) Mortality after spinal and general anaesthesia for surgical fixation of hip fractures. Anaesthesia 49:237-240

66.   Zuckerman JD, Skovron ML, Koval KJ et al (1995) Postoperative complications and mortality associated with operative delay in older patients who have a fracture of the hip. J Bone Joint Surg 77·1551-1556

GUIDELINES OF ACUTE AND CHRONIC PAIN MANAGEMENT

Chapter 24

Guidelines on acute postoperative pain management

G. Savoia, G. Scibelli, R. Gammaldi

In high-technology countries, the level of care in intensive care units or recovery units is high, whereas on many general wards the standards of acute pain therapy are low. "Standards" are derived from the sources that legitimately set the standards of knowledge and practice in the dominant medical care system. Standards are intended to be applied rigidly and in virtually all cases. Violation should trigger thoughts of malpractice. "Practice guidelines" aim at decreasing inappropriate variations in practice and reducing excessive expenses. They are appropriate for the majority of patients and should be followed in most cases. Guidelines are not intended to function as standards or absolute requirements.

"Options and recommendations" leave practitioners free to choose. They merely note the different interventions that are available. Table 1 furnishes a summary of published pain-related quality assurance / quality improvement standards or guidelines.

Ideally, guidelines are evidence-based. There is strong evidence, for example, that patient controlled analgesia (PCA) or epidural analgesia leads to greater patient comfort and patient satisfaction compared with conventional therapy (i.e., "as needed" or "at fixed hours" intramuscular injection of opioids). On the other hand, most studies have failed to show significant advantages in patient outcome (mortality, morbidity, hospital stay, etc.), as long as patient satisfaction per se is not assumed to be an "outcome". Tables 2 and 3 report some methods of measuring patient's satisfaction. Therefore, many areas within practice guidelines are not evidence-based, but are founded on experience of causal relationships (pathophysiology), on weighting potential risks and benefits, and on clinical feasibility. Ideally, postoperative pain treatment should be inserted into a quality assurance and changing practice program, such as described in Fig. 1 [1, 2].

Table 1. Summary of published pain-related QA/QI standards or guidelines [2]

Canadian Council of Health Facilities Accreditation – QA-Related Palliative Care Program Standards

- The Palliative Care Program has planned and conducted systematic activities for monitoring and evaluating the quality of patient care, including a plan for action(s) and follow-up to ensure that the action(s) is effective

American Pain Society's QA Standards on Acute and Cancer-related Pain

- Acute pain and chronic cancer pain are recognized and effectively treated
- Information about analgesics is readily available
- Patients are promised attentive analgesic care
- Explicit policies for the use of advanced technologies are defined
- Adherence to standards is mandatory

Agency for Health Care Policy and Research QA Guidelines

- General considerations
  - Institutional process of acute pain management begins with the affirmation that patients should have access to the best level of pain relief that may sagely be provided
  - Each institution should develop the resources necessary to provide the best and the most modern pain relief appropriate to its patients and should designate who and/or which departments are responsible for the required activities
  - Formal means must be developed and used within each institution to assess pain management practices and to obtain patient feedback to gauge the adequacy of pain control

- Key items to be included in an institutional QA program
  - Patient comfort and satisfaction with pain management
  - How those options are best applied
  - The range and appropriateness of options available within a particular institution
  - Minimizing side effects and complications related to pain control

Table 2. A comparison of the use of interviews versus questionnaires to obtain data on patient satisfaction [2]

Interview

- Sensitivity to patient opinions
- Flexibility in covering topics
- Rapport
- Clarification of ambiguous items or reasons for the items
- Respondent adherence
- More scope to follow up nonrespondents

Self-report questionnaire

- Standardization of items
- No interviewer bias
- Anonymity is maintained
- Low cost of data gathering
- Less need for trained staff

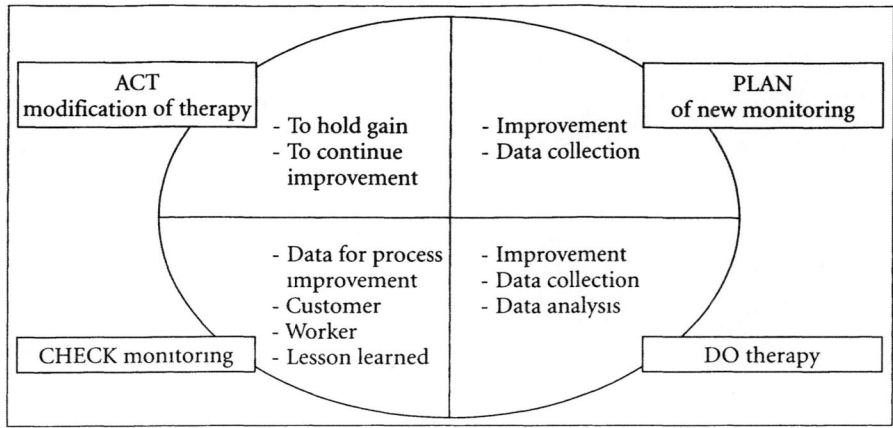

Fig. 1. Key aspects of the quality improvement action plan [2]

Table 3. Recommendations for assessing patient satisfaction with pain management [2]

1. Evaluate an episode of pain
2. Develop specific patient inclusion/exclusion criteria
3. Evaluate patient satisfaction with pain management and care providers using a descriptive numeric rating scale
4. Explore with patients incongruities in pain intensity ratings and the ratings of their level of satisfaction with pain management
5. Triangulate survey responses to determine the overall quality of pain management within an organization
6. Evaluate patients' expectations for pain and pain relief
7. Conduct inpatient and outpatient patient satisfaction surveys
8. Evaluate patient satisfaction with pain management across health care settings
9. Evaluate caregiver satisfaction with pain management
10. Link patient satisfaction data with patient outcomes (e.g., quality of life, mood, side effects and complications, functional status)
11 Evaluate the cost of patient satisfaction surveys of pain management
12. Conduct qualitative analyses of patient satisfaction with pain management and patients' opinions of factors that would improve the quality of pain management

ASA task force practice guidelines and ASRA consensus statement

The ASA Task Force strongly believes that "(…) the anaesthesiologist is in a unique position to provide leadership in integrating pain management into other aspects of perioperative care and thus improve this area of practice. In this leadership role, the anaesthesiologist can contribute further to quality of care by developing and directing institution-wide perioperative analgesia programs that include collaboration with and partecipation by others, when appropriate(…)" [3]. In the official agreement between the societies of anaesthesiologists and surgeons of Germany, particular emphasis was placed on an interdisciplinary approach, and a multidisciplinary pain service (guided by an anaesthesiologist or surgeon) was proposed [4].

The American Society of Regional Anaesthesia published a "consensus statement on acute pain management" as a synopsis of a consensus-style meeting held in the Spring of 1996 [5, 6]. Statements were as follows:

1. the combination of epidural opioids and local anaesthetics provides better pain control with fewer side effects than epidural or systemic opioids alone;
2. epidural analgesia is most effective when the site of injection is close to the affected dermatomes (i.e., thoracic epidurals for upper abdominal surgery);
3. epidural anaesthesia (intraoperative) and epidural analgesia (postoperative) reduce thromboembolic complications; are associated with a better recovery of gastrointestinal function; probably preserve immune function; probably reduce cardiovascular complications; inhibit endocrine metabolic stress responses to surgery; could help to shorten hospital stay, time of rehabilitation and return to work; and may reduce the incidence and severity of chronic pain syndromes.

Guidelines for monitoring respiratory depression include measuring the respiratory rate and assessing the degree of sedation. There is no evidence supporting the use of more sophisticated monitors. During neuraxial blockade, the sensory block level and hemodynamic stability should be assessed. Continuous techniques could be monitored by standard ward nursing care, supplemented by 12 h or intermittent rounds by pain management personnel.

Guidelines: purpose and contents

The principal purpose of guidelines is to maximize the results of health services, improving clinical practice and informing patients about different methods available. The guidelines may be used within a wide educational plan for physicians and nurses and to improve and ensure an adequate level of quality [7].

Practice guidelines are systematically developed recommendations that assist the practitioner and patient in making decisions about health care. These recommendations may be adopted, modified, or rejected according to clinical needs and constraints.

Practice guidelines are not intented as standards or absolute requirements. The use of practice guidelines cannot guarantee any specific outcome. Practice guidelines are subjects to revision from time to time, as warranted by the evolution of medical knowledge, technology, and practice. The guidelines provide basic recommendations that are supported by analysis of the current literature and by a synthesis of expert opinion, open forum commentary, and clinical feasibility data.

The purpose of guidelines for acute pain management in the perioperative setting is to facilitate the efficacy and safety of acute pain management in the perioperative setting and to reduce the risk of adverse outcomes. A number of adverse outcomes can result from undertreatment of postoperative pain. These include (but are not limited to) respiratory depression, brain injury, other neurologic injury, sedation, circulatory depression, nausea and/or vomiting, impairment of bowel function, pruritus, and urinary retention, extension of time spent in an intensive care unit and/or in hospital, and reduced patient satisfaction. In contrast, potential benefits of optimal postoperative pain menagement [8] are described in Table 4.

The ASA Task Force guidelines [3] provide that an individualized proactive plan (i.e., a predetermined strategy for postoperative analgesia) should be considered for all surgical patients. Activities that are commonly encompassed by proactive planning include (but are not limited to): 1) obtaining a pain history based on patients' experiences; 2) preoperative pain therapy when appropriate and feasible; 3) intraoperative procedures (i.e., wound infiltration), when appropriate and feasible; 4) intraoperative or postincisional preparation of patients for postoperative pain management (i.e., initiating epidural anaesthetic administration before the completion of surgery). Any treatment plan requires regular assessment and refinement based on the changing responses of individual patients.

The guidelines provide:
— education and training of hospital personnel;
— education and participation of patients and families in perioperative pain control;
— assessment and documentation of perioperative pain management;
— 24 h availability of anaesthesiologists;
— use of standardized institutional policies and procedures for ordering, administering, discontinuing, and transferring responsibility for perioperative pain management;
— use of three specific techniques for perioperative pain management:
  • PCA with systemic opioids;
  • EA (epidural analgesia) with opioids or opioid/local anaesthetic mixtures (or intrathecal opioids);

Table 4. Potential benefits of optimal postoperative pain managements [8]

* Improved patient comfort
  – Less physical and mental stress
  – Improved motivation and ability for active mobilization
* Pulmonary functions improved
* Less stress on cardiovascular system
* Thromboembolic complications reduced
* Less impairment of gastrointestinal functions
* Less urinary retention
* Less impairment of immunological functions
* Fewer septic complications
* Reduced mortality in high-risk patients
* Faster recovery after surgery
* Less chronic neuropathic pain
* Reduced health care costs

- RA (regional anaesthesia) techniques, including (but not limited to) intercostal blocks, plexus infusion, and local anaesthetic infiltration of incisions;
- a multimodality approach to perioperative pain management;
- an organized interdisciplinary approach to perioperative pain management;
- recognition and management of special features of paediatric perioperative pain management;
- recognition and management of special features of geriatric perioperative pain management;
- recognition of special features of perioperative pain management in emergency surgery patients.

McQuay and Moore [9] have furnished a meta-analysis on the treatment of postoperative pain. The rational approach to postoperative care is to use the highest quality evidence available. In the contest of postoperative care, this comes from systematic reviews of valid randomized trials. Several key decision nodes are explored. For pain relief, the simplest is that if patients can swallow, then the oral route should be preferred, and that non-steroidal anti-inflammatory drugs (NSAIDs), unless contraindicated, provide the best oral analgesia. The next decision node is prophylaxis versus "treat-as-necessary". In both pain relief and postoperative nausea and vomiting (PONV), the arguments for prophylaxis are not convincing. A third decision node is whether or not to use "peripheral" opioids. The evidence supports intra-articular, but not other routes.

Opioids and respiratory depression

Respiratory depression can occur in circumstances where the duration of an opioid's analgesic and respiratory depressant effects outlasts the duration of a painful stimulus. Even modest doses of opioids in awake subjects can have dramatic effects on the ventilatory response to hypoxemia. While depression of ventilatory responses to hypoxemia is of little consequence to most healthy subjects, the consequences can be severe in patients who may be dependent on hypoxic respiratory drive, such as those with chronic obstructive pulmonary disease (COPD) and long-standing hypercapnia.

While pain antagonizes opioid-induced respiratory depression, sleep can intensify the depressant effects of opioids. During normal respiration, subatmospheric pressure in the pharynx tends to draw the tongue against the palate, narrowing the airway. The finely coordinated contraction of the tongue (especially the genioglossus) and pharyngeal musculature helps to maintain airway patency and prevent snoring or inspiratory collapse of the airway. Sleep and opioids separately and in concert depress genioglossus and pharyngeal muscle tone and diminish airway protective reflexes. Critical incidents from opioid-induced respiratory depression appear to be more common in the hours from midnight to 6 a.m. Depression of level of consciousness is an extremely useful measure of the clinical effect in patients receiving opioids. Respiratory depression is almost always preceded by sedation or clouded senses [10].

Epidural opioid management

Epidural opioids are commonly used in Europe for the treatment of postoperative pain, particularly following major surgery. Although epidural opioids have been administered for more than 15 years, controversy still remains concerning the indications, agents, dose, and, in particular, the monitoring of patients.

Monitoring of epidural opioid analgesia requires the assessment of pain and the surveillance of incidence and severity of side effects [11].

Which parameters should be monitored for the assessment of side effects?

Respiratory parameters that could be monitored include arterial oxygen saturation (SaO_2), end-tidal carbon dioxide ($EtCO_2$), respiratory rate, and level of sedation. Pulse oximetric monitoring of SaO_2 cannot be recommended for two reasons. Firstly, depression of respiratory function may occur without arterial desaturation and, secondly, arterial desaturation could be due to ventilation perfusion mismatch unrelated to respiratory depression. However, patients receiving epidural opioids are prone to the development of hypoxemia episodes and oxygen supplementation (via a face mask or a nasal cannula) should be considered, particularly at night. End-tidal CO_2 or tissue PCO_2 would be appropriate parameters to monitor. No reliable technique is routinely available to achieve this in nonintubated patients breathing spontaneously.

Respiratory rate is a clinical parameter which is simple to monitor and a respiratory rate ≤ 10 breaths per minute is indicative of clinically significant respiratory depression requiring specific treatment, such as naloxone.

Respiratory depression related to epidural opioid administration does not occur suddenly but is a progressive event which is usually preceded by excessive sedation. Sedation monitoring uses a simple scale and should be part of routine nursing care as should respiratory rate and pain score assessment.

Regardless of whether patients receive epidural opioids in clinics or intensive care units, rapid access to resuscitation techniques is vital to ensure safety. Therefore, the placement of patients on a surgical ward during epidural opioid administration depends mainly on the number of nurses and on the organization of emergency care in a given institution. Conversely, the admission of a patient to an intensive care unit because of epidural opioid administration and the need for continuous monitoring is not necessarily justified if monitoring conditions are considered to be adequate on the ward [12].

Epidural analgesia includes opioids, local anaesthetics and α_2-agonists, but always requires a prevention planning of danger to patient derived by technical or drugs mismatches (Table 5) [8]. The real incidence of severe complications, such as epidural abscess, epidural hemorrhage, and anterior spinal artery syndrome, is very low (from 1:10 000 to 1:500 000), but their aknowledgment is mandatory for a rapid differential diagnosis (Table 6) [13].

Table 5. Sources of danger to patients during epidural analgesia [8]

- Too high dose of local anaesthetics
- Motor blockade
  - Mobilization impossible
  - Accidental fractures
  - Decubitus – sores at heels
- Autonomic nerve blockade
  - Hypotension
  - Urine retention
- Too high dose of opioid
  - Respiratory depression
  - Nausea/vomiting
  - Pruritus
  - Sedation
  - Urinary retention
- Epidural hematoma
  - Paraplegia
  - Arteria spinalis anterior syndrome
- Epidural infection
  - Epidural abscess
  - Meningitis
- Wrong drug!
- Cauda equina syndrome
- Nerve root damage
- Catheter migration
  - Intravenously
  - Subdurally
  - Into the subarachnoid space

Table 6. Differential diagnosis of epidural abscess, epidural hemorrhage, and anterior spinal artery syndrome [13]

	Epidural abscess	Epidural hemorrhage	Anterior spinal artery syndrome
Age of patient	Any age	50% over 50 years	Elderly
Previuous history	Infection	Anticoagulants	Arteriosclerosis/ hypotension
Onset	1-3 days	Sudden	Sudden
Generalized symptoms	Fever back pain	Sharp, transient back, and leg pain	None
Sensory involvement	None or paresthesias	Variable, late	Minor, patch
Motor involvement	Flaccid paralysis, later spastic	Flaccid paralysis	Flaccid paralysis
Segmental reflexes	Exacerbated – later obtunded	Abolished	Abolished
Myelogram/CT scan	Signs of extradural compression	Signs of extradural compression	Normal
Cerebrospinal fluid	Increased cell count	Normal	Normal
Blood data	Rise in sedimentation rate	Prolonged coagulation time	Normal

PCA: principles and complications

No serious complications during PCA were reported in the 1996 literature, apart from a warning of possible risk due to faulty extension sets. The incidence of respiratory depression varied between 0.2% and 1.2%. Two papers mentioned a slower bowel function recovery and longer hospitalization time with intravenous morphine PCA, compared with continuous epidural bupivacaine-morphine and with intramuscular morphine or ketorolac. The sources of danger to patients during patient-controlled i.v. morphine analgesia are described in Table 7 [8].

Who would have imagined how much was wrong with the management of simple postoperative pain? Would the concept of an acute pain service, and the newer international recommendations for adequate pain management have emerged without PCA experience? The 1996 literature confirms that PCA is still one of the best ways to achieve patient satisfaction and recuperation in the postoperative period. Furthermore, those who have no (or not enough) PCA devices

Table 7. Sources of danger to patients during patient-controlled i.v. morphine analgesia [8]

* Human errors
  - Drug prescription errors
  - Inappropriate prescribing
  - Drug-dilution errors
  - Computer programming errors
  - Errors when filling, installing, connecting
* Equipment malfunction
  - Pump or computer failure
  - Disconnections/syringe-cracks, gravity-infusion of entire content
* Nonpatient activation of bolus-demand button
  - Relatives
  - Nurses
  - Visitors or fellow patients
* Unanticipated drug-reactions
  - Interactions with hangover effects of anaesthesia
  - Unstable circulation with prolonged onset time
  - Postoperative renal failure
  - Accumulation of active morphine-glucuronides
* Continuous background infusion of morphine in adult patients
* Patient risk factor
  - Advanced age
  - Head injury
  - Sleep apnea syndrome
  - Obesity
  - Chronic respiratory failure
  - Hypotension
  - Hypovolemia
  - Renal failure
  - Hypothyroidism
  - Liver failure
  - Concurrent sedative medication

available can apply the "PCA principle". To do so involves trusting the patient, providing adequate monitoring and appropriate documentation, and, of course, raising the educational level of the staff on surgical wards [14].

Italian guidelines on postoperative pain management [15]

Introduction

An adequate treatment of postoperative pain is acknowledged to contribute significantly to the improvement of perioperative morbidity, considered as reduced incidence of postoperative complications, shorter hospitalization time, and reduced costs, especially for high-risk patients (ASA III-IV) undergoing major surgery. In a similar way, the risk/benefit ratio has to be taken into due consideration, since complications related to pain therapy cannot be completely eliminated.

It is desirable that in the next few years organization models, widely codified in other countries, be developed in Italy too, establishing units for the treatment of acute pain and the creation of skilled anaesthesiologists trained in the management of complex methods of postoperative pain treatment (such as epidural, patient-controlled analgesia), a difficult endeavor.

These organization models not necessarily have to be complex: new models at lower costs are founded on protocols which can be easily adopted in all departments by using simple evaluation forms of pain intensity and side effects and involving physicians and nurses in a process of permanent education and interactive management of postoperative pain.

Therefore, it is a very opportune time to make a series of recommendations for a rational approach to the management of postoperative pain, keeping in mind that suggested doses and advised drugs always have to be adapted to the clinical condition, and the intensity of actual pain in each patient and that the list of considered techniques is not exhaustive.

Plan of therapy

A correct plan of postoperative pain treatment should consider the following elements:
- expected incidence of intensity and duration of postoperative pain, in relation to site and kind of operation;
- expectations of the patient, conditioned by previous experiences and anxiety about surgery, requiring correct information about available techniques for pain therapy;
- an adequate preparation and the teaching of relaxation techniques, the adoption of cognitive strategies and copying techniques seem important and advantageous;
- the adoption of immediate instruments of pain "measurement" (such as ver-

bal scales and visual linear analogues) allows the adaptation of chosen techniques to the fluctuations of postoperative pain;
- the use of nonpharmacological techniques must be adapted to the patient's characteristics, in relation to intensity and duration of expected postoperative pain;
- as a priority simple instruments of pain measurement and documentation must be available and become routine procedure in all the departments.

Prevention of postoperative pain

It is current opinion that the adoption of preemptive analgesia techniques delays the onset of postoperative pain and reduces its intensity as well as prevents the priming of phenomena related to pain spinal memory. These methods may be systemic (NSAIDs and/or opioids) and/or locoregional (administration of local anaesthetics such as cream, infiltration of surgical area, peripheral and central blocks) carried out preoperatively, intraoperatively and before awakening, but realizing an adequate depth of analgesia before action of nociceptive stimuli.
The prevention requires measures so as to:
- ensure a comfortable position during the perioperative period;
- reduce surgical stress, limiting traction and stretching, taking care of hemostasis;
- avoid trauma during nursing maneuvers (intramuscular injections, aspiration, venous lines, medications, etc.).

The control of postoperative pain has to be included in a plan of treatment of "postoperative illness", providing at the same time multimodal analgesia, early mobilization, early enteral nutrition and active physiotherapy.

General principles of postoperative pain treatment

It is recommended:
- that the administration of drugs is adequate and in accordance to pharmacokinetic and pharmacodynamic principles;
- that continuous infusion techniques without flux control systems be avoided;
- the adoption of control measurements, by asking every treated patient to evaluate analgesia effectiveness and side effects related to pain therapy techniques (Table 8);
- to always keep in mind the residual effects of anaesthetic drugs, to avoid addictive effects and withdrawal intervals;
- to provide easy and effective instruments to ensure control, for use at home, too, of postoperative pain for day-surgery.

An adequate treatment of postoperative pain always requires planning of the anaesthesiologic work-load, so as to ensure the patients receive correct preoperative information about available techniques of pain therapy and that the staff is aware of how much postoperative time is needed for control and surveillance of patients undergoing postoperative pain treatment.

Table 8. Example of evaluation form for postoperative pain

Hours ➤	3	6	9	12	15	18	21	24
Resting VAS 0 ──➤ 10								
Incident VAS 0 ──➤ 10								
Blood pressure								
Heart rate								
Respiratory rate								
Pulseoximetry								
Sedation level* 1 ──➤ 6								
Bromage scale** 0 ──➤ 3								
High metameric level of loss of hot/cold sensorial discrimination C1- S5								
Nausea/vomiting								
Respiratory depression: R.R. <8/min; SaO$_2$ <85%								
Urinary retention								
Pruritus								

*Sedation levels according to Ramsey:
Level 1, anxiety and excitation of extreme degree; *Level 2*, cooperating, oriented and quiet patient; *Level 3*, patient executing orders on verbal command; *Level 4*, immediate reaction to external stimuli; *Level 5*, reduced reaction to external stimuli; *Level 6*, absent reaction to external stimuli; Kind of stimulus = light percussion of glabella or intense acoustic stimulus.
**Motor block in according to Bromage's Scale:
Level 0, absence of motor block; *Level 1*, impossibility to raise extended lower limb; *Level 2*, impossibility to bend knee; *Level 3*, total absence of movement

The techniques of postoperative pain therapy presently available can be scaled in three levels; each requires different planning of surveillance measures, considering available resources, pain intensity, adoption of respective surveillance levels, and ineffectiveness of inferior levels.

Level I

– Administration of paracetamol or NSAIDs at fixed times, with or without mild opioids;
– monitor paracetamol administration in case of liver failure; NSAIDs administration in case of positive anamnesis for gastric (gastric protection is absolutely necessary) and coagulation diseases, verified hypersensitivity to NSAIDs, simultaneous administration of other drugs affecting platelet aggregation, levels of seric albumin, asthma, and renal failure;
– controlled administration of major opioids within equivalent daily dose of 30 mg morphine; monitor reduced hepatic-renal clearance, late effects of anaesthetic drugs, reduced respiratory responses to hypoxia and hypercapnia, and extreme ages.
   It is recommended that effectiveness and side effects be monitored.

Level II

– PCA (patient controlled analgesia), i.v. with or without basal continuous infusion, within a restricted range (i.e., maximum of morphine in 24 h: 40 mg; bolus ≤1 mg; interval between boluses: 15 min);
– continuous infusion i.v. of NSAIDs and opioids at lower doses (i.e., morphine within 30-40 mg, petidine within 300 mg, tramadol within 400 mg in 24 h).
   It is recommended that effectiveness, side effects, sedation level, and respiratory rate be monitored.
– Techniques of continuous epidural analgesia by top-up or continuous infusion or PCA of local anaesthetics and/or opioids and/or clonidine within ranges of: morphine 6 mg/die, clonidine 300 μg/die, bupivacaine ≤0.125% 10 ml/h ropivacaine ≤2 mg/ml 10 ml/h;
– single dose of intrathecal morphine <0.5 mg.
   It is recommended that effectiveness, side effects, control of sedation level, respiratory rate and sensorial discrimination level be monitored, as a rule every 3-4 h. Physicians and nurses should receive information and training continuously, so as to recognize immediately and treat rapidly and efficaciously side effects and/or severe, even if uncommon, complications such as compartment syndromes, intrathecal migration of epidural catheter, epidural hematoma, and spinal ischemia.

Level III

– Continuous infusion of opioids at higher doses able to adapt patient to respiratory mechanical assistance;
– continuous epidural infusion of opioids (morphine >6 mg/die) and/or local anaesthetics (ropivacaine >2 mg/ml; bupivacaine >0.25%);
– PCA techniques within large range, via i.v. or spinal (maximum of morphine in 24 h>60 mg; bolus of 1-2 mg; intervals between boluses 5-10 min).

It is recommended that patients are hospitalized in a high-technology dependent "area or bed".

Acknowledgements. We thank the SIAARTI Study Group for Pain Therapy (Italian Society of
Anaesthesia, Analgesia, Resuscitation and Intensive Care) for raccomandation an the postoperative pain therapy

References

1. Wulf H, Neugebauer E (1997) Guidelines for postoperative pain therapy. Curr Opin
   Anaesthesiol 10·380-385
2. Miaskowski C (1994) Pain management: quality assurance and changing practice. Proceedings of the 7th World Congress on Pain. IASP Press, Seattle, pp 75-96
3 American Society of Anaesthesiologists Task Force on Pain Management, Acute Pain
   Section (1995) Practice guidelines for acute pain management in the perioperative setting. Anaesthesiology 82:1071-1081
4 BDA & BDC (1992) Agreement on the organization of postoperative pain management.
   Association of German Anaesthesiologists and of German Surgeons (in German)
   Chirurg 31.222-236
5 American Pain Society Quality of Care Committee (1995) Quality improvement guidelines for the treatment of acute pain and cancer pain. JAMA 274:1874-1880
6 Carpenter RL, Abram SE, Bromage PR, Rauck RL (1996) Consensus statement on acute
   pain management Reg Anaesth 21 (Suppl 6):152-156
7. FISM (Federazione delle Società Medico-Scientifiche Italiane) (1996) Raccomandazioni
   per la produzione, disseminazione ed implementazione di linee-guida di comporta-
   mento pratico. Milano, pp 1-24
8. Breivik H (1995) Benefits, risks and economics of postoperative pain management programmes. Baillieres Clin Anaesthesiol 9.403-422
9. McQuay H, Moore A (1997) The concept of postoperative care. Curr Opin Anaesthesiol 10:369-373
10. DuBose RA, Berde CB (1997) Respiratory effects of opioids. IASP Newsletter. IASP
    Press, Seattle, pp 3-5
11. Rawal N, Allvin R and the EURO Pain Study Group on Acute Pain (1996) Epidural and
    intrathecal opioids for postoperative pain management in Europe – a 17-nation ques-
    tionnaire study of selected hospitals. Acta Anaesthesiol Scand 40:1119-1126
12. Aguilar JL, Benhamou D, Bonnet F, Dahl J, Rawal N, Rubin A (1997) ESRA guidelines
    for the use of epidural opioids. Int Monitor 9(2):3-8
13. Wedel DJ, Horlocker TT (1996) Risks of regional anaesthesia – infectious, septic. Reg
    Anaesth 21:57-61
14. Lehmann KA (1997) Update of patient-controlled analgesia. Curr Opin Anaesthesiol
    10:374-379
15. Gruppo di studi SIAARTI per la terapia del dolore. Raccomandazioni per il trattamen-
    to del dolore postoperatorio Minerva Anestesiol 64(6):26-29

Chapter 25

Guidelines on chronic pain management

S. Ischia, G. Finco, E. Polati, L. Gottin

Chronic pain represents a topic of medicine to which an univocal and especially efficacious solution has not yet been found. The lack of unequivocally efficacious medical devices pressures physicians into searching for personal solutions which often have no clinical rationale and may expose the patients to useless, and sometimes increased, suffering. Moreover, many physicians attempt a pain therapy without adequate technical and scientific preparation. It is, therefore, of major importance to establish some guidelines for the treatment of chronic pain which are based on the demonstration of the efficacy of each device or, if this is not possible, on a physiopathologic rationale which suggests their use. The aim of this paper is to identify, based on the international literature and on our own clinical and scientific experience, criteria on which an adequate treatment of different types and clinical presentations of pain can be developed.

General considerations

First of all, a correct approach to pain entails adequate knowledge of the pain syndrome the patient has presented with, since each syndrome has peculiar pain characteristics and the response to a given treatment varies among different types of pain.

The identification of the etiological and physiopathologic mechanism of a disease enables one to understand which type of injury has hit the organism and its possible evolution. This might be useful to point the physician in the right direction for recognition of the patient's type of pain.

The therapeutic approach for nociceptive pain is completely different than for non-nociceptive pain since drugs usually effective for the former are absolutely useless for the latter. It seems that for non-nociceptive (neuropathic) pain anticonvulsant drugs [1] and microsurgical junctional dorsal root entry zone lesion (DREZ) [2], among the neurolesive techniques, are to date the most effective approaches.

The pharmacological response also differs for different types of nociceptive pain. For example, visceral colic type pain is better controlled by nonsteroidal anti-inflammatory drugs (NSAIDs) such as diclofenac and ketorolac, which also have an antispastic effect [3], whereas morphine, used at dosages that allow the patient an independent life with bearable side effects, is not able to abolish all types of nociceptive pain since cutaneous, neurogenic, and incident pain are poorly responsive to this drug [4, 5].

The timing of pain is another pain characteristic which has to be observed in order to understand how to dose therapy. Generally, for chronic pain a continuous therapy is mandatory with administration at fixed intervals. Nevertheless, in patients who experience sudden recrudescence of pain during the day, supplemental administration of drugs must be considered. These drugs must have a pharmacological profile with a rapid onset of action. Other pain syndromes are characterized by periods of remission of pain as, for example, cluster headache and arthritic cervico-brachial neuralgia in which pain treatment is limited only to the periods of occurrence of pain.

Many physicians still focus on pain intensity and consider this the only parameter for the definition of treatment. This may not always be correct, though, since pain intensity is only a quantitative and not a qualitative evaluation of pain. As mentioned above, the analgesic effect of drugs and other analgesic devices correlate with the qualitative characteristics of pain. Obviously, when a treatment is decided upon, the psychological-emotional effects on the patient must be considered. Sometimes, in fact, the beginning of a treatment which may impair the quality of life can have a negative influence on the psychological condition of a patient who is already psychologically debilitated. It is therefore necessary to analyze what effects the pain syndrome we have directed our attention to clinically may have on the patients. In this context, the varying different clinical experience reported in literature demonstrates how a patient's psychological behavior differs between acute and chronic pain conditions. Whereas anxiety in trying to identify the underlying disease prevails in acute pain, with chronic pain an attitude of weakness and suffering or a reaction of distress and anger evolves which compels the patient to search very intensely for a solution of his or her problem. This latter attitude is typical for patients suffering from neuropathic pain but it is not clear yet whether it is a consequence of a lacking pathological justification for the patient's often unbearable pain or whether it is the evolution of the disease itself interacting with the patient's normal psychological processes.

When defining guidelines for the management only those treatments which have been validated in the literature should be considered. This represents the main crucial point, since to date only a few pain treatments have demonstrated unequivocal and accepted clinical efficacy. Very frequently the validation of a certain treatment is based on the physician's own experience or on that of a single pain therapy center but, most importantly, has only been performed on a small number of patients without precise study protocols and with a high incidence of bias [6]. Here, the cost-benefit ratio of the different therapies in terms of pharmacoeconomy and patient safety must be considered.

Finally, the facility of each therapeutic procedure must be carefully evaluated, at least as regards the initial phases. Only in few pain therapy centers can all different types of therapy be performed. This is due to the availability of adequate devices and, therefore, to economic resources as well as to the presence of skilled physicians and nurses. The lack of interdisciplinary treatments may cause two types of inconveniences: first, deprive the patient of an effective treatment; second, abolish some effective analgesic techniques due to the lack of physicians able to perform them.

Guidelines for chronic malignant pain management

In the last 20 years the major World Health Organizations have focused their attention on defining and disseminating guidelines for malignant pain treatment which can be applied in every country in order to give each patient the chance to profit from an adequate pain treatment. Thus, a scale for the treatment of cancer pain was introduced by the World Health Organization (WHO) [7]. This treatment scale had the great advantage of helping physicians of any clinical discipline to approach cancer pain in an effective and rational manner. In fact, 70%-90% of the patients receive a sufficient pain relief. Nevertheless, the WHO scale only evaluates pain quantitatively without considering the qualitative component: pain intensity is the parameter that guides the choice of the therapy. The stronger the pain, the higher the potency of the drug or the more invasive the treatment chosen. This means that the patient often undergoes treatments which are not suitable for the type of pain he or she is experiencing before finding the most effective drug. It is, therefore, obvious that the type of pain must guide the therapeutic choice.

In general, cancer is caused by the infiltration of somatic and visceral structures. We are therefore confronted with continuous, sometimes intermittent, somatic and/or visceral pain for which the use of therapeutic devices listed on the first step of the WHO scale are justified: administration of the most effective NSAIDs for the specific type of pain, adjuvant drugs and weak opioids. But when pain assumes incidental characteristics or is neurogenic it might be useless to treat the patient with the sequence of drugs indicated by the WHO since the pain is poorly responsive to drugs available today. Even morphine only partially acts on these types of pain [4, 8], at least at dosages that permit the patient an adequate quality of life [9, 10]. It is therefore mandatory in these cases to offer the patient the possibility to decide for a neuroinvasive or neurolesive therapy. These are the only therapeutic options able to reduce all types of nociceptive pain. Neuroinvasive therapy in particular provides continuous and/or bolus administration of local anaesthetics, opioids, α2 agonists, competitive NMDA antagonists, cholinergic and other drugs into the epidural or subarachnoid space [11, 12]. In contrast, neurolesive therapies foresee the surgical interruption of the pain pathways at different levels, depending on the technique used. Today the neurolesive techniques most often performed are percutaneous cervical cordotomy and the DREZ lesion, which interrupt the pain pathways at the second neuron level [13]. The possibility of performing a percutaneous intervention and the lower incidence of side effects makes percutaneous cervical cordotomy the most widely used neuroablative technique, today [14].

The choice of neuroinvasive or neuroablative therapy is based on two completely different points of view. The choice of a neurolesive technique means a single medical procedure which is irreversible and therefore implies that the surgeon performing the procedure is able to guarantee a reliable result free of complications. This presupposes extensive experience in employing the technique. In contrast, deciding for a neuroinvasive technique means choosing a method where the physician's error is nearly always reversible and the patient can decide to interrupt the treatment at any time. Therefore, the medical procedure is a less dramatic decision.

Neuroinvasive therapy is indicated in patients who have no side prevalence of the pain, not even as regards the response to pharmacological therapy, those whose clinical condition is very poor, that is patients who have a reduced quality of life or are bedridden since these patients are more willing to accept an epidural catheter or an infusion pump and the side effects due to the method or the drug used.

In contrast, we believe that neurolesive therapy is preferable if unilateral pain is present or there is a clear side prevalence, if pain is incidental or neurogenic, if the patient's clinical condition is favorable and if life expectancy is good. For example, patients affected with Pancoast's syndrome or with cancer that causes other types of plexopathies are ideal candidates for early percutaneous cervical cordotomy. This way the percentage of patients who are pain free may reach 95% without any additional pharmacological therapy (personal data soon to be published).

A special situation is represented by the celiac pain which is typically present in pancreatic cancer: early performance of an alcoholic celiac plexus block is indicated [15, 16]. The neurolesive technique guarantees a complete pain relief up to death in 10%-24% of the patients as a single treatment and in 80%-90% of the patients if associated with other treatments [17]. Besides, analgesic drug consumption up to death and the incidence of drug-related adverse effects are lower [18, 19] and the patients' quality of life is improved [19].

Guidelines for chronic nonmalignant pain management

Nonmalignant chronic pain includes all those pain syndromes that do not originate from a neoplasm but which represent an enormous source of suffering for the patients. Patients who arrive at a pain therapy center mainly suffer from chronic nonmalignant pain, which is so intense that they are forced to reduce their social and working activity. Thus, it is useful to provide an adequate pain relief in order to reduce the social costs of the disease.

Yet, no ultimate pain treatments exist: there is no complete and permanent abolition of chronic nonmalignant pain. One can speak, therefore, about living with pain, or reducing pain, but this kind of impotence on the part of the physicians causes dissatisfaction and anger in the patient, which leads him or her to feel compelled to search for a personal solution, sometimes even suicide.

How should this type of pain be approached?

First of all, no false expectations of healing should be created. On the contrary, it is important to understand the psychological and emotional state of the patient and to interact with it. For this purpose, a constant and frequent contact between patient and physician might be useful so that the patient feels the presence of someone helping him. Moreover, therapy should be performed gradually so that the patient is more aware of the benefits, sometimes few, achieved by the administered drugs. Finally, the patient must be convinced to submit to the prescribed therapy constantly and regularly; there should be no intervals during the treatment.

Since there is no pharmacological nor neuroinvasive nor neurolesive means of treatment able to abolish all types of pain, a therapeutic diversification based on the characteristics of each pain syndrome can be observed.

One type of pain frequently seen in a specialized center is neuropathic pain. Examples are trigeminal neuralgia, atypical facial neuralgias, postherpetic neuralgia, phantom limb pain, and complex regional syndrome type I and II. For neuropathic pain the first-choice pharmacological treatment is anticonvulsant drugs [1] since they are the only ones that favorably interact with this type of pain. Tricyclic antidepressants in association with anticonvulsants [20, 21] as well as with α2 agonists [22] and TENS [23] may be useful.

Recently, three new anticonvulsants were used in clinical practice (gabapentin, vigabapentin, lamotrigine) which seem to offer better results than carbamazepine [24, 25] even if they seem not to reduce the incidence of side effects.

If the patient does not profit from the therapy with anticonvulsants, further therapeutic steps vary, depending on the presence or absence of a sympathetic component. If this component is present in a patient, regional intravenous sympathetic blocks with guanetidine [26] or bretylium [27], sympathetic blocks with local anaesthetic [28] or continuous epidural sympathetic blocks with local anaesthetic and clonidine [29] may be performed. In patients who have a positive response to any one of these blocks, alcoholic, surgical [30] or radiofrequency sympathectomy [31] is indicated. For patients who do not respond, the remaining therapeutic strategies are limited to the application of a spinal cord stimulator [32] or the subarachnoid administration of opioids or non-competitive NMDA antagonists [33].

Neuropathic pain however is still a controversial issue for two reasons. As many authors doubt the presence of a sympathetic component [34], and it is very difficult to develop guidelines for individual treatments on which all physicians and, primarily, patients agree.

In last years the idea of administering systemic, continuous opioids intravenously gained in importance even in patients suffering from neuropathic pain [35, 36]. With this therapeutic choice the physician is faced with the question of whether the administration of a drug which is believed to cause physical addiction and to alter the patient's health condition but which doesn't seem to have a specific action on nociceptive pain is indicated. The answer is not clear, yet. It seems that opioids are not addictive in patients with nonmalignant chronic pain nor do they affect the patient's health condition [37] but we still lack studies in a broad population of patients which could definitely convince those who disagree (maybe on principle) with this therapeutic strategy [38]. It is advisable to prescribe opioids only to those patients who did not benefit from any other means of therapy, in whom a short trial conducted in a hospital setting demonstrated adequate pain control and who have chosen spontaneously to undergo the treatment proposed by the family physician [37].

The guidelines for the treatment of chronic nociceptive pain are based on close cooperation among different medical disciplines such as pain therapy, orthopaedics, surgery, neurology, physiotherapy and pshichology. The physiotherapist is very important since the patients always tends to reduce physical activity especially in the painful part of the body and this may lead to an impairment in quality of life [39, 40].

The pharmacological approach considers the use of different types of drugs, not only analgesics. There is no doubt that NSAIDs' main role is to reduce many types of nociceptive pain but the need for prolonged use of these drugs may expose the patient to the risk of gastroenteric diseases. Therefore drugs such as paracetamol (acetaminophen) which do not have an anti-inflammatory action should be used which, moreover, is not always required [41].

The use of more than one NSAIDs simultaneously is absolutely useless; it is better to use different NSAIDs one after another until the most effective drug has been found.

For diseases such as arthritis, low back pain, muscular tension headache, or fibromyalgia the association of a muscular relaxant with other drugs may be useful since muscle contractions secondary to the posture of the patient are often present [40].

The use of corticosteroids for the treatment of chronic pain has not yet been accepted by all physicians. The only confirmed findings are, at least as regards diseases which cause chronic radicular pain, that the administration of corticosteroids via the subarachnoid route guarantees the patient a satisfactory pain relief with a variable time duration [42, 43].

Peripheral or central anaesthetic blocks do not seem to offer satisfactory results for the patient even if there is no doubt that a local anaesthetic temporarily causes the "interruption of sustained neural activity that produced and perpetuated the pain, relaxation of paraspinal muscle spasm, and resolution of accompanying reflex sympathetic dystrophy" [43, 44].

As for the use of opioids, one reference to what we previously said about neuropathic pain should be made. Of course, opioids would be indicated for nociceptive pain since they are able to control the type of pain much better even at dosages which do not expose the patient to important side effects. Nevertheless, further scientific studies in a broad patient population are needed before their use is accepted by the whole scientific community. Today, the so-called weak opioids are more frequently used. Codeine, in particular, which could be bought in pharmacies is safe at commonly used doses and taken by a large number of patients. Recently, tramadol was introduced on the European market, a drug with a selective agonist action on receptors of opioids which correlate to supraspinal analgesia – less so than morphine – but with a minor affinity to other receptors on which morphine usually acts [45]. Moreover, the analgesic action depends on its inhibitory action on norepinephrine and serotonin at the synapses, with an increased concentration of two neurotransmitters at the descending nervous pathway level where pain is modulated [46]. These pharmacodynamic characteristics and the low potency to induce action [47] make tramadol a possible, effective alternative to opioids in many patients suffering from chronic pain. In our experience, it should be administered in association with other nonopioid analgesic drugs.

Antidepressants play an important therapeutic role in many patients with nociceptive chronic pain. They have two effects: they modulate firstly the mood, which is nearly always changed by suffering, and, secondly, the pain, by the inhibition of serotonin and norepinephrine reuptake into the descending nervous pathways [48]. In fact, available data today do not demonstrate exactly the real efficacy of antidepressants in chronic pain management [20].

Finally, the patient may benefit from the use of so-called alternative methods. Techniques such as hypnosis [49], biofeedback therapy [50], and behavioral therapy [51] help perceive the presence of pain to a lesser extent. These should therefore be considered and signaled to each patient at any time during therapy.

References

1. Mc Quay HJ, Carroll D, Jadad AR, Wiffen P, Moore A (1995) Anticonvulsivant drugs for management of pain: a systematic review. Br Med J 311:1047-1052
2. Rosomoff HL, Papo I, Loeser JD, Bonica JJ (1990) Neurosurgical operations on the spinal cord. In: Bonica JJ (ed) The management of pain. Vol II. Lea and Febiger, Philadelphia, pp 2067-2081
3. Walfson AB, Yealy DM (1991) Oral indometacin for acute renal colic. Am J Emerg Med 9:16-19
4. Arner S, Arner B (1985) Differential effects of epidural morphine in the treatment of cancer-related pain. Acta Anaesthesiol Scand 29:32-36
5. Stein C (1997) Opioid treatment of chronic nonmalignant pain. Anesth Analg 84:912-914
6. Dickersin K (1990) The existence of publication bias and risk factors for its occurrence. JAMA 263:1385-1389
7. World Health Organization (1989) Cancer pain relief (2nd ed) World Health Organization, Geneva
8. Bruera E, MacMillan K, Hanson J, MacDonald RN (1989) The Edmonton staging system for cancer pain: preliminary report. Pain 37:203-209
9. Bruera E, Lawlor P (1997) Cancer pain management. Acta Anaesthesiol Scand 41:146-153
10. Hanks GW, Forbes K (1997) Opioid responsiveness. Acta Anaesthesiol Scand 41:154-158
11. Hogan Q, Haddox JD, Abram S, Weissman D, Taylor ML, Janjan N (1991) Epidural opiates and local anaesthetics for the management of pain. Pain 46:271-280
12. Lauretti GR, Lima ICPR (1996) The effects of intrathecal neostigmine on somatic and visceral pain: improvement by association with a peripheral anticholinergic. Anesth Analg 82:617-620

13   Ischia S, Gottin L (1996) Procedure neuroablative. In. Tiengo M, Benedetti C (eds) Fisiopatologia e terapia del dolore Masson, Milano, pp 473-484

14.   Ischia S, Gottin L, Polati E, Finco G, Zanoni L (1997) Role of neuroablative procedures for cancer pain management. December in New York· Current concepts in acute, chronic, and cancer pain management. New York, pp 229-231

15   Ischia S, Polati E, Finco G, Gottin L, Benedini B (1998) The role of neurolytic celiac plexus block in pancreatic cancer pain management. do we have the answer? Reg Anesth (in press)

16.   Lillemoe KD, Cameron JL, Kaufman HS, Yeo CJ, Pitt HA, Sauter PK (1993) Chemical splanchnicectomy in patients with unresectable pancreatic cancer. A prospective randomized trial Ann Surg 217:447-457

17.   Ischia S, Ischia A, Polati E, Finco G (1992) Three posterior percutaneous celiac plexus block techniques. A prospective, randomized study in 61 patients with pancreatic cancer pain. Anesthesiology 76:534-540

18   Mercadante S (1993) Celiac plexus block versus analgesics in pancreatic cancer pain Pain 52:187-192

19.   Polati E, Finco G, Gottin L, Bassi C, Pederzoli P, Ischia S (1998) Prospective randomized double blind trial of neurolytic coeliac plexus block in patients with pancreatic cancer. Br J Surg 85:199-201

20   McQuay HJ, Tramer M, Nye BA, Carroll D, Wiffen PJ, Moore RA (1996) A systematic review of antidepressants in neuropathic pain Pain 68.217-227

21.   Reig E, Vazquez de la Torre ML, del Pozo C (1996) New concepts for the treatment of neuropathic pain 7th International Symposium The Pain Clinic, Istanbul, pp 34-35

22.   Fusco BM, Alessandri M (1992) Analgesic effect of capsaicin in idiopathic trigeminal neuralgia Anesth Analg 74:375-377

23   Meyler WJ, de Jongste MJL, Rolf CAM (1994) Clinical evaluation of pain treatment with electrostimulation: a study on TENS in patients with different pain syndromes. Clin J Pain 10:22-27

24.   Tassinari CA (1998) Gabapentin: nuove acquisizioni e prospettive terapeutiche. Masson, Milano, pp 43-55

25.   Zakrzewska JM, Chaudhry Z, Nurmikko TJ, Patton DW, Mullens EL (1997) Lamotrigine (Lamictal) in refractory trigeminal neuralgia: results a double-blinded placebo controlled crossover trial. Pain 73:223-230

26.   Jadad AR, Carroll D, Glynn CJ, McQuay HJ (1995) Intravenous regional sympathetic blockade for pain relief in reflex sympathetic dystrophy: a systematic review and a randomized, double-blind crossover study J Pain Symptom Management 10·13-20

27.   Ford SR, Forest WH Jr, Eltherington L (1988) The treatment of RSD with intravenous regional bretylium. Anesthesiology 68:137-140

28.   Rowbotham MC (1995) Chronic pain: from theory to practical management. Neurology 45:S5-S10

29.   Yaksh TL, Progrel JW, Lee YW, Chaplan SR (1995) Reversal of nerve ligation-induced allodynia by spinal α2-adrenoreceptor agonists. J Pharmacol Exp Ther 272:207-214

30.   Herz DA, Looman JE, Ford RD, Gostine ML, Davis FN, VandenBerg WC (1993) Second thoracic sympathetic ganglionectomy in sympathetically maintained pain J Pain Sympt Manag 8:483-491

31   Rocco AG (1995) Radiofrequency lumbar sympatholysis. The evolution of a technique for managing sympathetically maintained pain. Reg Anesth 20:3-12

32.   North RB, Kidd DH, James C, Long DM (1993) Spinal cord stimulation for chronic intractable pain: experience over two decades. Neurosurgery 32 384-395

33.   Backonja M, Arndt G, Gombar KA, Check B, Zimmermann M (1994) Response

of chronic neuropathic pain syndromes to ketamine: a preliminary study. Pain 56:51-57

34. Cepeda MS (1995) Autonomic nervous system and pain. Curr Opin Anaesthesiol 8:450-454

35. Rowbotham MC, Reisner-Keller LA, Fields HL (1991) Both intravenous lidocaine and morphine reduce the pain of postherpetic neuralgia. Neurology 41:1024-1028

36. Jadad AR, Carroll D, Glynn CJ, Moore RA, McQuay HJ (1992) Morphine responsiveness of chronic pain: double blind randomised crossover study with patient controlled analgesia. Lancet 339:1367-1371

37 McQuay HJ (1997) Opioid use in chronic pain. Acta Anaesthesiol Scand 41:175-183

38. Schug SA, Large RG (1995) Opioids for chronic noncancer pain. (Clinical Updates) Pain 3:1-4

39. Twomey L, Taylor J (1995) Exercise and spinal manipulation in the treatment of low back pain. Spine 20:615-619

40. Deyo RA (1996) Drug therapy for back pain. Which drugs help which patients? Spine 21:2840-2850

41. Green LN, Winickoff RN (1992) Cost-conscious prescribing of non-steroidal anti-inflammatory drugs for adults with arthritis: a review and suggestions. Arch Intern Med 152:1995-2002

42. Castagnera L, Maurette P, Pointillart V, Vital JM, Erny P, Senegas J (1994) Long term results of cervical epidural steroid injection with and without morphine in chronic cervical radicular pain. Pain 58:239-243

43. Koes BW, Scholten RJPM, Mens JMA, Bouter LM (1995) Efficacy of epidural steroid injections for low-back pain and sciatica: a systematic review of randomized clinical trials. Pain 63:279-288

44. Benzon HT (1986) Epidural steroid injections for low back pain and lumbosacral radiculopathy. Pain 24:277-295

45. Vickers MD, O'Flaherty D, Szekely SM, Read M, Yoshizumi J (1992) Tramadol: pain relief by an opioid without depression of respiration. Anaesthesia 47:291-296

46. Raffa RB, Friderichs E, Reinman W, Shank RP, Codd EE, Vaught JL (1992) Opioid and nonopioid components independently contribute to the mechanism of action of tramadol, an 'atypical' opioid analgesic. J Pharmacol Exp Ther 260:275-285

47. Lee CR, McTavish D, Sorkin EM (1993) Tramadol. A preliminary review of its pharmacodynamic and pharmacokinetic properties, and therapeutic potential in acute and chronic pain states. Drugs 46.313-340

48. Botney M, Fields HL (1983) Amitriptyline potentiates morphine analgesia by direct action on the central nervous system. Ann Neurol 13:160-164

49 Barber J (1990) Hypnosis In: Bonica JJ (ed) The management of pain, vol 2. Lea and Febiger, Philadelphia, pp 1733-1741

50. Asfour SS, Khalil TM, Waly SM, Goldberg ML, Rosomoff RS, Rosomoff HL (1990) Biofeedback in back muscle strengthening. Spine 15:510-513

51. Turner JA, Clancy S (1988) Comparison of operant behavioral and cognitive-behavioral group treatment for chronic low back pain. J Consult Clin Psychol 56:261-266

Chapter 26

Terminal cancer illness: strategies and management

V.A. Paladini, B. Barbolan, L. Di Bello, A. Zamperoni

There is a relation between the way we live and the way we die. Each individual lives his or her life in a different way, with his/her own limits, disease, suffering and death. Each life is unique: the history of an individual with his/her family, socio-economic conditions, religion, spirituality, ethnic and racial background.

There is, therefore, a transcultural aspect and approach to the disease, to terminal therapy, to the last moments of life and the arrangements about how to deal with the body after death. Suffice it to recall the teachings of the Buddhist disciplines with their meditations on death and the hospice movement, which unlike euthanasia, aims at improving the quality of life of the patient and his/her family, giving meaning to the natural history of the individual, to life, to suffering and death. The social and economic organisational capacity of a country and the medical staff's knowledge of palliative care play a fundamental role in relation to the stande taken by the public on extreme measures such as euthanasia and assisted suicide. Probably, the scant knowledge on how to control symptoms, which are devastating for the patient, for the care-givers and family, pushes people towards these extreme choices [1]. A survey based on a questionnaire carried out on two sample groups of Japanese and Japanese-American physicians showed that the Japanese are much more oriented towards the use of therapeutic measures (transfusions, vasopressors and total parenteral nutrition) in terminally ill cancer patients for whom these measures are not effective. The patients of this group of physicians, although aware of their disease, often ask that measures not exclusively targeted at relieving symptoms be continued; frequently, physicians carry on these therapeutic measures to comply with the family's requests [2]. Social and economic factors leading to a lack of home care for the terminally ill patients play a decisive role in Japan [3]. Between the two extremes, i.e. the discontinuation of all therapies and therapeutic perseverance, there is the possibility of an ethical line pursuing the objective of the best possible quality of life and centred on the respect of the person as a whole [4]. In Italy, euthanasia is not legal. According to article 35 of the new code of medical deontology "Even if the patient asks for this, the physician is not to carry out treatments aiming at maiming the patient's psychic and physical integrity or making his/her life shorter or causing death"; on the other hand, according to article 36, the physician is recognised the faculty, "(...) in case of a disease with a surely unfavourable prognosis (...) at a terminal stage.." to "(...) confine his/her own work, if this is the patient's specific wish, to moral assistance and to a pain relieving therapy in order to spare the patient unnecessary pain, (...) while preserving the quality of life as much as possible".

The main principles discussed in palliative care are the following: breaking the bad news, developing a treatment plan and a death plan, and considering the discontinuation of artificial nutrition. During the last months or days of life, the path to follow is not easy but there is still a lot that can be done. This is a stage characterised by the crisis of the patient's life and the definition of the care-givers' objective of improving the patient's quality of life and giving support to his/her family. Patients carry with themselves their own history, with their own successes, failures, experiences, and illnesses. This is an extremely delicate stage: it means going back to the very beginning. This is why they deserve attention, tact and reflection; emotions are replaced by delicate feelings where patients become like children in need of care; this is the crucial time of life when knots loosen and life flows. Still, this stage deserves great attention because physical pain, or total pain rather, accompanies the patient's very existence. If the patient's family has not suffered a previous death, which is usually a very negative event causing family members to give up hope and regard their ill relative as if he/she were already dead, there is a magnification of emotions and affections, and everything is lived gradually, day by day. If the relationship between the patient and his/her family has never been good, this may be the time when their relationship can improve, so that any sense of guilt after the patient's death can be dispelled. Family members feel as if they are crushed by a load and therefore need emotional support, guidance, encouragement and help in decision-making.

This issue concerns strategies cancer including a creative aspect of how to approach a terminally ill cancer patient; sometimes carers learn to orient some of their actions towards patients and their families in a creative way, using unexpected resources, comparable to a work of art.

The discussion involves topics such as guidelines, current controversies, and pain management methods as well as new drugs, new acquisitions in terms of mechanisms of action, the accompanying symptoms [5, 6], hydration and nutrition, haemorrhage and transfusion, and convulsions. We shall also deal with the delicate psychotherapeutic support to patients and their families during the terminal stage of their illness. Topics include the trials performed on pain, notably the opioid doses used in North America and Europe, as well as the rotation and titration of the same.

With regard to hydration, nutrition and transfusion there are no guidelines; we shall report our opinion as well as the data of the literature.

Pain and its treatment: guidelines and controversial points

Pain evaluation takes into account aetiology and pathophysiologic mechanisms. A recent prospective study examined 2 266 patients referred to the pain service of a German university hospital. Of these patients 98% suffered pain, in 77%

very strong or severe; 4 542 painful syndromes were identified (39% with two sites, 31% with three or more sites and 30% with one site). The lumbar, abdominal, chest, lower limb, cervical regions and the head were most frequently involved.

Intestinal and airway cancer most frequently caused pain in the primary site, whereas bone pain was more frequent in breast, airway and genitourinary cancer. Pain of the soft tissues and neuropathic pain were diagnosed in patients with cancer of the head or neck; the incidence of visceral pain was greater in cancer of the gastrointestinal tract. In most cases, pain was continuous, fluctuating and non-fluctuating: in 12% of the cases it was associated with paroxysms; in 17% it had been present for more than 6 months, in 44% from 1 to 6 months, and in 36% for less than a month [7].

Attention should be paid to incident pain, which is severe and short and may recur suddenly many times over the day, triggered by movements or positions, micturition or defecation, or cough. It tends to decrease by remaining still. A distinction has to be made between incidental pain and breakthrough pain, a type of incidental pain which is difficult to predict and treat, as it is not correlated to triggering factors. Incidental pain can be controlled by locoregional techniques, such as epidural infusion of local anaesthetics and opioids; ropivacaine does not lead to a motor block and is, therefore, the local anaesthetic of choice since it makes ambulation possible. If pain is qualitatively different, adjuvant drugs will have to be given too. For the treatment of breakthrough pain, rapid-release opioids are indicated [8].

From a clinical point of view, pain can also be classified as responsive, semi-responsive or resistant to opioids. Resistance can be due to the use of low doses or to poor drug absorption. Pain of the soft tissue due to muscular infiltration, bone metastases, neuropathic pain, and pain due to increased endocranial pressure and incidental pain can present a limited response to opioids, while pain due to muscle spasm, secondary to bone metastases, is the only really opioid-resistant form [9]. All of this is controversial.

Processes modifying sensitivity to exogenous opioids include the following: loss of receptors following peripheral axonotmesis, increased activity of anti-opioid substances, such as cholecystokinins and adenosine, or the development of central mechanisms reducing responsiveness to opioids [10, 11].

The effectiveness of opioids in neuropathic pain is controversial: some studies showed a limited pain reduction with high opioid doses. Indicated drugs include antidepressants, anticonvulsants, ketamine, some local anaesthetics and the antagonists of N-Nethyl-D-Aspartate (NMDA) receptors.

Drug therapy plays a fundamental role in the treatment of cancer pain and can be associated with physiotherapeutic, psychotherapeutic, surgical, radiotherapeutic, chemotherapeutic, hormone-therapeutic and neuroablative treatment.

The well-known World Health Organisation (WHO) ladder proposes a pharmacological approach by steps, taking into account pain intensity; the subdivision between weak and strong opioids is conventional and does not respond to strictly clinical criteria: for instance, oxycodone, regarded by some as a medium-strength opioid, has turned out to be effective in the treatment of severe pain as well. A study carried out between 1983 and 1992 considered 2 118 cancer patients treated according to the WHO ladder: the route of administration during the days of treatment was enteral in 82% of the cases and parenteral in 9%; non-opioid analgesics (NOA) were used on 11% of the days of treatment, strong opioids on 49%, and weak opioids on 31%; on 37% of the days coanalgesics were associated, in 15% antidepressants, in 13% anticonvulsants and in 13% corticosteroids. This shows the clear prevalence of the non-invasive route in the pharmacological treatment of cancer pain [12]. In our retrospective study of 1986, 227 cancer patients were treated: 89% of them with opioids and adjuvant drugs and 71% with opioids. The mean survival rate was 91.8 days, hospital deaths accounted for 96% [13]. In the treatment of cancer pain the most updated aspects are the recently introduced analgesics, the new routes of administration and new formulations. The present trends concerning opioids should be recalled, with special attention to their toxicity and rotation. In the pharmacological field there are tendencies contrary to those of the past and controversies on the use of NOAs and their possible rotation with the aim of reducing adverse effects.

More prospective and short-term trials have been conducted than retrospective ones on pain; clinical practice does not match research and vice versa.

Clinical experience evaluates the risks and benefits of a method or a drug and supplements or, rather, verifies the knowledge acquired by controlled clinical studies. Research and practice only communicate with great difficulty and slowly; the guidelines are sometimes neglected and not complied with although they should transmit to each physician scientific information after it has been selected and critically interpreted in a simple form and in terms of recommendations of clinical conduct. The difficulty and the limits of the prospective studies concern the ethical aspects of pain and its treatment and the evaluation of the risks and benefits over a vast population; often, the population at risk is excluded from the studies. Retrospective studies provide information about the practical application underlining the interindividual difference: how drugs are used in different settings; and how many prescriptions are in line with the indications; and how to interpret the remarkable range of behaviours. In the case of well-known drugs, widely used among the general population, adverse effects are known; for new drugs this information is not very accurate. One example concerns NOAs, which are known for their analgesic and anti-inflammatory efficacy; however, they have not been studied as regards approved clinical indications or the different dosages.

With regard to the individualised therapy, some pharmacokinetic elements should be clarified. The main therapeutic effect and the adverse effects depend on the drug concentration in blood, described as "blood concentration curve". In the curve, attention should be paid to the maximum concentration peak, the time of permanence in the therapeutic window and the values outside that window. From the blood, the drug goes to the tissues where it carries out its specific dynamics until it reaches steady state. When the blood goes through the liver, the exchange takes place with the hepatocytes performing the metabolic function. The lower the metabolic activity, the higher the amount of drug that, after each liver passage, goes back to the tissues; more administrations induce accumulation and increase the analgesic effect as well as any unwanted effects. The risk is to exceed the therapeutic window and to reach toxic or even lethal concentrations. The semi-elimination time (t/2), or half-life, indicates the time required for the concentration to be halved and provides us with useful information on drug behaviour. Some factors can protract the elimination time; they are related to the excretory metabolic activity of the liver and the kidney. The longer the time interval between adminstrations, the lower the accumulation. A shorter semi-elimination time is matched by a lower accumulation (with equal intervals between dosages). By halving both the time interval between doses and the dose itself, a better stabilisation of the blood concentration can be achieved, thereby reducing oscillation (this can be a useful posologic tool to improve efficacy or to obtain a reduction in unwanted effects). It is, therefore, important for the physician to consider, before changing a drug, whether its administration is correct and suitable for the patient and whether blood concentration is optimal and within the therapeutic window. For morphine there is no one standard effective dose; analgesia and side effects must be individualised and monitored, especially during the pharmacological adjustment phase. In the following paragraphs, dose titration will also be discussed. Unlike weak opioids, the dosage can be continuously increased to the maximum tolerated dose, since for strong opioids such as morphine, hydromorphone and methadone, there is no ceiling effect and the dose-response ratio is linear. The ceiling effect – above which a dosage increment does not increase analgesia – and the therapeutic window occur with some antidepressants and buprenorphine.

Old and new opioids

Trials carried out in North America and Europe have shown that opioid doses are very different. The aetiopathogenesis, the initial and final doses of the drug, treatment duration, and pharmacological associations are seldom reported. The difference can be especially observed between prospective and retrospective studies as well as between North America and Europe. Little has been written on their analgesic efficacy, which is taken for granted, and much more about side effects. In Europe the mean doses/day of oral morphine are between 52 mg (Minotti 1997) and 108 mg (Boureau 1992), while in North America the mean doses/day, always orally, range between 87 (Warfield 1991) and 2 415 mg (Lichtblau, 1996); the mean dosage of i.m. or i.v. morphine per day is between 100 mg and 35 000 mg (3% of patients) (Coyle 1989). With regard to the opioid rotation from morphine to methadone, again orally, the mean morphine consumption/day is 1 165 mg, the range 85-24 027 (Lawlor 1998).

Lawlor's retrospective study concerns a sample of 14 patients for whom Edmonton's staging is the prognostic index for analgesia in cancer pain: stage 1 (good prognosis), stage 2 (intermediate prognosis), and stage 3 (poor prognosis; patients with neuropathic pain, incidental pain, tolerance, psychological problems, alcohol or drug abuse). The study and the rotation occur because of poor analgesia and toxic side effects. Morphine is rotated with methadone and methadone with morphine. The mean pre-rotation dose/day for morphine is 1 165 mg while the methadone dose is 60 mg. The authors conclude that the correlation between the morphine dosage before rotation and the morphine-methadone ratio dose shows a high positive correlation. This suggests great caution ın the morphine-methadone rotation to confirm the underestimated potency and toxicity of the latter, which is potentially lethal, so much so as to suggest a revision of the equianalgesıc conversion tables.

Opioid analgesics can be classified according to different criteria:
— in terms of analgesic potency, they can be divided into weak and strong;
— in terms of action on the receptor into agonists, antagonists, partial agonists and agonist-antagonistand;
— in terms of origin into natural, semi-synthetic and synthetic.

Many authors include oxycodone among the weak opioids, although it is effective even in severe pain. Buprenorphine is regarded as a weak opioid for the presence of a ceiling effect; it has greater affinity for the receptor than the pure agonist and can replace it in the receptor site; if administered alone, it has an agonist effect.

The administration routes are: oral, buccal, sublingual (buprenorphine), rectal (morphine, oxymorphone and hydromorphone), transdermal (fentanyl), intranasal (butorphanol), oral transmucosal (fentanyl in breakthrough pain under study), subcutaneous, intravenous, epidural, intrathecal and cerebral intraventricular (Table 1).

The oral route for opioids, NOAs and adjuvant medications is the first choice, when possible. The opioid dose has to be "titred", taking into consideration the progress of the disease and the onset of tolerance. Additional doses with rapid-release formulations are to be envisaged if breakthrough pain develops. Considering the plasma steady-state of morphine, the total morphine dosage should be increased by 50%-100% every 24 h in patients with uncontrolled severe pain. The increase of the daily opioid dosage is by 25%-50% in uncontrolled moderate pain to reduce the risk of overdose. The opioid dose should be reduced by 25%-50% in patients with side effects and in patients not needing additional doses for breakthrough pain [14]. Switching to another route of administration or other opioids requires the use of conversion tables. In case of tolerance, another opioid can be administered, with doses equal to 50%-75% of the equianalgesic dose, because cross-tolerance is incomplete. The painful syndrome must always undergo a second assessment before switching to another opioid. If analgesia is insufficient or if it is impossible to use the oral route of administration, an alternative route will be needed, giving priority to the noninvasive, rectal or transdermal routes, and as an alternative the subcutaneous or the intravenous route. Spinal administration through a catheter with a reservoir or a pump and neuroablation techniques should be reserved for selected cases.

Among the weak opioids, tramadol and codeine deserve to be mentioned.

Tramadol acts selectively on the μ receptor, inhibits noradrenaline re-uptake and increases the intrasynaptic serotonin concentration [15]. Protein bonding is low (20%), metabolism is hepatic, and elimination mainly occurs through the kidneys, with a 5- to 7-h half-life. Tramadol posology is to be adjusted to the intensity of pain and individual sensitivity: the daily 400 mg dose should not normally be exceeded. As in the case of other opioids, after protracted administration, sweating, giddiness, nausea, vomit, dry mouth, sleepiness and obnubilation have been reported. In the Italian Information Bulletin on Drugs of February 1998, cases of convulsions were described "the incidence of which increases at doses higher than the recommended ones; however, cases were also reported inside the therapeutic interval. Tramadol administration can increase the risk of convulsions in patients taking tricyclic anti-depressants, inhibitors of serotonin re-uptake, MAO inhibitors, neuroleptics, other drugs reducing the convulsive threshold". In case of overdose, naloxone is regarded as the treatment of choice. "Adverse reactions have been reported, classifiable as correlated to the development of addiction, in patients with a present or remote clinical history of opiate abuse or addiction. Tramadol, therefore, should not be used in opiate addicted patients or in patients that have recently been taking high opiate doses, even if for therapeutical purposes, since they can develop withdrawal symptoms typical of the other opiate" [16]. In cancer pain, tramadol is a drug on the second step of the WHO ladder. According to a study, tramadol has been the drug of choice for long-term treatment in moderate and severe cancer pain, because of the relation between analgesic efficacy and side effects [17].

Codeine is one of the most outstanding drugs of the second step. The latest commercial preparations, in effervescent tablets, contain codeine and paracetamol: the association gives rise to a greater and long-lasting analgesic effect than its individual components. Effervescence allows the immediate solubilisation of active substances. The contact of carbon dioxide with the walls of the digestive tract induces a reactive treatment of blood circulation, accelerating drug extraction from the intestinal content. The analysis of plasma paracetamol concentrations shows, at equal doses, that the maximum concentration is achieved faster and that the effervescent form has a greater bioavailability than the anhydrous form. The solubilisation of active substances favours the scattering of the active ingredient in the gastric environment, thereby preventing any risks of ulceration. According to our experience, in patients treated with codeine until their death, there was no onset of tolerance.

Morphine, together with fentanyl, is the most used strong opioid in cancer pain. Its bioavailability, orally, ranges between 35% and 75% following the metabolism of the first liver passage. Kidneys also play an important role in metabolism. The bonding with plasma protein is weak: 35% with albumin and 6% with γ-globulins. A limited amount goes beyond the hemato-encephalic barrier and through the placental barrier and is found in maternal milk. Potentially, the dosage can be increased indefinitely to obtain the desired level of analgesia, because in the case of morphine there is no ceiling effect manifesting itself through

Table 1. Administration routes of opioids. (Modified from [73])

	Route	Equianalgesic Dose (mg)	Duration (h)	Plasma half-life (h)	Comments
Opioids agonists					
• Morphine	IM	10	4-6	2-3.5	Standard for comparison; also available in slow-release tablets
	PO	60	4-7		
• Codeine	IM	130**	4-6	3	Biotransformed to morphine
	PO	200**	4-6		
• Oxycodone	IM	15	3-5	–	Short acting; available alone or as 5-mg dose in combination with aspirin and acetaminophen
	PO	30	4-5		
• Heroin	IM	5	4-5	0.5	Illegal in U.S.: high solubility for parenteral administration
	PO	60	4-6		
• Levorphanol	IM	2	4-7	12-16	Good oral potency, requires careful titration in initial dosing because of drug accumulation
	PO	4			
• Hydromorphone	IM	1.5	4-5	2-3	Available in high-potency injectable form (10 mg/ml) for cachectic patients and as rectal suppositories; more soluble than morphine
	PO	7.5	4-6		
• Oxymorphone	IM	1	4-6	2-3	Available in parenteral and rectal-suppository forms only
	PR	10	4-6		
• Meperidine	IM	75	4-5	3-4	Contraindicated in patients with renal disease; accumulation of active toxic metabolite normeperidine produces CNS excitation
	PO	300**	4-6	12-16	
• Methadone	IM	10		15-30	Good oral potency; requires careful titration of the initial dose to avoid drug accumulation
	PO	20			

(cont.)

Table 1. (cont.)

	Route	Equianalgesic Dose (mg)[*]	Duration (h)	Plasma half-life (h)	Comments
Mixed agonist-antagonist opioids					
• Pentazocine	IM	60	4-6	2-3	Limited use for psychotomimetic effects
	PO	180[**]	4-7		
• Nalbuphine	IM	10	4-6	5	Not available orally; less severe psychotomimetic effects than pentazocine; may precipitate withdrawal in physically dependent patients
	PO	–			
• Butorphanol	IM	2	4-6	2.5-3.5	Not available orally; produces psychotomimetic effects; may precipitate withdrawal in physically dependent patients
	PO	–			
Partial agonist					
• Buprenorphine	IM	0.4	4-6	?	Not available in U.S.: no psychotomimetic effects; may precipitate withdrawal in tolerant patients
	SL	0.8	5-6		

IM, intramuscular; *PO*, oral; *PR*, rectal; *SL*, sublingual

[*] Based on single-dose studies in which an intramuscular dose of each drug listed was compared with morphine to establish the relative potency. Oral doses are those recommended when changing from a parenteral to an oral route. For patients without prior narcotic exposure, the recommended oral starting dose is 30 mg for morphine, 5 mg for methadone, 2 mg for levorphanol, and 4 mg for hydromorphone

[**] The recommended starting doses for these drugs are listed in Table 5

partial agonists. Opioids have favourable effects on pain, but also cause adverse effects. The impairment of cognitive functions in long-term therapies is the consequence of very high dosage neurotoxicity.

Morphine neurotoxicity ıs related to the metabolic processes mainly taking place in the liver, to a lesser extent in the kidneys and in the brain, with the formation of morphine-3-glucuronide (M3G) and morphine-6-glucuronide (M6G). M6G is a selective agonist for μ and δ receptors with a potency 45 times greater than that of morphine and plays an important role in the mechanisms of morphine toxicity, while M3G has a low receptor affinity and has shown to have no analgesic action. High M6G levels in the cerebrospinal fluid, following long-term therapy with morphine, are probably responsible for the greater analgesia as against that obtained after a single administration. Penetration of M6G inside the central nervous system is limited by its high hydrophilicity. Metabolites are excreted with urine and all forms of kidney failure, even the mild forms in elderly patients, can lead to an accumulation of the same. This applies in particular to M6G, where blood concentration can exceed those of morphine, thereby allowing the drug to pass through the hemato-encephalic barrier because of a mass action with a protracted analgesic effect and risk of neurotoxicity [18]. The protracted use of opioids at very high doses can cause important cognitive deficits, psychomotor agitation, hallucinations, nausea and vomiting; important convulsive episodes, characterised by multifocal myoclonias, have been observed. In these cases, opioid rotation has been proposed. In a study carried out at the Edmonton General Hospital in 191 patients under protracted therapy with opioids showing neurotoxic symptoms, 80 patients were subjected to pharmacological rotation with two or three types of opioids with an improvement of symptoms in 73% of cases [19]. For drug rotation, hydromorphone, oxycodone, transdermal fentanyl and sublingual buprenorphine are indicated at equianalgesic doses. Some authors even suggest methadone.

Rapid-release morphine is available in tablets, water solution and syrup. The solubility limit is 30-40 mg/ml. Peak plasma concentrations are reached in 1 h and their action lasts for about 4 h. Advantages include low cost, good tolerability and efficacy with wide therapeutic range and low toxicity risks. Rapid-release morphine is also used in the treatment of incident pain and breakthrough pain, at doses equivalent to or equal to 50% of that administered every 4 h. This formulation is useful in the cases in which, in the absence of previous therapies, the ideal dosage of morphine is to be determined in view of starting the rapid-release formulation.

The titration of the daily dose of morphine is carried out by administering rapid-release morphine at 4-h intervals; if incidental pain sets in, the patient can take an additional dose equal to the previous doses. After a few days the effective daily dose for that patient can be calculated by evaluating the mean daily dose taken. There is no standard dose; the dosage is always individualised. Usually to begin with, a low 5- to 10-mg dose is administered every 4 h.

Slow-release morphine tablets (SRMT), made up of two phases – an external hydrophilic one and an internal lipophilic one – allows the release of the active ingredient progressively and gradually, avoiding plasma peaks. The administration is scheduled every 12 h. The plasma peak is reached in 2-4 h and tends to remain unchanged until the beginning of the seventh to eighth hour. One of our studies of 1990, concerning 13 cancer patients, evaluated the kinetics of slow-release morphine at a 30 mg dose twice a day for 5 days, while monitoring the VAS and morphine blood concentration on the fifth day. Although observing a progressive VAS reduction in the first 6 h concomitantly with the increase of plasma morphine concentrations, a linear correlation between VAS and morphine levels was not found. Analgesic efficacy peaked in the fourth hour. Its effect gradually decreased from the fourth to the sixth hour, subsequently dropping more markedly. Three patients, two with jaundice and one with kidney failure, were excluded from the study since they showed considerable bradypnoea and sleepiness; they were treated with naloxone. Blood concentrations were greater than 100 µg/ml [20].

In addition to this, there are the sustained-release morphine gelatinous capsules containing microgranules with a water-proof polymer coating. The aim is to obtain stable and constant plasma morphine levels: in fact, while the plasma peak of oral morphine in syrup or solution is reached in 30-90 min and then rapidly declines, its release with the new formulation is controlled by the polymer coating and the absorption phase is longer, although the metabolism and the excretion phases remain unchanged. The content of the gelatinous capsules, administered every 24 or 12 h to patients with swallowing difficulties, can be mixed with food, and administration can be performed through a nasogastric cannula. For patients who have never taken opioids, the initial dose is 40 mg every 24 h or 20 mg every 12 h [21-23].

In a double-blind randomised study, the administration of sustained-release morphine in microgranules every 12 h, was compared with the administration of morphine sulphate solution every 4 h, in 24 patients with moderate or severe cancer pain. During the study, the morphine sulphate dose was titred to obtain the optimal analgesic effect. Pain intensity was evaluated by VAS for 7 days. The results of the two formulations on pain control did not show statistically significant differences, with the same incidence and severity as the side effects.

The subcutaneous administration of morphine is indicated if the patient vomits and in the terminal phases. It is more convenient than the intravenous route and can also be performed at home. The morphine dose to be administered subcutaneously is limited by its solubility; an excessive volume of infused fluid leads to a risk of accumulation in the infusion site. The speed of infusion is 1-2 ml/h; morphine subcutaneous infusion is compatible with other drugs such as metoclopramide, haloperidol, midazolam, while it is not compatible with chlorpromazine, phenytoin and diazepam. Subcutaneous infusion is contraindicated in the presence of generalised oedema, rashes, local pain or sterile abscesses, if there are haemocoagulation disorders or poor peripheral vascularisation.

Intravenous administration of morphine is the best choice for the control of acute-onset severe pain and/or in the terminal stages.

There are no indications for the intramuscular administration of morphine, since the subcutaneous route is as effective and less painful.

The rectal route can be used as an alternative to the oral one, although absorption is slower; spinal administration is indicated in selected case of severe and diffuse pain and in visceral pain. The latter is administered every 6-12 h or in continuous infusion, epidurally at a dose equal to 20% of the systemic 24 h dose and subarachnoidally at a 2% dose.

Morphine has been administered surgically by the cerebral intraventricular route in cases of untreatable severe pain in the terminal stages. It has also been administered by a catheter introduced in the cervical subarachnoid space, pushed up to the *foramen magnum* or in the posterior cranial fossa [24].

The buccal route requires biconvex tablets to be introduced between the gingival mucosa and the upper lip; absorption depends on the extension of the contact surface between the tablet and the mucosa as well as on the amount of saliva [25].

Morphine has also been used by nasal aerosol, at a dose of 5 mg in 5 ml of physiologic solution, with a 6-8 h analgesia, and by absorption through the ganglion sphenopalatinum by means of a nasal tampon, soaked in morphine diluted with distilled water [26]. Morphine can be injected intra-articularly, into the knee, or perinervously in the periphery [27].

A case report has recently studied the analgesic efficacy of morphine hydrogel at 0.08% topically in neoplastic ulcerations, assuming that the septic state and the cytokine activation would reduce the opioid response systemically [28].

Fentanyl is a synthetic opioid with a short-lasting analgesic action and a potency 75-125 times that of morphine. The low molecular weight, high potency and liposolubility of fentanyl indicate this drug for the transdermal therapeutic system (TTS) which was introduced in the past few years. This system releases the drug within a constant range comprised between 25 and 100 µg/h. Available for clinical administration for the first time in the USA in 1991 and, later, in 1994 in the Russia, fentanyl TTS is currently used in Europe for cancer pain. A patch is applied at concentrations of 25, 50, 75, 100 µg/h at 72 h intervals. Studies on its pharmacokinetics by Portenoy et al. [29] showed that, after the first application, stable blood concentrations of fentanyl are reached from the 15th-24th hour, with a mean serum concentration of 2.15 ng/ml and a 21 h half-life. Similarly, other authors [30-32] have observed that blood concentrations stabilise in the last hours of the first application of fentanyl TTS with a half-life between 16 and 25 h. About 50% of the total dose is absorbed within 24 h, while more than 80% is absorbed before 48 h. By titring fentanyl, after removing the transdermal system, its half-life is longer than via other routes because of its absorption from cutaneous deposits. The individual variability in serum concentrations reflects the combinations of the individual differences in the kinetics of elimination and transdermal absorption [29]. Korte et al. [33] studied the analgesic efficacy of fentanyl TTS in relation to the currently recommended doses: in a group of 39 patients with poorly controlled or uncontrolled cancer pain VAS (Visual Analogue Scale) was evaluated before beginning the therapy and in the following days three times a day for 28 days, by titring fentanyl on a daily basis. A significant reduction in pain symptoms appeared after 24 h with an effective analgesia within 48 h and an increment of the initial dose between the first and the fourth week. No side effect was so severe as to require discontinuation of the treatment.

A personal experience on fentanyl TTS in cancer pain, in the terminal stage

We studied a sample of 29 patients, hospitalised with advanced cancer and treated with fentanyl TTS, 20 males (68.9%) and nine females (31%), whose average age was 64.2±11.2 SD (range 45-84).

Patients presented with a neoplastic pathology with the following proportions: oral cavity cancer in ten patiens (34.4%); gastroenteric cancer in eight patients (27.6%); genitourinary cancer in four patients (13.8%); breast cancer in three patients (10.3%); lung cancer in two patients (6.9%); prostate cancer in one patient (3.4%); and probable osteosarcoma in one patient (3.4%). The therapy included: bland opioids (tramadol, codeine) and nonsteroidal anti-inflammatory drugs (NSAIDs) in five patients (17.2%); strong opioids (temgesic, morphine) in four patients (13.8%); NSAIDs in three patients (10.3%); NSAIDs and antidepressants in three patients (10.3%); major opioids and NSAIDs in three patients (10.3%); major opioids, minor opioids and NSAIDs in three patients (10.3%); minor opioids, NSAIDs and antidepressants in two patients (6.9%); minor opioids in one patient (3.4%); major opioids, NSAIDs and antidepressants in one patient (3.4%); minor opioids and antidepressants in one patient (3.4%); not defined in two patients (6.9%); and absent in one patient (3.4%).

Initial VAS, before the treatment, had a median value of 90 (range 50-100), (Table 2). On the second day, VAS had a median value of between 0 and 30 (range 0-100): in 15 patients (51.7%) VAS was 0; in the remaining 14 patients

Table 2. Conversion from oral morphine to transdermal fentanyl with the ratio of 100:1. (Modified from [91])

Oral morphine (mg/day)	Fentanyl TTS (mg/day)	Fentanyl TTS (µg/h)
30-90	0.6	25
91-150	1.2	50
151-210	1.8	75
211-270	2.4	100
271-330	3.0	125
331-390	3.6	150
391-450	4.2	175
451-510	4.8	200
511-570	5.4	225
571-630	6 0	250
631-690	6 6	275
690-750	7.2	300

TTS, transdermal therapeutic system

(48.2%) VAS was between 30 and 100. On the tenth day, the median VAS value was 0 (range 0-50): VAS was 0 in 20 patients (68.9%) and in the remaining nine (31%) it ranged between 20 and 50.

In addition to fentanyl TTS, all patients received induction with oral or parenteral morphine for 24 h. All patients were treated with anti-inflammatory drugs, antidepressants and some of them even with anti-convulsants. The initial dose of fentanyl TTS used on the sample was: 25 µg/h in five patients (17%), 50 µg/h in 19 patients (64.6%), and 75 µg/h in five patients (17%).

The final dose of fentanyl TTS of the 15 patients who died within 10 days (range 1-10 days) was 25 µg/h in four patients (26.6%), 50 µg/h in eight patients (53.3%), and 75 µg/h in three patients (20%). The final dose of fentanyl TTS of 14 patients, who died after the tenth day (range 15-204 days), was: 25 µg/h in one patient (7.1%), 50 µg/h in ten patients (71.4%), 75 µg/h in one patient (7.1%), and 100 µg/h in two patients (14.2%). The duration of the treatment of the sample [29], expressed in days, was a mean of 18.9±38.4 days (range 1-204).

With regard to side effects, constipation was not significant and, when it was, it concerned patients with subocclusive states due to gastrointestinal cancer. Two patients (6.8%) developed confusion and hallucinations: the first patient was a 71-year-old woman with pancreatic cancer, as of the eighth day of administration of 50 µg/h. It was sufficient to reduce the dose to 25 µg/h and administer bromazepam at low doses "as needed" to eliminate both confusion and hallucinations. The second patient, an 81-year-old woman with ovarian cancer metastasised in the lungs and bones, presented with confusion on the tenth day which was also in her medical history following spinal anaesthesia with local anaesthetic and fentanyl. These symptoms disappeared by reducing the fentanyl dose from 50 to 25 µg/h.

During hospitalisation, 15 patients died (51.7%), the remaining 14 patients (48.2%) were discharged and treated at home with morphine, according to the conversion table. At present, of the 14 patients, four patients are alive (13.8%).

In conclusion, in our sample of terminally ill patients, fentanyl TTS proved to have good control of pain as of the second day, with an increment of efficacy on the tenth day (Table 3). Side effects were mild and controllable.

Recently, studies have been carried out on the therapeutic action of intravenous fentanyl in neuropathic pain, traditionally described as refractory to opioids. Dellemijn and Vanneste [34] used a double-blind study, administering fentanyl, diazepam and saline solution in 53 patients with neuropathic pain of different aetiology. The data show that fentanyl is superior to both diazepam and placebo, since it plays a selective role, not correlated to the effects on the patient's mood.

Hydromorphone, a strong opioid and a receptor agonist of semi-synthetic origin, is the traditional alternative to morphine in the case of onset of neurotoxic symptoms. It comes in a controlled-release formulation to be administered every 12 h. Its analgesic efficacy appears to overlapping with that of morphine [35].

Table 3. Fentanyl TTS in cancer pain: VAS, doses and duration of treatment

Total patients	29
Age (years)	Average 64.2±SD 11.2 (range 45-84)
VAS before treatment	Median 90 (range 50-100)
VAS 2nd day	Median 0-30 (range 0-100)
VAS 10th day	Median 0 (range 0-50)
Initial dose: fentanyl	25 μg/h: 5 pts (17%); 50 μg/h: 19 pts (64.6%); 75 μg/h: 5 pts (17%)
Final dose: fentanyl 15 pts within 10 days	25 μg/h: 4 pts (26%); 50 μg/h: 8 pts (53.3%); 75 μg/h: 3 pts (20%)
Final dose: fentanyl 14 pts after 10 days	25 μg/h: 1 pts (7.1%); 50 μg/h: 10 pts (71.4%); 75 μg/h: 5 pts (7.1%); 100 μg/h: 2 pts (14.2%)
Duration of treatment	Average 18.9±SD 38.4 (range 1-204)
Days of sample	29

TTS, transdermal therapeutic system; *VAS*, visual analogue scale; *pts*, patients

Oxycodone, regarded as a weak opioid by some authors and as a strong opioid by others, available in an immediate and controlled-release oral formulation, can be also administered by the parenteral, rectal and subcutaneous route. It is demethylated to noroxycodone, which does not have any pharmacological property, and to oxymorphone, a potent agonist which only forms in small amounts. A study has compared the analgesic efficacy, the adverse effects and the time necessary to obtain an adequate analgesia by means of a slow-release oxycodone as compared to slow-release morphine. Good analgesic efficacy has been achieved with both substances. With oxycodone there has been a greater incidence of vomiting with morphine and constipation. The notion of an "effective period" is important: oxycodone is more effective if administered as a first drug: this may be due to the action on κ and not on μ receptors, with an agonist-antagonist mechanism typical of weak opioids [36].

Buprenorphine, considered to be a strong opioid by some and a weak opioid by others owing to its partial agonism, is a widely used drug, even during opioid rotation.

Finally, according to various studies, morphine has a stimulating, suppressing or even no effect on the immune system; hydromorphone and oxycodone do not seem to affect the immune response, tramadol has an immunostimulating effect [37, 38].

Considerations on non-opioid analgesics

Contrary to the WHO guidelines, providing for the use of (NOAs) in all the three steps of cancer pain treatment, patients receive inadequate analgesia, because drugs are not prescribed for them, because there is no priority in the prescription and because there is no collaboration with the experts about pain [14, 39, 40]. NOAs are potent analgesics if the dose-effect ratio is considered. A retrospective study carried out on 1 070 patients with cancer, treated according to the WHO guidelines, showed that an appropriate combination of drugs is effective and safe in the treatment of cancer pain [41].

While in the past the guidelines indicated the use of high doses of NOAs at close intervals [42] (Table 4), with important side effects, recently new attention has been paid to NOAs alone or in association with corticosteroids, antidepressants and anticonvulsants [43]. Their use in the treatment of painful syndromes has increased over the past few years, although there has been a more limited and selected use. This is ascribable to the side effects developing during protracted treatment and, in particular, owing to the high doses used.

This has led to a reduction of doses, the synthesis of new molecules and new formulations. There are two classifications (Table 5), (non-steroidal anti-inflammatory drugs, new molecules and propacetamol are included). NOAs are effective in the treatment of bone metastases, since these are associated with bone de-

Table 4. Effective doses of nonopıoids for cancer paın. (Modıfied from [42])

Generic name	Dose (mg)	Interval of administration during day
Acetylsalıcylıc acıd	750-1 250	Every 3 h
Salicylamıde	750-1 000	Every 3 h
Phenacetın	400-600	Every 3 h
Paracetamol	600-800	Every 3 h
Phenazon	500-1 000	Every 3 h
Propyphenazon	450-800	Every 3 h
4-Amınophenazon	450-800	Every 3 h
Noramıdopyrın methansulfonate-sodıum (metamızol)	750-1 000	Every 3 h
Mofebutazon		
monophenylbutazon	200-400	Every 4 h
phenylbutazon	200-400	Every 4 h
oxyphenbutazone	100-200	Every 4 h
Mefenamıc acıd	500	Every 3 h
Flufenamıc acid	200	Every 4 h
Indomethacın	50-75	Every 4 h
Benzydamın	100	Every 4 h
Ibufenac		Every 4 h
Ibuprofen	200-400	Every 3 h
Naproxen	250-500	Every 3-4 h
Nıflumic acıd	250-500	Every 3-4 h
Alclofenac	500-1 000	Every 4 h
Nefopam	60-120	Every 3 h

Table 5. Classifications of drugs

Classification 1
• Antiphlogistics
  – Steroids
  – NSAIDs (old and new generation)
  – Antihistaminics
  – Immunosuppressors

Classification 2
• Non-opioid analgesics (NOAs)
  – Salicylic derivatives: acetylsalicylic acid
  – Pyrazolonic derivatives: phenylbutazon, metamizol, aminophenazon and derivatives
  – Phenylanthranilic acid derivatives: flufenamic, mefenamic and niflumic acid
  – Arylacetic acid derivatives: indomethacine, diclofenac, nabumetone and sulindac
  – Arilpropionic acid derivatives: ibuprofen, ketoprofen, fenoprofen and naproxen
  – Oxicam derivatives: pyroxicam and tenoxicam
  – Paraminofenol derivatives: phenacetine and paracetamol (acetaminofen)
  – Others: nimesulide, ketorolac

New molecules
• Meloxicam, nabumetone and propacetamol

struction by tumoral prostaglandins [44-46], in the infiltration of the soft tissues, in postsurgical pain and in serosites [14].

Furthermore, some authors have found that NOAs have a ceiling effect for analgesic efficacy (once they have reached the maximum dose they are no longer effective and toxicity increases). They, therefore, suggest discontinuing the treatment and using other NOAs, choosing the drugs correlated to the symptoms at the lowest dose by the least invasive route and at fixed times. The rotation method is introduced, as in the case of opioids.

In order to optimise administration, new formulations have been developed, depending on the type of absorption: direct (intravenous) or indirect (systemic or local). The systemic system provides for an oral, sublingual and rectal administration; the local system provides for a continuous release depot form by the transdermal, subcutaneous and intramuscular routes. The oral and subcutaneous routes are the most convenient. The sublingual form is used when swallowing is impaired; it provides a more rapid absorption in the first hour of administration and also has a local tolerability; the rectal route is indicated in the presence of nausea and vomiting refractory to the therapy or intestinal malabsorption and other factors requiring other administration routes [39]. The Task Force recommends the use of analgesics by the rectal or the transdermal route before using more invasive systemic therapies. The oral, effervescent formulation provides easy use, rapid absorption, excellent tolerability and safety.

Many types of pain are controlled by analgesics, but at the cost of many side effects [43]. Their use should be confined to medium-moderate pain. The dosage approved by the Food and Drug Administration (FDA) shows that patients with a body weight below 50 kg cannot take certain NOAs at the suggested analgesic doses, owing to the possible onset of side effects [39] (Table 6). A meta-analysis of the randomised control trials has evaluated the efficacy and safety of NOAs in the treatment of cancer pain, thereby proving the exis-

Table 6. Dosage of NSAIDs for adults and children[a]. (Modified from [39])

Drug	Body weight ⩾50 kg	Body weight <50 kg
• **Acetaminophen and over-the-counter NSAIDs**		
– Acetaminophen[b]	650 mg every 4 h or 975 mg every 6 h	10-15 mg/kg every 4 h or 15-20 mg/kg every 4 h (rectally)
– Aspirin[c]	650 mg every 4 h or 975 mg every 6 h	10-15 mg/kg every 4 h
– Ibuprofen	400-600 mg every 6 h	10 mg/kg every 6-8 h
• **Prescription NSAIDs**		
– Choline magnesium trisa-lycylate[d]	1 000-1 500 mg 3 times/day	25 mg/kg 3 times/day
– Choline salicylate[d]	870 mg every 3-4 h	Not approved by FDA
– Diflunisal[e]	500 mg every 12 h	Not approved by FDA
– Etodolac	200-400 mg every 6-8 h	Not approved by FDA
– Fenoprofen calcium	300-600 mg every 6 h	Not approved by FDA
– Ketoprofen	25-60 mg every 6-8 h	Not approved by FDA
– Ketorolac tromethamine[f]	10 mg every 4-6 h to a maximum of 40 mg/day	Not approved by FDA
– Meclofenamate sodium[g]	50-100 mg every 6 h	Not approved by FDA
– Mefanamic acid	250 mg every 6 h	Not approved by FDA
– Naproxen	250-275 mg every 6-8 h	5 mg/kg every 8 h
– Naproxen sodium	275 mg every 6-8 h	Not approved by FDA
• **Parenteral NSAIDs**		
– Ketorolac tromethamine[h]	60 mg initially, then 30 mg every 6 h (i.m. dose should not exceed 5 days)	Not approved by FDA

[a] Only NSAIDs that have been approved by the Food and Drug Administration (FDA) for use as simple analgesics are shown; clinical experience has been gained with other drugs as well. Dosages given per kilogram are per kilogram of body weight
[b] Acetaminophen lacks the peripheral anti-inflammatory and antiplatelet activities of the other NSAIDs
[c] Aspirin is the standard with which other NSAIDs are compared; it inhibits platelet aggregation and may cause bleeding. Aspirin is contraindicated in children who have fever or viral disease because of its association with Reye's syndrome
[d] These drugs may have minimal antiplatelet activity
[e] Administration of diflunisal with antacids may decrease absorption
[f] For short-term use only
[g] Coombs-positive autoimmune haemolytic anaemia has been associated with prolonged use of meclofenamate
[h] Ketorolac has the same toxic gastrointestinal effects as oral NSAIDs

tence of a dose-response relationship between analgesia and dosage, although not statistically significant; the *trend* of incidence of the side effects increases proportionally to the increment of the dose and the number of doses. Recent studies have shown that the administration of individual or multiple doses of weak opioids, associated and not associated with NOAs, are not more analgesic than the individual NOA [46]. Several studies have been carried out to evaluate the efficacy of the new molecules (nabumetone, meloxicam and propacetamol) [47-49] in relieving post-operative pain or pain due to rheumatoid arthritis, in comparison with the old NOAs, but few studies exist about the use of propacetamol in cancer pain and none at all about nabumetone and meloxicam.

Patients with cancer often do not take acetylsalicylic acid because of the high gastropathy incidence and the inhibition of platelet aggregation for the risk of haemorrhage.

Many NOAs, by inhibiting the cyclo-oxygenase enzyme, block the production of the substances responsible for the inflammation, inhibit chemotaxis of the cells involved, antagonise bradykinin, stabilise the lysosomal membranes and, according to recent studies, also act at a central level by modulating pain through the descending inhibiting system [44]. They are well-known for their anti-inflammatory, antipyretic and analgesic properties of varying extent according to their respective molecules.

Over the past few years, the most studied NOAs in cancer pain treatment include diclofenac, ketorolac, naproxene, paracetamol, indomethacine, and diflunisal.

Finally, corticosteroids are used in the treatment of refractory, continuous, pyrotic, lancinating, neuropathic bone pain and pain due to medullary compression caused by a malignant lesion; in pain due to malignant lesions of the brachial and lumbosacral plexus; in myofascial pain; in inflammatory diseases; in cerebral edema and increase of intracranial pressure; in the infiltration of soft tissues; in nervous compression or infiltration; and visceral distension [14].

Desametazone, prednisolone and deflazacort are the most frequently used molecules in the treatment of cancer pain. Deflazacort, widely used in our country, is effective for a shorter time than methylprednisolone and its anti-inflammatory activity is about 10-20 times that of prednisolone. Its effects last more than those of the other glycocorticoid drugs at equiactive doses, and the side effects are more limited than with methylprednisolone, even in terms of induced osteoporosis [50]. Doses range between 6 and 90 mg, according to indications and severity.

New molecules

According to a Medline and Embase search, there are no articles on the use of new molecules in cancer pain treatment in the world literature. The activation of the enzyme-converting arachidonic acid into PG, COX1 cyclo-oxygenase leads to the synthesis of PGI-2, which is cytoprotective on the gastric mucosa and regulates renal flow and natriuresis. COX-2 activation brings about the production of PG and other mediators responsible for the inflammation [48, 49].

The new, synthesised drugs acting selectively on COX-2 have fewer side effects, despite possessing a powerful antiphlogistic and antalgic action. There are numerous clinical studies showing the efficacy and tolerability of meloxicam compared with other NSAIDs for the treatment of benign chronic pain [49]; however, at present in the literature there are no trials for their use in cancer pain. It would be interesting to study these new molecules in cancer pain to evaluate the actual efficacy and to define their use according to the WHO ladder.

Prevention of gastroduodenal lesions and NSAIDs

By comparing omeprazole (20 or 40 mg/day orally) with ranitidine (150 mg/day orally) for the prevention of gastroduodenal ulcer in a double-blind study involving 541 patients treated with NSAIDs, ranitidine was found not to be effective in the prevention of gastric ulcer induced by NSAIDs (by direct endoscopy), although it prevents duodenal ulcer. Omeprazole prevents both [51]. In another double-blind study carried out on 935 patients treated with NSAIDs, the efficacy of omeprazole (20-40 mg/day orally) was compared with that of misoprostol (200 μg/four times a day) in the prevention of gastric lesions (erosions and ulcers). Omeprazole turned out to be more effective in healing NSAID-induced lesions than misoprostol; however, both of them have a comparable efficacy in preventing the onset of a gastric ulcer; misoprostol is better in preventing gastrointestinal complications associated with the use of NSAIDs (erosions) [52]. The omeprazole therapy is associated with a lower drop-out rate as it is better tolerated. Nevertheless, prophylaxis is necessary in patients requiring long NSAID treatment and after assessing the risk factors (age, medical history, type and dose of administered NSAIDs, associated therapy with warfarine or glucocorticoids) [53].

Adjuvant medications

Psychotropic drugs (neuroleptics, benzodiazepines, antidepressants, and anticonvulsants) are used to strengthen the analgesic action [6]. Some of them have a sedative effect, others a hypnotic effect and yet others a stimulating effect. The mechanism action of some of them is well-known, that of others complex and not completely clear. Neuroleptics are used in some emergencies, such as psychomotor agitation and hallucinations; benzodiazepines and their derivatives are used for sleep disorders, ansiolysis and, in some cases, for convulsions and panic attacks. A depressive syndrome is the most frequent emotional response in patients with pain. Antidepressants, in particular tertiary structure tricyclic antidepressants, potent inhibitors of the re-uptake of serotonin – a neuromediator involved in the analgesic action of anti-depressants – have shown a powerful analgesic efficacy and have been used since 1960 [54]. The therapeutic options in neuropathic pain are numerous and not always satisfactory; the advent of new drugs is, therefore, desirable. There are no drugs indicated for neuropathic pain, but there are adjuvant analgesics, i.e. drugs with analgesic properties that do not have analgesia as a first indication: many drugs have been studied: tricyclic antidepressants, anticonvulsants, local anaesthetics, sympatholytics, anti-arrhythmics, ketamine and, among the opioids, morphine and fentanyl [54-58]. Indeed, the use of the latter is very controversial [34, 59].

The development of research has subsequently led to the synthesis of other "typical" tricyclic antidepressants and, in the last decade, the "anti-depressants of the second generation" or "atypical" with different pharmacological and chemical characteristics. All antidepressants, except mianserine, whose working mechanism is not completely clear, block the aminic pump, an active transport system located in the presynaptic membranes of the nerve endings, thereby inhibiting the re-uptake of monoamines, noradrenaline, serotonin and dopamine: the antidepressant effect is thought to be correlated to the action of the amine pump. This property is probably responsible for the most common unwanted effects. Although inhibiting the uptake, the most recent antidepressants do not have an affinity for receptors and selectively block only serotonin or catecholamine uptake. Antidepressants are used in neuropathic pain related or not related to cancer; in cancer pain they are used in association with non-narcotic analgesics and with opioids. The typical tricyclic antidepressants have been used and studied most in pain treatment, although they have shown, in addition to analgesia, rather significant side effects related to the anticholinergic activity, their potential cardiotoxicity, their antiadrenergic activity, and their antihistaminic action. Only some antidepressants, especially the tertiary-structure tricyclic and the serotoninergic antidepressants, have an inherent analgesic efficacy (already evident in the first day of therapy). Over the past few years, the analgesic action has been proved to be separate from the antidepressant action [54]. Recently, in animals, it has been found that serotoninergic antidepressants, i.e. chlorimipramine and amitriptyline, have an intrinsic analgesic action; they strengthen the antinociceptive effect of morphine and increase the concentration of β-endorphins [60, 61]; in the association with opioids there is a pharmacological strengthening according to some authors, a synergetic action according to others. Recent experimental animal studies have identified further mechanisms of action: chlorimipramine appears to carry out a peripheral antiedemigenic activity, probably due to the inhibition of polymorphonucleate chemotaxis, while for fluoxetine the activity is mediated by the central mechanisms of the hypothalamus-adrenal axis [62, 63]. There is no evidence that the most recent antidepressants have a greater analgesic effect than the tricyclic ones [64].

Many authors have used them in the treatment on cancer pain, neuropathic pain and the depressive syndrome associated to it [65]. It has been demonstrated that the descending pathways of the trunk have an inhibiting function on the pain impulse; serotonin is the mediator which increases the pain threshold. Injury of the serotoninergic pathways blocks the action of morphine, the analgesia

Table 7. Typical and atypical tricyclic antidepressants: doses in depression and chronic pain [54]

Drugs	Depression (mg/day)	Chronic pain (mg/day)
• **Typical**		
– Imipramine	100-200	50-75
– Amitriptyline	100-200	25-100
– Desipramine	100-200	50-75
– Nortriptyline	75-150	50-100
– Protriptyline	15-40	
– Trimipramine	75-250	50-100
– Chlorimipramine	30-50	–
– Dothiepin	75-150	–
– Doxepin	100-200	25-100
• **Atypical**		
– Amoxapine	200-300	100-200
– Maprotiline	200-300	50-100
– Nomifensine	100-200	–
– Trazodone	150-200	50-200
– Mianserin	30-60	–
– Viloxazine	150-300	–
– Amineptine	200-300	–
– Zymelidine	200-300	–
– Fluoxetine	20	20

of which is due to the release of serotonin. Antidepressants are known to modulate serotoninergic and/or serotoninergic and/or noradrenergic tone in the CNS and release β-endorphins in the hypothalamus [60]. Many antidepressants and have a three-level modulating effect: they modify mood, improve the quality of sleep, and have an analgesic action.

The analgesic doses suggested in the literature for neuropathic pain range between 25 and 200 mg/day orally, i.e. they are lower than the doses used in depression (Table 7). The median analgesic dose of amitriptyline is 75 mg/day (range 25-150 mg/day); the analgesic effect appears as early as the second, third day [54, 64]. According to their characteristics, antidepressants can be classified into activating, intermediate and sedative (Table 8). At our institute the analgesic activity of some antidepressants has been studied. Fluoxetine was also studied, at doses of 40 mg/day orally, associated with NOAs, in cancer pain with nerve infiltration in 20 patients with multifoci, VAS equal or greater than 5 and mood disorders. These data showed that in patients suffering from cancer pain, the use of fluoxetine, associated with opioids, anti-inflammatory drugs and lorazepam, significantly reduced the intensity of pain during treatment, eliminating it completely in three patients. Pain was reduced already on the third day. The plasma concentration of fluoxetine effective for analgesia is lower than 200 ng/ml. The depression index had decreased slightly at the end of treatment, while the previ-

Table 8. Characteristics of antidepressants

- **Activating**
  - Amineptine
  - Minaprine
  - Viloxazine
  - Desimipramine
  - Rubidium salts
  - I-Mao
- **Intermediate**
  - Nortriptyline
  - Imipramine
  - Clomipramine
  - Dothiepin
  - Fluoxetine
  - Sertraline
- **Sedative**
  - Trimipramine
  - Amitriptyline
  - Mianserine
  - Trazodone
  - Dibenzepine
  - Doxepin
  - Fluvoxamine
  - Paroxetine
  - Sertraline

ously high anxiety was considerably reduced after the therapy. On the whole, there was an increase in the participation in family activities, deambulation and the use of means of transport; the side effects, which were more frequent and mild, included sleepiness, xerostomia, giddiness, sweating and tremors. In patients suffering from cancer pain, opioids, if used alone, have little effect in the advanced stage with metastases and neuropathic pain; in these cases the association with NOA and psychotropic agents is common. The extent of pain reduction confirms of this.

Through the interaction with the ionic channels or the neurotransmitter receptors, anticonvulsants act on neuropathic pain through two general mechanisms: they reduce the excessive discharge of altered neurons and the diffusion of excitation from abnormal foci. Phenytoin, carbamazepine (which in rats has been found to have an anti-inflammatory effect with the same characteristics as the tricyclic anti-depressants) [66], and valproic acid are the most commonly used drugs in neuropathic cancer pain. These molecules are characterised by pharmacological interactions of clinical importance and by unwanted side effects (hypotension, depression in the atrioventricular conduction, confusion, nausea, vomiting, constipation, thrombocytopenia, and leucocytopenia) which may even lead to the discontinuation of the therapy. The most recent of these, gabapentine, approved about 3 years ago in the USA has shown some peculiar features. Gabapentine appears to modulate the GABA-ergic system by increasing in vitro the activity of the glutamic-acid-decarboxylase (GAD), a key enzyme in GABA synthesis; this led us to believe that gabapentine may increase GABA synthesis [67]. In terms of pharmacokinetics, it reaches the plasma peak in 2-3 h; at therapeutic doses there is a linear correlation between plasma concentration and dosage. It does not bind with plasma proteins, it is not metabolised, and, therefore, there is a smaller kinetic variability and a lower risk of pharmacological interaction. It does not cause induction and enzyme inhibition in the liver; there is no kinetic interaction with other anti-epileptics; plasma clearance can be correlated to creatinine clearance; and excretion is renal. The good tolerability of this drug in association with other drugs has contributed to its use in the USA and in Italy, where it is becoming "the front-line drug for the treatment of all types of neuropathic pain" [56]. There are no controlled guidelines, data or studies.

The first data reporting the efficacy of gabapentine in neuropathic pain refer to small case studies (painful neuropathies, diabetic neuropathies, sympathetic-reflex dystrophy, post-herpetic neuralgia, deafferentation neuropathy, painful erythromelalgia, and multiple sclerosis) [55]. These are preliminary experiences: to date, only two placebo-controlled studies have been carried out to check its efficacy and tolerability in the therapy of diabetic neuropathy and in post-herpetic neuralgia [68]; however, there is no literature about its specific use in neurologic cancer pain. According to our experience, not confirmed by controlled studies, at doses of 900-1 200 mg, gabapentine is already effective in the modulation of neuropathic cancer pain. From the clinical point of view, it appears to be more effective than diphenyldantoine and to have fewer side effects than carbamazepine.

Pamidronate and metabolic radiotherapy

Bone metastases are more frequently observed in patients affected by breast, prostate, lung, kidney and thyroid cancer. The activation of osteoclasts is the key point in the pathophysiology of osteolytic metastases, although osteoblastic metastases are possible. Biphosphonates (di-sodium-clodronate and the most recent pamidronate) are used to inhibit ectopic calcifications and bone resorption. The mechanism of action of pamidronate mimics the physiochemical action of pyrophosphate, a substance physiologically present in biological tissues with the function of preventing the formation of calcium phosphate crystals in soft tissues and avoiding their dissolution in the skeleton. Pamidronate is a biphosphonate whose central atom of oxygen has been replaced with carbon, thereby making it stable. With regard to its mechanism of action, this is probably based on the inhibition of bone resorption by binding to the bone surface, making the latter less available to osteoclastic activity; by inhibiting recruitment of osteoclast precursors; by preventing the migration of osteoclasts towards the bone; by altering osteoclast morphology; and by inhibiting prostaglandin E2, interleukin 1 and proteolytic enzymes [69, 70]. The intravenous route is preferred, with a 60- to 90-mg dose by infusion every 3-4 weeks. Pamidronate is not a cytotoxic agent and does not seem to affect survival; the oral route of administration has also been studied. At present, there is no clinical trial comparing the activity of the various biphosphonates or analysing the cost-benefit ratio [71]. Clinical studies in patients with mainly lithic bone metastases or in multiple myeloma have shown that pamidronate prevents or delays complications in the skeletal system (hypercalcaemia, pathologic fractures, medullary impairments, need of radiotherapy, and orthopaedic surgery) and decreases bone pain, thereby allowing the use of analgesics to be reduced. Compared with the side effects of the previous biphosphonates (increase in blood phosphates and kidney failure due to calcium biphosphonate precipitation and formation of its aggregates), the side effects of pamidronate are considered to be limited and temporary (symptomatic hypocalcemia and fever appear within 48 h from infusion).

With regard to bone metastases, in palliative care the use of radiotherapy pursues three main objectives: anantalgic effect, the prevention and cure of pathologic fractures, and the prevention of secondary paralysis and medullary suffering. The most recent radiotherapic technique include radioisotopes, which, administered intravenously, concentrate around the lesion where the osteoblastic reaction is greatest. Radiometabolites are osteotropic and not oncotropic, which means that their anti-cancer activity can only be hypothesised: in some patients with prostate carcinoma treated with strontium-89, there is evidence of a significant reduction of the specific prostate antigen and of alkaline phosphatase, which appears to have a cytotoxic effect on neoplastic cells [72]. Many radioisotopes have been proposed up to now: phosphorus-32, strontium-89, rhenium-186, samarium-153, and tin-117. Rhenium, samarium, and tin are still at an experimental stage, while strontium is currently the only radiopharmaceutical approved by the FDA in the USA and registered in Italy. The antalgic effect takes place in 80% of patients with a limited medullary inhibition after 5 weeks after the beginning of the therapy, with a recovery of platelet synthesis within the 12th week and white-cell synthesis within the six month of treatment.

Other drugs

Ketamine at subanaesthetic doses has recently been evaluated in cancer pain for its analgesic properties. Its analgesic action seems to be mediated by the inhibition of the NMDA receptor. Its main indication is neuropathic pain, especially hyperalgesia and allodynia. It is administered orally or subcutaneously in continuous infusion [57].

Again with regard to neuropathic pain, special attention is paid to the study and research of antagonists on NMDA receptors for glutamate. The receptors, located in the nervous system along the nociceptive afferent pathways, play a role in hyperalgesia, hyperpathia and allodynia, which are often associated with nervous damage. In addition to ketamine, a similar blocking action is carried out by dextromethorphan, methadone and pethidine. Finally, some local anaesthetics such as lidocaine and mexiletine, by their blocking action on the sodium channels, bring

Table 9. Adjuvant analgesics. (Modified from [43])

Class (examples)	Usual indications

• Anticonvulsants
  – Phenytoin
  – Carbamazepine
  – Clonazepam
  – Valproate
	Neuropathic pain, particularly lancinating pain

• Antidepressants
  – Amitriptyline
  – Nortriptyline
  – Imipramine
  – Desipramine
  – Trazodone
	Neuropathic pain

• Local anesthetics
  – Lidocaine
  – Mexiletine
	Neuropathic pain

• Corticosteroids
  – Deflazacort
  – Dexamethasone
  – Prednisone
	Tumor invasion of neural tissue, elevated intracranial pressure, spinal cord compression, additional effects (mood elevation et al)

• Antihistaminics – Hydroxyzine	Coanalgesic, antiemetic

• Muscle relaxants
  – Orphenadrine
  – Carisoprodol
  – Methocarbamol
  – Chlorzoxazone
  – Cyclobenzaprine
	Occasionally useful for musculoskeletal pain

• Neuroleptics
  – Methotrimeprazine
  – Fluphenazine
	Neuropathic pain

• Other drugs for neuropathics pain
  – Baclofen
  – Clonidine
  – Calcitonin
  – Capsaicin, topical
	Neuropathic pain

• Drug action on bone
  – Biphosphonates (pamidronate)
  – Calcitonin
  – Radiopharmaceuticals (Strontium-89)
	Bone pain

• Anticholinergics
  – Scopolamine
  – Glycopyrrolate
	Visceral pain due to bowel obstruction

• Psychostimulants
  – Caffeine
  – Methylphenidate
  – Dextroamphetamine
	Decrease sedation due to opioid analgesia

about a state of inhibition of the nervous transmission, thereby reducing the membrane hyperexcitability typical of the neuropathic syndrome [58] (Table 9).

Invasive techniques

Invasive techniques are reserved for selected cases of painful syndromes that would otherwise be uncontrollable, in the not very advanced stages: spinal, peridural, subarachnoid and cerebral intraventricular analgesia obtained with opioids or anaesthetics and opioids, the chemical or physical neurodamaging techniques, such as the block of the coeliac plexus and surgical cervical chordotomy or percutaneous chordotomy by radiofrequency (hot). Mention should be made of cryoanalgesia [73], palliative surgery, fixation of pathologic fractures or the implant of arthroprostheses for articular metastases, laser disobstruction and positioning of a tube in oesophageal cancer, and bypass surgery in the intestines, biliary and urinary tracts.

Currently debated associated symptoms

Convulsions

Convulsive seizures can be observed in 20%-30% of cancer patients; furthermore, they can appear in patients using high opioid doses. In some countries, opioid rotation is employed to prevent this symptom. Neurosurgery and radiotherapy are pointless if they do not change life expectancy. A diagnostic procedure has to be followed to rule out any metabolic, toxic, pharmacological causes, vascular alterations or infections.

Haemorrhage and transfusions

Overt haemorrhage is observed in 14% of terminally ill cancer patients [74], while light continuous bleeding can affect 23.8% of them [75]. These two complications are pathophysiologically different since they induce acute or chronic anaemia. The causes have to be assessed, the transfusion programme, if required, discussed with the patient and the evaluation should include the Karnofsky index, the cognitive state, life expectancy, the trend of blood losses in the short and medium term, the haemopoietic synthesis capacity, and the state of hydration and nutrition [76].

The cause of the anaemia has to be looked for and, when possible, treated by means of palliative radiotherapy for superficial ulcers, haemoptysis, haematuria, oesophageal and bronchial lesions; tranexamic acid administered systemically or topically; astringent solutions containing aluminium, sucralphate paste topically; haemostatic medication; or laser therapy, diathermocoagulation, cryotherapy, or embolisations in bronchial and renal haemorrhage. Any symptoms and signs ascribable to anaemia and other concomitant causes will have to be determined: syncope, dyspnoea, tachycardia, angina, postural hypotension, transient ischaemic attacks, pallor, and lethargy. An important loss of blood volume in a short period of time implies haemodynamic alteration. In this situation, before any transfusion, volemic replacement should be performed. If anaemisation is chronic, it is necessary to define whether it is symptomatic (Fig. 1). By reducing dyspnoea or asthenia, the quality of life definitely improves [77].

If the cardiac function is limited because of a pre-existing cardiopathy or factors related to neoplasia (chemotherapic factors, mediastinal obstruction) or if there is a reduction in the ventilation-pulmonary perfusion ratio, the haemoglobin deficit will increase the symptoms.

In the presence of acute haemorrhage, before organising transfusion support, it is necessary to stop the blood loss, if possible, in addition to evaluating the prognosis and the Karnofsky index.

It should also be stressed that, in the last days of the patient's life, transfusion does not show any favourable influence on the symptoms (dyspnoea, asthenia).

Nutrition and hydration

At an advanced stage, the programming of nutrition and hydration support is always subject to the patient's consent and the family's opinion and then it depends on the patient's history, the local and systemic pathophysiology of the disease, physical examination, survival, level of consciousness, and Karnofsky index [78, 79].

However, it is unrealistic to think that symptoms such as asthenia and thirst will disappear thanks to hydration and diet in the last days of life [80, 81].

In a study carried out by Ellershow et al. in 1995 on a sample of 82 terminally ill cancer patients, the relation between thirst, dry mouth and state of dehydration was evaluated. No significant association was found between the level of hydration and these symptoms [82].

It is fundamental to make sure that palliative measures such as artificial saliva and ice cubes are available. For maintenance hydration, it is possible to use the hypodermal or the intravenous route [83, 84]; we recommend the administration of 1.5-2 l/day of maintenance solution during the last days of life.

Before programming any supplementary nutrition it is important to take general assistance measures (oral cavity hygiene, curing ulcers and infections, artificial saliva, and gastroprotectors). There are many alternative routes of administration: the least invasive one is to be preferred.

The most physiologic forms of nutrition should have priority, compatible with the gastrointestinal absorption capacity and canalisation: the enteral oral route, the nasogastric cannula or percutaneous enterogastrostomy (PEG) or parenteral support nutrition using a catheter.

It is hardly ever possible to meet the nutritional requirements of a terminally ill cancer patient. A study we carried out in patients at an advanced stage of disease showed that a supplementary nutrition based on proteins and calories led

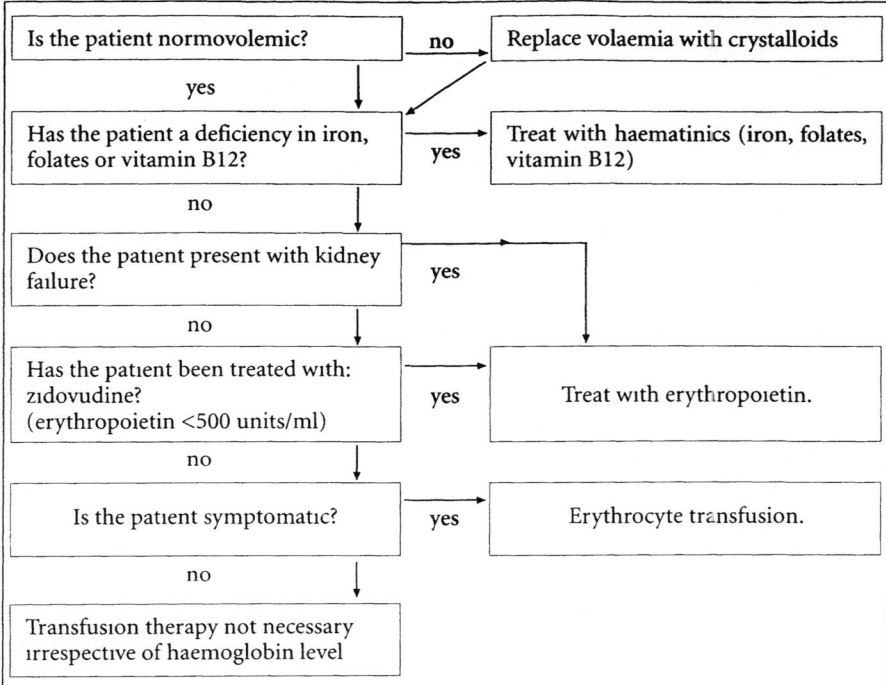

Fig. 1. Elective erythrocyte transfusion in patients with persistent anaemia: a treatment strategy. (Modified from [77])

to an improvement of the quality of life, measured by the Karnofsky index, and the muscular strength measured by dynamometry. Patients were able to take care of themselves, walk, and there was a reduction of asthenia and an improvement in mood [85].

During the last moments of the patient's life, family members often exert psychological pressure on the care-givers for them to protract hydration and nutrition, in the belief that the patient's general condition might improve.

Psychotherapy

Psychotherapeutic techniques can be used not only for analgesic purposes; in association with other techniques, they also modulate pain by interfering with perception, meaning, feelings and/or behaviour. They do not involve a high risk; however, they are more time-consuming than other methods. In the psychotherapeutic approach, guiding, explorative and support techniques are used.

– Guiding techniques have the aim of changing acquired behaviours or convictions and include cognitive therapy, behavioural therapy and cognitive-behavioural therapy.

– Explorative techniques, such as psychodynamic therapy, psychoanalysis, hypnoanalysis and guided imagination are used in the case of intrapsychic conflicts.
– Support techniques consist of information, praising and reassuring procedures.

Our approach in the cancer patient is mainly individual, cognitive, affective and behavioural and remains so even in the advanced and very advanced stages. In the very advanced stage, we implement group techniques with the patient's family by providing cognitive and affective support. Counselling is also provided on an individual basis [86-90].

We conclude by quoting a text taped during a group meeting. The son of a deceased patient of ours, says:

"After suffering that attack on Tuesday, he changed completely ... I mean, he was really a completely different person ... he was another person altogether, his personality had changed, he was ... well, I don't know ... he no longer had all that rage inside him. I mean, lately, in the past three months I think he had been accumulating a lot of rage and fear. This is what I think. You could really see it in his face ... and after this attack, no trace of this was left on his face, no rage or fear. He seemed like an enquiring person, he was ... puzzled. He would start many sentences by saying 'I don't understand... I wonder why...' he looked just like someone who was wondering ... I don't know ... it was as if it was difficult for him to tell the difference between life and death at that moment ... He seemed to take very little interest in whether he was alive or not ... and the therapies were the only thing that could make him angry, he would say they were useless. He got very angry about transfusions ... He received a transfusion that Wednesday, the day he died, and said that it was a waste of blood, that he didn't want it ... he said that staying in hospital was pointless and that he wanted to go home ... he wanted to go to the seaside at Barcola where he would feel better ... he also said that he would find the sea and the sunshine there ...".

References

1. Meier DE, Emmons CA, Wallenstein S et al (1998) A national survey of physician-assisted suicide and euthanasia in United States. N Engl J Med 338:1193-1201
2. Asai A, Fukuhara S, Lo B (1995) Attitudes of Japanese and Japanese-American physicians towards life-sustaining treatment. Lancet 346:356-359
3. Tanida N (1995) Commentary on attitudes of Japanese physicians towards life-sustaining treatment. Lancet 346:970-971
4. Sgreccia E (1992) Linee etiche per l'assistenza medica al malato terminale. Min Anestesiol 58:581-585
5. Paladini VA, Peressin P, Contin F (1990) Principi di terapia dei sintomi nel cancro avanzato. Gi Med Crit Ter Antalg e Cure Palliative 2:26-31
6. Paladini VA, Peressin P, Contin F (1990) Psicosi nel paziente con cancro avanzato: diagnostica e Terapia. Gi Med Crit Ter Antalg Cure Palliative 2:32-38
7. Grond S, Zech D, Diefenbach C, Radbruch L, Lehmann KA (1996) Assessment of cancer

pain: a prospective evaluation in 2266 cancer patients referred to a pain service. Pain 64:107-114

8. McQuay HJ (1997) Opioid use in cancer pain. Acta Anaesthesiol Scand 41:175-183
9. Twycross R (1997) Cancer pain classification. Acta Anaesthesiol Scand 41:141-145
10. Xu XJ, Puke MJC, Verge VMK et al (1993) Up-regulation of cholecystokinin in primary sensory neurons is associated with morphine insensitivity in experimental neuropathic pain in the rat. Neurosci Lett 152:129-132
11. Xu XJ, Wiesenfeld-Hallin Z (1991) The threshold for the depressive effect of intrathecal morphine on the spinal nociceptive flexor reflex is increased during autotomy after sciatic nerve section in rats. Pain 46:223-229
12. Zech DFJ, Grond S, Lynch J et al (1995) Validation of World Health Organisation guidelines for cancer pain relief: a 10-year prospective study. Pain 63:65-76
13. Paladini VA, Antonaglia V, Scalia M et al (1986) Pharmacological therapy in advanced cancer pain. In: Gullo A (ed) APICE. Trieste, p 34
14. Levy MH (1996) Pharmacologic treatment of cancer pain. N Engl J Med 335:1124-1132
15. Driessen B (1992) Interaction of the central analgesic, tramadol, with the uptake and release of 5-hydroxytryptamine in the rat brain, in vitro. Br J Pharmacol 105:147-151.
16. Bollettino d'informazione sui farmaci. Ministero della Sanità, anno 5°, n.1, gen-feb 1998
17. Tawfik MO (1990) Tramadol hydrochloride in the relief of cancer pain: a double-blind comparison against sustained release morphine. Pain 8(Suppl 5):377
18. Christrup LL (1997) Morphine metabolites. Acta Anaesthesiol Scand 41:116-122
19. De Stoutz ND, Bruera E, Suarez-Almazor M (1995) Opioid rotation for toxicity reduction in terminal cancer patients. J Pain Symptom Manage 10:378-384
20. Paladini VA, Mocavero G, Saltarini M et al (1990) Livelli ematici ed analgesia della morfina a lento rilascio nel dolore da cancro. G Med Crit Ter Antalg Cure Palliative 2:39-48
21. Gourlay G, Cherry D, Cousins M (1986) A comparative study of the efficacy of oral methadone and morphine in the treatment of severe pain in patients with cancer. Pain 25:297-312
22. Toner G, Cramond T, Bishop J et al (1993) Randomized double-blind, phase III crossover study of a new sustained-release oral morphine formulation, Kapanol capsules. 7th World Congress on Pain, Paris
23. Paul D, Standifer K, Inturrisi C, Pasternak G (1989) Pharmacological characterization of morphine-6beta-glucoronide, a very potent morphine metabolite. J Pharmacol Exp Ther 251:477-483
24. Mocavero G (1986) Techniques and results of the injection of opioids into the cerebral ventricle through a cervical catheter. In: Gullo A (ed) Advances in Anaesthesia, Intensive Care and Pain Therapy Postgraduate Course. Trieste, p 71
25. Bell MDD, Mishra P, Weldon BD, Murray GR, Calvey TN, Williams NE (1985) Buccal morphine – a new route for analgesia? Lancet 1:71
26. Mocavero G (1989) Le nuove tecniche in terapia antalgica. La somatostatina, la morfina e la lidocaina somministrate mediante aerosol nasale, instillazione oculare e sul ganglio sfeno-palatino danno analgesia. G Med Crit Ter Antalg Cure Palliative 1:190-193
27 Mocavero G (1981) Analgesia selettiva con morfina perinervosa. Incontri di Anestesia, Rianimazione e Scienze Affini 16:1-3
28. Krajnik M, Zylicz Z (1997) Topical morphine in malignant cutaneous pain. Abstracts of the Fifth Congress of the European Association for Palliative Care, London, p S34
29 Portenoy RK, Southam MA, Gupta SK et al (1993) Transdermal fentanyl for cancer pain Anaesthesiology 78:36-43
30. Holley FO, van Steennis C (1988) Postoperative analgesia with fentanyl: pharmacoki-

netics and pharmacodynamics of constant-rate i v. and transdermal delivery. Br J Anaesth 60:608-613

31. Plezia PM, Kramer TH, Linford J, Hameroff SR (1989) Transdermal fentanyl: pharmacokinetics and preliminary clinical evaluation. Pharmacotherapy 9:2-9

32. Gourlay GK, Kowalski SR, Plummer JL et al (1989) The transdermal administration of fentanyl in the treatment of postoperative pain. Pain 37:193-202

33. Korte W, de Stoutz N, Morant R (1996) Day-to-day titration to initiate transdermal fentanyl in patients with cancer pain: short- and long-term experiences in a prospective study of 39 patients. J Pain Symptom Manage 11:139-146

34. Dellemijn R, Vanneste JAL (1997) Randomized double-blind active-placebo-controlled crossover trial of intravenous fentanyl in neuropathic pain. Lancet 345:753-758

35. McDonald CJ, Miller AJ (1997) A comparative potency study of a controlled release tablet formulation of hydromorphone with controlled release morphine in patients with cancer pain. Abstracts of the Fifth Congress of the European Association for Palliative Care, London, September, p S37

36. Heiskanan TY, Kalso E (1997) Controlled-release oxycodone and morphine in cancer related pain. Pain 73:37-45

37. Sacerdote P, Bianchi M, Manfredi B et al (1997) Effects of tramadol on immune responses and nociceptive thresholds in mice. Pain 72:325-330

38. Sacerdote P, Manfredi B, Mantegazza P, Panerai AE (1997) Antinociceptive and immunosuppressive effects of opiate drugs: a structure-related activity study. Br J Pharmacol 121:834-840

39. Agency for Health Care Policy and Research (1994) New clinical-practice guidelines for the management of pain in patient with cancer. N Engl J Med 3:651-655

40. Ahmedzai S (1997) Pain control in patients with cancer. Eur J Cancer 33:S55-S62

41. Grond S, Zech D, Schug SA, Lynch J, Lehmann KA (1991) The importance of non-opioid analgesics for cancer pain relief according to guidelines of the World Health Organization. Int J Clin Pharmacol Res 11:253-260

42. Bonica JJ, Ventafridda V (1979) Advances in pain research and therapy. Raven, New York, pp 255-262

43. American Society of Anaesthesiologists Task Force on Pain Management, Cancer Pain Section (1996) Practice guidelines for cancer pain management. Anaesthesiology 84:1243-1257

44. Payne R (1997) Mechanism and management of bone pain. Cancer 80:S1608-S1612

45. Portenoy RK (1992) Cancer pain: pathophysiology and syndromes. Lancet 339:1026-1035

46. Eisemberg S, Berkey CS, Carr DB (1994) Efficacy and safety of nonsteroidal anti-inflammatory drugs for cancer pain: a meta-analysis. J Clin Oncol 12:2756-2765

47. Farhat F, Savoyen MC, Jair C (1995) Efficacité du propacetamol sur la doleur postoperatoire selon deux modés d'administration intraveineuse. Cah Anaesthesiol 43:351-356

48. Friedel HA (1993) Nabumetone. A reappraisal of its pharmacology and therapeutic use in rheumatic diseases. Drugs 45:131-156

49. Engelhardt G (1996) Pharmacology of meloxicam, a new nonsteroidal anti-inflammatory drug with an improved safety profile through preferential inhibition of COX-2. Rheumatology 35(Suppl 1):4-12

50. Markham A, Bryson HM (1995) Deflazacort. A review of its pharmacological properties and therapeutic efficacy. Drugs 50:317-333

51. Yeomans ND, Tulassay Z, Juhasz L et al (1998) A comparison of omeprazole with ranitidine for ulcers associated with nonsteroidal anti-inflammatory drugs. N Engl J Med 338:719-726

52. Hawkey KJ, Karrash JA, Szczepanski L (1998) Omeprazole compared with misoprostol for ulcers associated with nonsteroidal anti-inflammatory drugs. N Engl J Med 338:727-734

53. Twycross RG (1993) Advances in cancer pain management. J Pharmacol Care Pain Symptom Control 1:5-30

54. Paladini VA, Mocavero G (1990) Gli antidepressivi nella terapia del dolore. Tergestum, Trieste

55. Tassinari CA (1998) Gabapentin: nuove acquisizioni e prospettive terapeutiche. Masson, Paris

56. Galer BS Treatment of neuropathic pain: use of "adjuvant" analgesic. Vol 122. American Academy of Neurology, 49th Annual Meeting pp 43-47

57. Shima Y, Yanagisawa H, Aruga E (1997) Neuropathic pain: treatment with low dose ketamine. Abstracts of the Fifth Congress of the European Association for Palliative Care, London, p S32

58. Dickenson AH (1997) NMDA receptor antagonists; interaction with opioids. Acta Anaesth Scand 41:112-115

59. Arné S, Meyerson BA (1998) Lack of analgesic effects of opioids on neuropathic pain and idiopathic forms of pain. Pain 33:11-23

60. Sacerdote P, Brini A, Mantegazza P, Panerai AE (1987) A role for serotonin and beta-endorphine in the analgesia induced by some tricyclic antidepressant drugs. Pharmacol Biochem Behav 26:153

61. Panerai AE (1988) Il concetto di potenziamento in farmacologia. Min Anestesiol 54:123

62. Panerai AE, Bianchi M (1966) Farmacologia degli analgesici: gli antidepressivi, nuovi aspetti del loro meccanismo d'azione. Proceedings 18° Congresso Nazionale Associazione Italiana per lo Studio del Dolore (AISD), pp 55-58

63. Sacerdote P, Bianchi M, Panerai AE (1997) In vivo and in vitro clomipramine treatment decreases the migration of macrophages in the rat. Eur J Pharmacol 319:287-290

64. McQuay HJ (1977) Antidepressants and chronic pain. Br Med J 314:763-765

65. Walsh TD (1983) Review. Antidepressants in chronic pain. Clin Neuropharmacol 6:271

66 Bianchi M, Rossoni G, Sacerdote P, Panerai AE, Berti F (1995) Carbamazepine exerts anti-inflammatory effects in the rat. Eur J Pharmacol 294:71-74

67. Taylor CP (1995) Gabapentin: mechanisms of action. In: Levy RH et al (eds) Antiepileptic drugs. Raven, New York, pp 829-841

68. Backonja M, Hes MS, La Moreaux LK, Garofalo EE, Koto EM (1997) Gabapentin (neurontin) reduces pain in diabetics patients with painful peripheral neuropathics: results of a double-blind placebo controlled clinical trial. American Pain Society, 16th Annual Scientific Meeting Program Book, p 108

69. Hortobagyi GN, Theriault RL, Porter L et al (1996) Efficacy of pamidronate in reducing skeletal complications in patients with breast cancer and lytic bone metastases. N Engl Med 335:1785-1791

70. Lipton A, Glover D, Harvey H et al (1994) Pamidronate in the treatment of bone metastases: results of 2 dose-ranging trials in patients with breast or prostate cancer. Ann Oncol 5(Suppl 7):S31-35

71. O'Rourke N, MacCloskey E, Houghton F et al (1995) Double-blind, placebo-controlled trial of oral clodronate in patients with bone metastases J Clin Oncol 13:929-934

72. Blake G (1986) Strontium-89 therapy: strontium kinetics in dissemination carcinoma of the prostate. Eur J Nucl Med 12:447-454

73. Foley KM (1985) The treatment of cancer pain. N Engl J Med 11:84-95

74 Regnard CFB, Tempest S, Toscani F (1994) Manuale di medicina palliativa. CIS, Milano

75. Olivo R, Paladini VA, Perotto A et al (1988) L'assistenza domiciliare al malato con dolore

da cancro. Assistenza ınfermıerıstıca. Recent Advances ın Anaesthesıa, Intensıve Care and Pain Therapy Postgraduate Course. Trıeste, pp 343-348

76. Ashby M, Stoffel B (1995) Artıfıcıal hydratıon and alımentatıon at the end of lıfe: a reply to Craig. J Med Ethıcs 21:135-140

77. Quarta Cırcolare Informatıva sul buon uso deı concentratı erıtrocıtarı Anno 1992. Polıclınıco San Matteo, Pavia

78. Margarıt O, Paladını VA, Iuretıgh C (1992) Anamnesi, valutazione, fabbısognı e prıncıpı terapeutıcı in terapia del dolore e cure pallıatıve. II Corso residenzıale a cura dı Paladını VA, APICE. Trıeste, pp 302-316

79. Paladini VA, Margarit O, Lugnanı F (1996) La nutrızıone domıcılıare nella fase avanzata della malattıa neoplastıca: organızzazıone dell'équıpe dı cura. In: Paladını VA (ed) La nutrızıone domıcılıare nel paziente con cancro avanzato. APICE. Trıeste, pp 1-6

80. Bozzettı F (1996) Guidelınes on artıfıcıal nutrıtion versus hydratıon ın termınal cancer patient. Nutrıtıon 12:163-167

81. McCann RM, Hall WJ, Gruth-Juncker A (1994) Comfort care for termınally ıll patıents. The appropriate use of nutrition and hydration. JAMA 272:1263-1266

82. Ellershow JE, Sutcliffe JM, Saunders CM (1995) Dehydratıon and the dyıng patıent. J Paın Symptom Manage 10:221-228

83. Dunphy K, Finlay I, Rothbone G, Gılbert J, Hıcks F (1995) Rehydratıon ın pallıatıve and termınal care: ıf not- why not? Palliat Med J 9:221-228

84. Dunlop RJ, Ellershow JE, Baınes MJ et al (1995) On wıthholdıng nutrıtıon and hydratıon ın the termınally ıll: has palliative medıcıne gone too far? A reply. J Med Ethics 21:141-143

85. Paladını VA, Margarit O, Lugnani F (1996) La nutrızıone ıntegratıva dı supporto, per via orale, nel cancro avanzato. In: Gullo A (ed) La nutrızıone domıcılıare nel pazıente con cancro avanzato. APICE. Trieste, pp 51-63

86. Paladını VA, Mocavero G (1993) Psıcologıa del dolore. Trattato encıclopedıco di anestesıologıa, rıanımazıone, terapia ıntensıva. In: Belluccı G, Damıa G, Gasparetto A (eds) Terapıa antalgıca. Vol. 5. Pıccın Nuove Librerıe, Padova, pp 1-16

87. Morant R, Paladını VA, Cruz Y, Roson Fiorentino F (1990) Language communıcatıon between physıcıan and patıent. In: Gullo A (ed) Recent Advances ın Anaesthesıa, Pain, Intensıve Care and Emergency. Trieste

88. Paladıni VA (1998) Prıncıpı dı psicologıa e psıcoterapıa del dolore cronıco. In: Tıengo M (ed) II Corso Superıore dı aggiornamento ın fısıopatologıa e terapıa del dolore. Mılano, pp 125-145

89. Paladını VA, Cusın SG, Cattaruzza I et al (1985) Dolore cronıco e angoscıa dı morte attraverso ıl Rorschach. Min Anestesıol 51:557-559

90. Paladını VA, Cusın SG, Cattaruzza I et al (1986) Ansia e depressione nel dolore cronıco. Mın Anestesıol 52:321-324

91. Donner B, Zeus M, Tryba M et al (1996) Dırect conversıon from oral Morphıne to transdermal fentanyl: a multıcenter study ın patıents with cancer paın. Paın 64:528

COST-EFFECTIVENESS OF LOCO-REGIONAL ANAESTHESIA

Chapter 27

Cost effectiveness of anaesthesia/analgesia

Q. Piacevoli, F.S. Mennini, F. Palazzo, E. Ferrari Baliviera

The economical assessment of biomedical technologies is a well-established praxis in every industrialized country due to the need to keep health expenditure within a given percentage of the gross national product (GNP).

As economists and all other specialists concerned in health economics know very well, health expenditure has in general maintained a growing trend higher than the GNP increase. Together with the need for a financial control of expenditure, also the assessment of the results of medical actions has long since become indispensable and, to this purpose, the techniques commonly known as cost-benefit analysis proved to be particularly adequate.

The assessment of results has taken great advantage from a discipline called since 1992 Evidence-based Medicine (EBM) [1]; this discipline originated from an alteration of the paradigm of the basic principles of the clinical epidemiology developed two decades before [2]. The importance of this discipline, which is not new to those scientists who base medicine on the acquisition of objective and verifiable data [3], lies in that it gives many of the data necessary also for the economical assessment, and particularly so for the technique known as cost effectiveness.

Cost-assessment

The Office of Technology Assessment (OTA), an American Government body, defines as "biomedical technology" not only drugs and devices, but also all the procedures and the organizative supports used by physicians [4]. Therefore, anaesthesiologic routines are biological technologies and are assessable in terms of both costs and results. As it is well known, the anaesthesiologic routines can be parted in three groups: general, regional and local. Since indications are not exactly identical for all of them, the comparison between costs and results should always be limited to those patients who can be given indiscriminately all the three kinds of anaesthesia – or two of them when the analysis involves only a partial comparison, as in our study (general anaesthesia versus regional anaesthesia). Indications vary according to both diseases and their severity.

The elements to be used for cost assessment are: the time spent by the various specialists (and, among them, particularly the anaesthesiologists), drugs and other consumable stores and the devices. In the case of inpatients, it is moreover important to consider the mean hospitalization time, discriminating between ICU patients and regular bed patients. Mean hospitalization time is not only an important cost component but also an indicator of the outcome, though rough it may be. As a matter of fact, supposing that no unjustified prolongations exist – and this is usually the case, at least in those countries where systems similar to the Diagnosis Relate Group's (DRG) are used, as the Italian "Raggruppamenti Omogenei di Diagnosi" – a shorter hospitalization means a faster improvement of patient's conditions. But the results of the various actions should be assessed by means of indicators that take into account also the health improvement in population.

Firstly, the mortality rate that indicates the risk of fatal events either directly – since one type of anaesthesia can cause a higher death percentage than another – and indirectly since an anaesthesiological alternative (general anaesthesia) can be more invasive, as it involves also the respiratory and the cardiovascular system, and therefore lead to a worsening of the main disease.

Secondly, a given type of anaesthesia could be more preferable than others since it causes fewer complications. The consequence of an inadequate choice reflects negatively, not only in terms of greater risks for patients' safety and longer hospitalization, but also for what concerns the recovery time (longer postoperative course after discharge) and the effects on patient's health. All those aspects are usually defined as effectiveness and can be assessed by means of EBM.

Evidence based medicine

The EBM technique was developed when the discussions about "health expenditure beyond control", and therefore the discussions about limiting and reducing the resources to be allocated to this sector, became a prioritary matter. Through EBM physicians tried to give an answer to these demands with the aim of explaining to the "third paying part" (be it either the welfare state or the social security institutions, or the insurance companies), and above all to the community, the consequences of their actions, mainly from the effectiveness point of view, but also, and indirectly, from the economical one.

EBM underlying philosophy implies that [5]:
- all clinical decisions are to be based on the evidence of the scientific data available;
- the type of evidence to be looked for is determined by the clinical problem;
- statistic and epidemiologic criteria are to be used;
- the conclusions drawn from the data are useful only when used for therapy;
- the results obtained by a given treatment must be continuously re-assessed.

Anyway, EBM method does not imply a comparisons between costs and results; it focuses exclusively on these latter. Its usefulness in cost-benefit comparison techniques is nevertheless unquestionable since it gives the basis for a correct evaluation of effectiveness. But criticism arose well soon: first of all, the support given to population pragmatic trials – versus controlled clinical trials –

as the sole instrument for the most reliable assessment of the therapeutic advantages in terms of public health; in other words, to base the assessment of efficacy on effectiveness (it must be explained that unlike anglophone people, Italians use the word "efficacy" without discriminating between the results obtained in a clinical trial and those obtained on population).

Secondly, the possibility exists that most studies focus on drugs only (that are financed by industries) disregarding any other form of nonpharmacological treatments. This does not mean to deny that industries (since ever charged to be the main responsible for the continuously increasing health expenditure in all countries) are also committed in offering products of unquestionable efficacy. There exist the risk of parting the technologies in two categories: A-rate and B-rate, the first, unlike the other one, being subject to accurate assessment.

Finally, the use of EBM techniques shows that only few medicosurgical treatments are statistically better than their alternatives, whilst this judgement usually came from the experience of physicians only. And on this same basis EBM itself re-evaluated the judgement of physicians springing from their experience – provided that they are considered to be trustworthy. In other words, this does not mean to deny the authoritativeness of some experts when compared with "objective" methods such as EBM, but rather to get over the authoritarism ("the doctor said it!") that was dominating before the development of less biased assessment methods [6].

Cost-benefits analysis

Having said this, we must now define in detail the cost-benefit techniques. First of all it is to be noted that the cost-benefit analysis, in the true sense of the word, is not an assessment method used in medicine. Apart from very few studies based on the "human capital" approach – whereby benefits are assessed with reference to the patient's productive capacity – and on the "willingness to pay" that, more precisely, defines the value of the results obtained towards market price (wherever it exists), there is a certain reluctance to "monetize" health benefits. This reluctance is not only limited to the majority of physicians, but involves also many economists; given the practical difficulties and the theoretical resistance to use methods that depend on the individual income – with the consequent discriminations against the poorest, that is against those who should be more protected by the welfare state – other techniques have been preferably developed, such as cost-effectiveness analysis (CEA) and cost-utility analysis (CUA).

We have already mentioned the cost-effectiveness technique and its indicators. We can now only add that in many CEA studies the result was assessed also considering the potential years of life gained (PYLG). These indicate the decrease in mortality in a different way, keeping into consideration also the age and not only the event "death" per se.

The CUA technique introduces the problem of quality into the economical assessment of the results. For instance, by means of the quality adjusted life years (QALYs) also the quality of life after the various alternative treatments is assessed, in addition to the duration of life [7]. This obviously advantages those treatments for which a statistical evaluation of longer survival is not possible, but, on the contrary, it is possible to verify an increase in life quality.

Several indicators have been used to assess the quality of life (among them we can mention: the Rosser's scale, the multiattribute utility and the standard gamble method or the time trade off method) by which the quality of life is evaluated on the basis of the preferences indicated by some experts (physicians or other health providers), by patients themselves (or by their relatives) and by the community (the citizen not directly involved by the disease being considered).

But here again an important question arises that concerns both effectiveness and a strictly ethical matter. To this purpose we can refer to the most important debate taking presently place in Italy, a controversy that has brought this problem far beyond the borders of medicine and economy: the so-called Di Bella's multitherapy.

The problem we are talking about has not been dealt with by the literature; it rather originates from a series of meetings of some specialists in economical assessment in medicine. Some of them believe that different treatments must at least have equal efficacy, and this is what physicians, pharmacologists and, above all, institutions ("the paying third") tend to believe. Cost increments are therefore advantageous when they guarantee an increase in efficacy: this is the principle adopted for example by the Italian Commissione Unica del Farmaco (CUF - Sole Drug Committee) when choosing the drugs to be included in the "Fascia A" (A cathegory) (i.e. drugs that are fully reimboursed to patients).

According to the economical principle known as "consumer's sovereignity", the preferences indicated by the patients and their relatives could make acceptable the choice of methods that showed lower efficacy in scientific tests but better quality of life according to the patients' (and their relatives') opinion. Even at the risk of overestimating the efficacy itself, and well aware of the fact that some treatments are less effective than others, the choice depends on patient's decision. There seems to exist a trade-off between efficacy and quality (as assessed by the patient) on an indifference curve where certain reductions in efficacy can be substituted with an increase in quality.

This is undoubtedly a questionable point of view but no exact indications can be found in the literature that contradict it demonstrating that patient's preferences are to be subordinated to efficacy. CUA should therefore be considered as a technique to be used to improve the assessments made through CEA – as it adds further information about quality of life – or whenever the greater efficacy of a treatment can or could be demonstrated.

As to regional anaesthesia, that is more expensive since it requires a longer preliminary administration time than general anaesthesia, no sufficient elements exist to prove a higher efficacy. Regional anaesthesia, which is less invasive and more easily accepted by the patients (apart from those who specifically ask for general anaesthesia in order to avoid being awake during the operation), has therefore better quality, in spite of a small additional cost.

Through the CUA method it is also possible to demonstrate the suitability of regional anaesthesia in delivery (obstetrical analgesia); in this case the alternative is not general anaesthesia but rather "to do nothing". The suitability of epidural obstetrical analgesia can be therefore demonstrated by comparing its higher cost against the increases in comfort (i.e. utility) for the mother, even with no evident increases in efficacy.

As demonstrated by our study (to be published) the Italian tariff system grants no additional reimbursement for epidural analgesia in labor. It would be therefore necessary to update the DRG granting system according to the results given by the economical assessments made through cost-effectiveness techniques and particularly CEA and CUA.

Conclusive remarks

As previously said, the "economical" assessment of anaesthesiological procedures shows several difficulties. In particular, the lacking of objective scientifical data proving the real superiority of one technique compared with another (given the same type of disease to be treated), in terms of results, is a sufficient cause of the impossibility to draw exact guidelines in order to save resources.

From an analysis of the international literature of the last three years about the cost-benefit analysis of regional anaesthesia, no decisive data can be found, and the existing works are not homogeneous for what concerns both the choice of the efficacy indicators and the type of cost considered (drugs only, operating theatre utilization time, etc.).

Moreover, as pointed out by Balas et al. [8], after a review of the clinical studies published in the last 30 years and including the key words "costs", "cost-benefits", "cost analysis", "cost control" and "saving", apart from generical statements about costs, no real data (i.e. figures) are mentioned and even in those works where costs are somehow quantified, expenditure data are often generical and incomplete.

In order that an anaesthesiologic technique be considered more advantageous than another, it should theoretically be equally effective and safe, less expensive and easily accepted by both patients and anaesthesiologists. Bothner et al. [9] have processed the data they collected during a five-month research on 282 patients in a university hospital traumatologic ward, for a project of the German Society of Anaesthesia and Intensive Care aiming at defining quality parameters in anaesthesiology. They found no meaningful differences in the postoperative outcome quality of the patients who had undergone two different types of anaesthesia: general and regional anaesthesia (parameters assessed by the anaesthesiologists).

Anyway, the patients that underwent regional anaesthesia showed a higher subjective comfort ($p<0.0001$) during the postoperative period. These data suggest therefore how important the "patient factor" is when assessing, even from an economical point of view, an anaesthesiological technique.

Sabate et al. [10] demonstrated that in oncologic coloproctologic surgery the choice between general anaesthesia and regional anaesthesia (epidural) does not affect, positively or negatively, neither the patient outcome nor the hospital general costs (intervention plus hospitalization).

In contrast, data can be found in vascular surgery confirming the advantage, in terms of cost-effectiveness, of regional anaesthesia when compared with general anaesthesia. Godin et al. [11] have demonstrated that patients undergoing an intervention of carotid endoarterectomy in regional anaesthesia (cervical plexus block) showed a faster discharge time than patients operated in general anaesthesia; moreover, a these authors have demonstrated a saving of about $2 480 per patient for the regional anaesthesia group, when compared with the general anaesthesia group ($p<0.0001$). Of course mortality and morbidity rates of the two groups were identical. Also according to the work group of the vascular surgery ward of the San Raffaele Hospital in Milan [12], the choice of regional anaesthesia for this type of intervention not only offers relevant clinical advantages (collaborative patients and optimal control of the neurological conditions during the intervention), but also contributes to cost reduction (even if a monetary assessment of the quota to be charged to anaesthesia is lacking).

Intravenous regional anaesthesia is indicated in outpatient hand surgery: even if its cost is dramatically lower than that of general anaesthesia (about $24 60 versus $448 66), it is not always (11% of all cases) equally effective in assuring a good level of intraoperative analgesia [13].

In the reduction of distal fractures of the radius, a peripheral anaesthesia combined with sedation seems to be the most effective solution in terms of time, results, costs and acceptance by the patients, in comparison with the peripheral block alone and/or the general anaesthesia [14].

Regional anaesthesia is used also in case of outpatient kneee arthroscopy; even if it requires a longer procedure for the preparation of the patient, it is however less expensive than general anaesthesia if one considers the cost of the drugs to be used and the time of stay in the recovery room ($450 versus $527); clinical efficacy and complications are almost equal for both procedures. But, according to some authors [15] only local anaesthesia has a cost-effectiveness ratio higher than that of the other two procedures, with good acceptance by the patient.

The concern about the discovery of anaesthesiologic procedures allowing also a saving in economical resources is making the interest in the regional anaesthesia grow more and more. Molliex et al. [16] collected 24 cases of outpatient nasal surgery performed through the block of the nasociliary nerve and of the infraorbitary nerve: the clinical efficacy of such a procedure resulted to be optimal, while the limits of this technique were represented by the long duration of intervention (more than 60 minutes); the acceptance of this technique by patients was excellent. Even if the authors did not consider the cost of this procedure, it can be intuitively assumed that it was lower than that of general anaesthesia.

In obstetrics too, regional anaesthesia is more and more used for both Caesarian section and obstetric analgesia [17, 18]: the clinical assumptions are well known and the beneficial effects of analgesia on the mother during spontaneous labour are now demonstrated; there is still a lack of larger-scale studies demonstrating a better cost-advantage ratio for regional anaesthesia versus general anaesthesia.

References

1. Evidence-based Medicine Working Group (1992) Evidence-based medicine: a new approach to teaching the practice of medicine. JAMA 2:2420-2425
2. Liberati A, Penna A, D'Amico R, Telaro E (1997) La evidence-based medicine: origini e prospettive. Tendenze Nuove, pp. 6-10
3. Davidoff F, Case K, Fried PW (1995) Evidence-based medicine: why all the fuss? Ann Int Med 122:727
4. Office of Technology Assessment (1978) Assessing the efficacy and safety of medical technologies. OTA-H-75. Government Printing Office, Washington
5. Mordini E Etica ed evidence-based medicine. Bollettino FOMCeO, Roma
6   Sackett DL, Rosemberg W, Gray M et al (1996) Evidence-based Medicine: what it is and what it is not. Br Med J 312.71-72
7. Weistein MC, Fineberg HV (1984) L'analisi della decisione in medicina clinica. Franco Angeli, Milano
8. Balas EA, Kretschmer RA, Gnann W et al (1996) Interpreting cost analysis of clinical interventions. JAMA 279:54-57
9. Bothner U, Schwiek B, Steffen P et al (1996) Perioperative monitoring of the course of anesthesia, the postanesthesia visit and inquiry of patient satisfaction. A prospective study of parameters in process and outcome quality in anesthesia. Anaesth Intensiv Med not Fallmed Schmerzther 31:608-614
10. Sabate A, Perha MJ, Vila C et al (1997) Analysis of cost minimization of epidural anesthesia compared with general anesthesia in oncologic coloproctologic surgery. Ann Med Int 14:291-296
11. Godin MS, Bell WH, Schwedler M et al (1989) Cost effectiveness of regional anesthesia in carotid endoarterectomy. Am Surg 55:656-659
12. Melissano G, Castellano R, Mazzitelli S et al (1997) Safe and cost-effective approach to carotid surgery. Eur J Endovasc Surg 14:164-169
13. Chlivers CR, Kinahan A, Vaghadia H et al (1997) Pharmacoeconomics of intravenous regional anesthesia vs general anesthesia for outpatient hand surgery. Can J Anaesth 44:1152-1156
14. Funk L (1997) A prospective trial to compare three anesthetic techniques used for reduction of fractures of the distal radius. Injury 28:209-212
15. Lintner S, Shawen S, Lhnes J et al (1996) Local anesthesia in outpatient knee arthroscopy: a comparison of efficacy and cost. Arthroscopy 12:482-488
16 Molliex S, Navez M, Baylot D et al (1996) Regional anesthesia for outpatient nasal surgery. Br J Anaesth 76:151-153
17 Wulf H, Stamer U (1998) Current practices in anesthesia for Caesarian section in German University Clinics. Result of a survey in the year 1996. Anesthesist 47:59-63
18. Oyston J (1995) Obstetrical anaesthesia in Ontario. Can J Anaesth 42:1117-1125

Main symbols

ACTH	Adrenocorticotropin
AMPA	Alpha-Amino-3-Hydroxy-5-Methyl-4-Isoxazoleproprionate
APN	Acute Pain Nurse
APS	Acute Pain Services
β-LPH	β-Lipotropin
BDNF	Brain-Derived Neurotrophic Factor
γ-MSH	Melanocyte-Stimulating Hormone
CCK	Cholecystokinin
CEA	Cost-Effectiveness Analysis
CFA	Complete Freund's Adjuvant
C_{max}	Concentrations
CNS	Central Nervous System
COPD	Chronic Obstructive Pulmonary Disease
COX	Cyclo-Oxygenase Enzyme
CREB	Ca^{2+}/cAMP-Response Element Binding
CRPS	Complex Regional Pain Syndromes
CSE	Combined Spinal Epidural
CUA	Cost-Utility Analysis
CUF	Commissione Unica del Farmaco
CVS	Cardiovascular System
DAG	Diacylglycerol
DREZ	Dorsal Root Entry Zone Lesion
DRG	Diagnosis Relate Group's
EBM	Evidence-Based Medicine
ECM	Extracellular Matrix
EMG	Electromyogram
ESRA	European Society of Regional Anaesthesia
$EtCO_2$	End-Tidal Carbon Dioxide
F-actin	Filamentous actin
FDA	Food and Drug Administration
FNF	Femoral Neck Fracture
FRC	Functional Residual Capacity
FVC	Forcel Vital Capacity
GA	General Anaesthesia
GABA	γ-Amino-Butyric Acid
GABA	γ-Aminobutyric Acid
GAGs	Glycosaminolgycans
GNP	Gross National Product

HETEs	Hydroxyeicosatetraenoic Acids
IASP	International Association for the Study of Pain
IFs	Intermediate Filaments
IgG	Immunoglobulin G
IgSF	Immunoglobulin Superfamily
IP3	Inositol-1,4,5-trisphosphate
LAAs	Local Anaesthetic Agents
LRA	Locoregional Anaesthesia
LTs	Leukotrienes
M3G	Morphine-3-Glucuronide
M6G	Morphine-6-Glucuronide
MAPs	Microtubule-Associated Proteins
MIP	Maximum Inspiratory Pressure
MVD	Microvascular Decompression
NACS	Neonatal Adaptive Scores
NFs	Neurofilaments
NgCAM	Neuron-glia Cell Adhesion Molecule
NGF	Nerve Growth Factor
NMDA	N-Methyl-D-Aspartate
NOA	Non-Opioid Analgesics
NS	Nerve Stimulation
NSAIDs	Nonsteroidal Anti-Inflammatory Drugs
NT-3	Neurotrophin-3
NT-4/5	Neurotrophin 4/5
OTA	Office of Technology Assessment
OTM	Oral Transmucosal Delivery
PAG	Periacqueductal Grey
PCA	Patient-Controlled Analgesia
PGa	Proteoglycans
PGs	Prostaglandins
PIP2	Phosphatidylinositol-4, 5-bisphosphate
POMC	Pro-Opiomelanocortin
PONV	Postoperative Nausea and Vomiting
PYLG	Potential Years of life gained
QALYs	Quality Adjusted Life Years
RA	Regional Anaesthesia
RFT	Radiofrequency thermorhizotomy
RPTKs	Receptor Protein Tyrosine Kinases
RPTP	Receptor Protein Tyrosine Phosphatase
RVM	Rostral Ventral Medulla
SaO_2	Oxygen Saturation
SCR	Skin Conductance Reactions
SP	Subtance P
SRMT	Slow-Release Morphine Tablets
TAG-1	Transiently Expressed Axonal Glycoprotein-1
TENS	Transcutaneous Electrical Nerve Stimulation
THR	Total Hip Replacement
TN	Trigeminal Neuralgia
VAS	Visual Analogic Scale
VMH	Ventromedial Hypotalamus
WHO	World Health Organization

Subject index